A
COMPROMISED
GENERATION

*The Epidemic of Chronic Illness
in America's Children*

Beth Lambert

With Victoria Kobliner MS RD

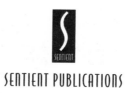

SENTIENT PUBLICATIONS

First Sentient Publications edition 2010
Copyright © 2010 by Beth Lambert

A paperback original

Cover design by Kim Johansen, Black Dog Design
Book design by Timm Bryson

Library of Congress Cataloging-in-Publication Data
Lambert, Beth, 1976-
 A compromised generation : the epidemic of chronic illness in America's children / Beth Lambert ; with Victoria Kobliner. – 1st Sentient Publications ed.
     p. cm.
 Includes bibliographical references.
 ISBN 978-1-59181-096-4
 1. Chronic diseases in children–United States. 2. Chronic diseases in children–Prevention. I. Kobliner, Victoria. II. Title.
 RJ380.L36 2010
 618.92'044–dc22

                         2009047602

Printed in the United States of America
10 9 8 7 6 5 4 3 2 1

SENTIENT PUBLICATIONS
A Limited Liability Company
1113 Spruce Street
Boulder, CO 80302
www.sentientpublications.comA Limited Liability Company

TO DIANA AND ALL THE OTHER MOTHERS . . .

who instinctively knew that something wasn't right.

CONTENTS

ACKNOWLEDGEMENTS

Many generous people donated their time, knowledge and wisdom to the production of this book. I would like to thank the many (too many to name) physicians, researchers, clinicians, teachers, school nurses, parents and other experts who were interviewed during the research phase. I would especially like to thank Dr. Nancy O'Hara, Dr. Gail Szakacs, Dr. Lauren Stone, Vicki Kobliner, Gail Vanark, and Dr. Toby Watkinson, all dedicated healthcare practitioners committed to healing children with chronic illnesses. Thank you for always taking time out of your busy days to answer my many questions and to provide me with an informal education on all things pertaining to chronic illness. To Dr. Leo O'Connor, thank you for your support and guidance with this project.

I would also like to thank Kris Lowe and Mona Strassburger, my first editors. Thank you for providing me with solid grounding and guidance throughout the development of this book. Thank you to Dr. Allison Bloom, my medical editor, for excellent medical advice and perspective. I must also acknowledge the many "mommies" who contributed to this book either by sharing their children's illness and recovery stories or by reading the manuscript and providing feedback. To Tori, thank you for staying on this journey with me regardless of how far down the rabbit hole it took us. Of course, this book

would not have been written were it not for the eternal encourage-
ment and support of my husband Greg and the rest of my family. I
would especially like to thank my mother and father, Diana and
Charles, for believing in me and believing in the importance of this
message.

FOREWORD

When I started teaching children with autism twenty-five years ago, it was a rare illness. More than fifteen years ago, when I was a general pediatrician, autism affected 1 in 10,000 children. Now even conservative estimates are 1 in 150. Also, it's not just autism (ASD) which has increased by 6,000 percent. Attention deficit hyperactivity disorder (ADHD) has increased 400 percent, asthma by 300 percent, allergies by 400 percent and diabetes (IDDM) by 103 percent. Why such meteoric increases? It's not just genetics. Genetics don't cause epidemics. As Francis Collins and others have said, "Genetics loads the gun and environment pulls the trigger."

As Beth Lambert so eloquently expresses in this book, we are raising a generation of sick children—children with allergies and asthma; children with gut problems, diarrhea, constipation, and bloating; and children with neurodevelopmental delays, to name a few of the issues. More and more parents and increasing numbers of physicians are concerned about the tremendous increases in ASD, ADHD and other disorders. Why is this happening, we ask?

As Beth describes, due to a multitude of factors, including increasing exposure to toxins in our environment, our food and our vaccines, our children's ability to handle these toxins is limited. Their immune systems and their guts are unable to handle these exposures and they are developing allergies, autoimmune problems and toxicities (both neurologic and systemic) as a consequence.

This book is an invaluable resource examining, evaluating and explaining the problems our children face and the possible treatment options. When we are confronted with a sick child with unexplained rashes, stomach problems or sleep disturbances, we often need to look beyond traditional medicine. When we are presented with a child with cognitive delays, neurologic issues or behavioral problems, we often need to look beyond traditional medicine. We often need to look at dietary changes, nutrient supplementation and other natural interventions. As parents, we need to pursue all promising avenues.

As physicians, we need to listen to parents. We need to hear what they are experiencing – the abnormal stools, the difficult sleep patterns, the recurrent rashes and the behavioral and cognitive problems that ensue. We need to figure out the connections between these immune, gut and sleep problems and the resultant cognitive, neurologic and behavioral issues. We need to recover this lost generation. Beth shows us why this is happening, why the gut and the brain are connected and how to treat this lost generation of children.

Scientific research has only begun to look at the myriad of problems facing this generation of children. Through the research and practical applications that Beth puts forth, we can understand each child's needs and teach both parents and professionals how to care for these children so that they can reach their fullest potential.

All of our children are gifts. Some are wrapped in many layers of wrapping paper, layers of immune, gut, sleep and detoxification problems. Layers that we need to unwrap one by one to see the true gift of each of our children inside. This book will help you understand these layers and discover how to "unwrap" your child.

This book is a gift.

Thank you Beth, for the gift.

—Nancy H. O'Hara, MD

Introduction

If our American way of life fails the child, it fails us all.

                    —PEARL S. BUCK

Over the last several decades, we have become a society obsessed with children's health, wellness and safety. We do things with our children today that people fifty years ago would have found strange, perhaps even laughable. We measure our children's height, weight, and head circumference every month during infancy to ensure that each child is on track. We use baby monitors to listen to our infants' every peep as they sleep—and we put them all to sleep on their backs. We protect our children from infectious diseases, including sexually transmitted diseases, through the most comprehensive vaccination program in the

world. We sanitize their surroundings. We have stringent laws outlin-
ing which car seats or bike helmets must be worn to prevent injury.
We have developed crime-stopping protocols like Amber Alerts on
highways and Safe Havens on city streets. In many localities, parents
have been arrested for leaving their children alone in a car for even a
few brief moments. Children left unattended at home afterschool
were once called latchkey, now they are called neglected. There is
more anxiety today about the well-being of children than at any other
time in American history.

Yet, somehow, for all of this concern about our children's health
and safety, we seem to be overlooking what appears to be the most
widespread and potentially devastating crisis in children's health of
the modern era: More American children are suffering from diagnosable chronic illnesses than at any other time in our history. Asthma,
autism, ADHD, allergies, juvenile diabetes, celiac disease, obesity,
and many other illnesses are growing at unprecedented rates, and we
do not know why.

This phenomenon is not limited to children diagnosed with particular illnesses. Many children considered to be healthy or normal are
showing signs of chronic immunological impairment and unhealthy
physiological imbalances. The signs are common, everyday occurrences like runny noses, constipation, or temper tantrums. These are
easy to dismiss, as they occur in most children intermittently. What
sets these signs apart from normal childhood experiences is that they
are chronic, unrelenting, and persistent. While many parents are
tuned in to these signs, intuiting that there is something wrong with
their children, many others dismiss these signs as harmless or incon-
sequential. Sometimes it is just easier to accept our pediatrician's most
heartfelt reassurances that all is well. But all is not well.

HEALTHY KIDS, SICK KIDS

Jamie is a bright and sensitive three-and-a-half-year-old girl, who by
all accounts seems perfectly healthy and typical. Jamie's mom, Kath-

leen, however, knows that something isn't right with her daughter, despite reassurances from the pediatricians and numerous specialists that Kathleen has brought Jamie to see. Jamie is chronically constipated. She has had difficulty with bowel movements since she was nine months old and will cry and tantrum to avoid having to "go." She has developed a true fear of going to the bathroom, as it hurts her to do so. Jamie has also developed some significant behavioral problems or abnormalities, including excessive tantrums, crying and sadness, as well as acute sensitivity to normal noises like the vacuum cleaner, or hammering. She will cover her ears and yell for the noise to stop. She also demonstrates a high level of anxiety, paranoid feelings that people are "looking at her," and some aggressive behavior toward her one-year-old sister.

Kathleen has taken Jamie to multiple pediatricians, multiple gastroenterologists, and is now waiting to see a child psychiatrist who specializes in bowel-related trauma and anxiety. Each doctor has given her the same response: diet changes and Miralax (a laxative) and "wait and see what happens." Jamie has been on Miralax for over a year, despite the fact that the prescribing information explicitly states that it should not be given for more than seven days. Yet, the many doctors that Jamie has been to see offer no other solutions. Kathleen keeps asking, "What is the root cause of my daughter's constipation?" and the doctors shrug their shoulders and tell her to just continue with the Miralax. But for how long? Jamie's condition does not seem to be improving and Kathleen is worried about the impact of chronic Miralax usage and that her daughter's behavioral problems (which she *knows* are related to the constipation) do not seem to be improving. Kathleen desperately wants help for Jamie but feels abandoned by her many medical doctors. Kathleen is still looking for answers.

Kim is the mother to five beautiful, active and seemingly healthy children between the ages of two and eight years old. Her middle three children, Larsen, Kaelin and Tristan, are triplets. During the winter of the triplets' second year, their grandmother commented to Kim that her kids always seemed sick. Someone in their family (most often the triplets) always had a runny nose, cold, fever, bronchiolitis, wheezing, or some other ailment. Her children also struggled with occasional loose stools and tummy aches. The triplets were put on chronic nebulizer treatments to help with the wheezing, and occasional courses of antibiotics were prescribed throughout their early years, but nothing seemed to help alleviate their symptoms. Currently, they are all taking Singulair (a common asthma medication). Kim took the triplets to see every type of specialist, from ear nose and throat specialists (ENT) to naturopaths, trying to figure out what was wrong with her children. There were no diagnoses to fit these children, yet Kim felt that something about their immune systems simply was not working. Kim is still looking for answers.

Shefali is a hard working and beautiful eight-year-old honor student and the middle of three girls. When Shefali was about five years old, her mother, Padma, noticed a sudden, inexplicable weight gain. Padma took her daughter in for blood work to discover that she had hypothyroidism, a condition where the thyroid does not produce enough of the hormone necessary for basic metabolic activities in the body. Repeated visits to pediatricians and endocrinologists resulted in Shefali's treatment with Synthroid, a synthetic thyroid hormone medication. Around the time that Shefali began treatment with Synthroid, Padma noticed that she developed quite severe seasonal allergies (hay fever) despite no one in Padma's family or her husband's family having had any history of allergies. The seasonal allergies seemed to precipitate chronic respiratory and sinus infections that were usually treated with antibiotics. Shefali typically receives eight to ten courses of antibiotics per year just to manage these infections.

After multiple courses of antibiotics, Shefali developed wheezing and asthmatic symptoms that she now manages with albuterol, delivered by a nebulizer. Doctors recommended that Shefali begin treatment with Singulair and Pulmicort—both asthma medications, but Padma has resisted because she is concerned about overmedicating her daughter. Currently, on a daily basis, Shefali takes thyroid medication, albuterol, antihistamines, and antibiotics (if she is experiencing an acute lung or sinus infection). Shefali has difficulty sleeping through the night, she is constantly coughing and congested, and just recently, her hay fever symptoms have worsened so that she is constantly sneezing and rubbing her itchy eyes. Despite many pharmaceutical interventions, Shefali seems to be getting worse, not better. It is a testament to this child's character and tenacity that she is able to maintain her honor student status, despite her many health challenges. Padma, herself a trained medical professional, has become fed up with conventional western medicine's drug-driven "band-aid" approach to disease management. She wants to get at the root of her daughter's chronic illness, but all her many doctors can do is provide her with more drugs. Padma is still looking for answers.

Tori, mother of four children ages one to seven, began to notice that something wasn't right when her oldest child, Ethan, started snoring at age three. Ethan is a completely normal kid in most ways, intelligent with a great sense of humor, but he has always struggled with a variety of bizarre health issues. Around the time that she noticed the snoring, Tori began to pick up on other symptoms like unusual bowel movements—he would be constipated for days with no bowel movement, then he would sit on the toilet for an hour with diarrhea, only to repeat the process all over again four or five days later. Other abnormalities included toenails that were thick and malformed, and pretty severe hay fever, with itchy eyes and a constantly running nose. He spent a good portion of his preschool years on Benadryl. She also noticed that when he drank milk, his ears would get red and hot. His lymph nodes were chronically swollen and he would experience episodes of fevers a couple times a month. Ethan even developed a tic. Yet, Ethan's doctors all classified him as healthy and normal physically.

Tori took Ethan to see ENTs, gastroenterologists, allergists, and even a highly respected infectious disease specialist. None of the doctors could provide Ethan with a diagnosis or an explanation for what was causing his health problems. He tested negative for allergies, infectious diseases, GI disorders and many other commonly recognizable ailments. Finally, Ethan's adenoids and tonsils were removed, but no significant improvements were seen in his symptoms. Eventually, Ethan developed asthma, which was managed, although not effectively, with medications. Tori's other children, Emily, Kate, and the youngest, Macy, also began to demonstrate symptoms of ill health. Emily had chronic ear infections, Kate developed rashes, a distended belly, and chronic sinusitis, and Macy, just a baby, had severe eczema, reflux, and choking and regurgitation of food, and developed the bizarre behavior of always sticking her tongue out. Frustrated by her medical doctors' inability to help her children, Tori sought help elsewhere, with alternative practitioners. Tori is still looking for answers.

What all of these women have in common is that they have sharp instincts that tell them that something just isn't right with their children's health, and they are not willing to be dismissed by pediatricians who reassure them that their children are "typical," "normal," or "healthy." A parent knows when their child is not well, and these women refuse to accept that chronic diarrhea, chronic constipation, chronic colds and wheezing and the many other symptoms are normal. They are right. The symptoms exhibited by their children are not normal. And there are many children like them across this country. These children are sick and need help, but our medical system is failing them. There are no established diagnoses for these children because the syndrome of symptoms that they exhibit is unique to each child, and the symptoms are seemingly benign (if exhibited intermittently), and thus not recognized as clinically meaningful. Pediatricians and parents have not been trained to see these early signs of chronic illness as problematic. Pediatricians in particular—hardworking, busy professionals—see children with much worse conditions, such as leukemia, autism, cystic fibrosis and other debilitating illnesses—they cannot be expected to take every case of constipation or swollen glands seriously.

Fifty years ago, it made sense for a pediatrician or a parent to dismiss the occasional case of sniffles, constipation, and eczema. These are not severe childhood illnesses and can be caused by any number of transient and benign factors (e.g., eating too many processed foods can cause constipation—eating more fiber will clear it up). Today, however, the circumstances have changed, and the fact that so many children experience these symptoms chronically (without abatement) should serve as a red flag alerting us to some kind of fundamental biological or physiological breakdown in the bodies of these children.

The signs of illness in children today are so ubiquitous that they have become the new normal, but ask grandmothers of today if children were like this fifty years ago and they will tell you that something is radically different about their grandchildren's generation. Every day, we as parents dismiss critical health symptoms in our children, but these symptoms should make us aware that something about their physical health is off. Following is a brief list of some of the irregular symptoms exhibited by many American children today. It is a catalogue compiled by vigilant parents who see some of these signs in their children and their children's friends on a daily basis. Although they are common, they are not normal when exhibited chronically. Scan through the list. Do your children, or children that you know, exhibit any of these symptoms with persistence?

- One or two red cheeks after eating
- Red or hot ears after eating
- Chronic runny nose or cough
- Chronic mouth breathing
- Chronic or recurrent ear infections
- Chronic or recurrent sinus infections
- Chronic or recurrent strep infections
- Patches of red, dry, scaly skin (eczema) on face, hands, elbows, knees or other parts of the skin
- Frequent diaper rashes in babies, especially red rings around the anus or redness of the vaginal area
- Vaginal or anal itching or probing
- Cradle cap or excessive scaling and dandruff on the scalp
- Thinning hair or hair loss
- Cavities and excessive tartar, or bad breath despite proper dental hygiene

- Frequent daytime wetting in an already potty-trained child
- Nighttime bedwetting well into the grade school years
- Nocturia, frequent waking to go to the bathroom
- Dark circles or bags surrounding the eyes, "droopy" eyes
- Excessive drooling in children too old to drool
- Colic, excessive crying or irritability in babies
- Frequent temper tantrums (multiple times a day)
- Frequent crying, sadness, anxiety, anger (multiple times a day)
- Esophageal reflux, babies who chronically spit up or regurgitate after eating
- Mood swings
- Skin pallor
- White coating on the tongue
- Chronic thrush infections
- Unusual fingernail or toenail formation
- Frequent loose stools, diarrhea
- Undigested food routinely found in stool
- Infrequent stooling, constipation (only going once every few days, or straining with a bowel movement)
- Excessive gas, flatulence
- Chronically discolored stools: white, yellow, or black
- Floating stools, or dry stools ("rabbit pellets")
- Tummy aches
- Distended pot belly
- Persistent toe-walking (always walking on tip-toes)
- Delays in crawling, walking, talking
- Gross motor delays—difficulties completing age-appropriate physical tasks (e.g., jumping or climbing)
- Sideways glancing—looking out of the sides of the eyes instead of making direct eye contact
- Sensory defensiveness: covering the ears from everyday sounds like vacuum cleaners or telephone rings; shielding the eyes from bright lights; sensitivity or revulsion to common smells; avoidance of certain textures like sand, wetness, certain fab-

rics; over sensitivity or emotional reaction to tags in clothing, seams in socks, hair brushing; avoidance of kisses, hugs, or other forms of affection

- Sensory-seeking behaviors: always looking to crash into people, objects
- Pressure-seeking behavior: trying to push the belly or body against objects, the floor, tables
- Head banging
- Tongue hanging out of the mouth
- Failure to thrive, growth delays
- Arm flapping
- Low muscle tone
- Excessive hyperactivity
- Chronically swollen lymph nodes
- Obsessive or compulsive type behaviors—constant hoarding of toys, possessions
- Lining up toys, constantly opening and closing doors, turning switches on and off, or other repetitive behaviors
- Persistent aggressive behavior
- Persistent noncompliant or oppositional behavior
- Tics (verbal or physical)
- Recurrent urinary tract infections
- Chronic vaginal infections
- Chronic athlete's foot, ringworm or other fungal skin infections

Perfectly normal and healthy children may exhibit a few of these symptoms occasionally. This is not a concern. All children exhibit occasional temper tantrums, hoarding of toys, constipation, hyperactivity, and many more of the aforementioned symptoms. However, it is *not* normal when children exhibit any of these symptoms chronically or with particular intensity and severity, despite conventional treatment approaches (e.g., diet and behavioral modifications). It is precisely because these are normal child behaviors that they are often dismissed.

Many physicians and parents dismiss these symptoms in children, even when they severely compromise quality of life or a child's ability to learn, because they do not understand what is causing the symptoms, nor do they have many effective tools to address the symptoms. Neither parents nor pediatricians know what to make of children who exhibit these symptoms chronically because there is no medical or historical precedent for these types of problems. Thousands of parents are left searching for answers and for ways to heal their children. There are answers, but they are complicated, and it takes time and a willingness to buck medical convention before they can be elucidated.

This book documents the growing epidemic of chronic illnesses and chronic poor health in American children and how some pioneering researchers and health care practitioners are getting to the bottom of this crisis. For the purposes of this book *chronic childhood illness* refers to the condition of children who are unhealthy, either with diagnosed illnesses like autism or ADHD, or those children who exhibit particular symptoms, like chronic diarrhea, excessive tantruming behavior or chronic ear infections. Even children believed to be healthy or normal but who exhibit any of the aforementioned symptoms chronically can be considered among the children affected by the epidemic of chronic illness. Your child does not have to have a disease or a diagnosis to be considered chronically ill, it is just that as a society, we do not yet recognize or understand that many normal and healthy children are actually quite unhealthy under the surface.

Perhaps the most visible epidemic is that of autism. The factors that may contribute to the etiology of autism are likely the same factors that are making other children sick, either severely as in the case of multiple sclerosis, or mildly, as in the case of chronic sinusitis. We will look at the statistics behind the epidemic, and provide a scientific explanation for the epidemic, as well as an explanation of the cultural factors that precipitated this unfortunate trend. The final chapters of this book offer hope, as there are ways to heal children who are sick, and ways to prevent others from getting sick. Many children have recovered from chronic illness, including children with severe disabilities like autism. These children's recovery stories tell us that chronic illnesses are *not* determined by genetics alone, as some doctors and medical researchers would have us believe. By making changes to our environment, we can heal sick children.

There is something unique about modern western society that is making an entire generation of children susceptible to chronic illness. This is what is described in the following pages. This generation of children is truly *a compromised generation*. Their health is compromised, their ability to learn is compromised, and the future, for them, and for all of us, is in jeopardy. Every day our children battle a variety of individual health problems that we did not have to contend with as children. Up until this point they have struggled on their own because neither parents nor doctors understood that specific environmental influences in their lives were making them chronically sick. This is slowly changing, but our children need more help. We need to educate ourselves to the environmental factors making them sick so that we can begin to reverse this horrible trend. Let the learning and the healing begin.

NOTE FROM THE AUTHOR

It should be noted that I am not a medical professional. I am a parent, a former teacher, and a former healthcare researcher and consultant. The scientific and medical evidence presented in this book is taken straight from the medical literature and from interviews with medical experts. The research conducted for this book is thoroughly documented in my endnotes, as I wanted to leave a breadcrumb trail so that others interested in this topic can research it for themselves. My hope is that this book will land on the desks of those who are medically trained so that they can evaluate the research that I have compiled, and build on it. We all need to start asking questions and stop just taking the word of the medical establishment, such as the American Academy of Pediatrics or the Centers for Disease Control, who continue to assure us that all is well with America's children. It is not. I also hope that this book provides some support and guidance to parents who instinctively feel that something is not right with their children's health.

When requested, the names of certain interviewees were changed to protect their privacy or maintain anonymity. Changed names are indicated with asterisks.

Finally, some topics in this book are considered quite controversial, such as autism and vaccination. It is my hope that the book will motivate people to better educate themselves on these topics, so that we can have open, honest, and progressive conversations rather than arguments and circular debates.

chapter 1

Sick Kids

🌱

THE ALARMING STATISTICS

Kids get sick. In fact, children are particularly susceptible to sickness as they are often grouped together indoors for prolonged periods of time practicing poor hygiene and swapping germs with one another. Their developing immune systems are ripe for infection in this setting. This is why, on average, children typically suffer from three to eight colds a year. Infection is simply a part of childhood. The good news is that modern medicine, health and sanitation practices, nutrition and childhood immunization programs have all helped to reduce the threat of truly serious childhood infectious diseases. The *bad* news is that modern medicine, health and sanitation practices, nutrition and childhood immunization programs have also significantly increased the risk for developing *chronic* disease. Many of the same forces that saved millions of lives over the course of the twentieth century are, astonishingly, also causing millions of children to suffer from incurable, and therefore chronic, disease. American children today are confronting health challenges that have never before been seen. Chronic noninfectious illnesses in children are growing at unprecedented, and truly confounding, rates. Diseases like autism, diabetes or celiac disease used to be extremely rare among children, but today, these illnesses, and many more, are touching the lives of almost every community in America.

Walk into the office of any school nurse in America and he or she will tell you what chronic childhood illness looks like today. Inhalers, nebulizers and Epi-pens; psychiatric evaluations and discipline reports; Ritalin, Adderall and Strattera. This is a glimpse into American childhood in the twenty-first century. Most veteran teachers will report that children of today just aren't the same as children of even thirty or forty years ago. To be sure, much has changed in the lives of American children, but these teachers report that the differences go beyond the impact of latchkey and video games. There are physical and behavioral signs that children are sick. Dark circles under the eyes, red cheeks and eczema so common in children today are all classic physical features of allergies and environmental sensitivities. Hyperactivity, inattention, defiance, and noncompliance are all behaviors commonly seen in America's classrooms. These behaviors often can have a *biological* basis. Obesity, an indication of metabolic dysfunction, is at an all-time high in American children. Over one-third of American children are classified as either obese or overweight, and this represents a tripling in prevalence since the 1970s.[1]

Diane Armstrong, a New Jersey school nurse for thirty years, has seen many sick children over her career, but in her opinion, today's children are not only sicker, their illnesses are not always well managed:

> The children who have asthma, for instance, . . . some of these kids
> are *just so sick*, and their asthma can lead to more severe infections.
> . . . If their asthma is not attended to right away, their whole immune
> system is affected by it. Kids are staying home sick with asthma and

missing school. When I see a kid sick with asthma, I call up the parents and tell them "your child is wheezing and you need to get them to the doctor" . . . but they can't always get there, and this goes on for weeks. Some of these kids are just so hard to treat. *They are really sick.*

Linda McMahon, a middle school science teacher from Bernardsville, New Jersey, with forty years of teaching experience, describes how children have changed over the course of her career:

When I first started teaching in 1968, most all students scaled my bar of expectations with ease. Today in 2009, more than half of my students would prefer to crawl under the bar or avoid it altogether. After-school scheduling, family pressures, curricula for which they are not ready, poor eating habits, and chronic health issues (for example, allergies to everything)—all these things are contributing to the steady decline of school performance.

Linda also noted that she began to see a radical change in her students over the last ten to twelve years. Many of these children are ignored while their behavior is attributed to poor parenting and others are given a psychiatric diagnosis such as depression, borderline personality disorder, bipolar disorder, oppositional-defiant disorder, or conduct disorder. Many of these children are then prescribed psychotropic medications, which may exacerbate existing physiological dysfunctions, ultimately intensifying behavior and conduct problems. Something is fundamentally wrong with these children: it is observable, you can talk about it, yet no one is able to explain exactly what is going on.

Behavioral problems in school are, by all accounts, on the rise.[2] Most educators, psychologists and other mental health professionals believe that social factors are to blame for the increasing rates of behavioral problems. In one review study published in 2005, the investigators listed the major risk factors believed to predispose children to significant behavioral disorders. These factors include: child characteristics (such as temperament, attachment, cognition, language development), parent

characteristics (such as maternal depression, parental stress, harsh discipline and maternal education), and sociodemographic risk factors
(such as ethnicity, family conflict, and community violence). To be
sure, these social factors are important forces that shape and contribute to problem behaviors in children. What is interesting about
this report (and others like it) is that no mention of the *physical* health
of the children is made at any point in the analysis. There seems to
be the assumption that physical health is somehow not relevant to a
child's psychological or behavioral well-being.[3] Is it possible that many
of these behaviors are caused, or at least exacerbated by, physically
impaired health? The last time you had a sinus infection, a migraine
headache, or a hangover, were you able to behave like your normal,
adorable, friendly self? It might be time to reassess whether social factors are indeed solely responsible for the increase in behavioral problems. Some of these children just may be chronically ill but with
underrecognized conditions.

Other professionals who work with very young children agree that
they have seen noticeable differences in children's health over the last
decade or so. Carrie* is a grandmother of twelve children and has
been working at her local YMCA day care center for more than fourteen years. She works with the children of over a hundred families in
her community. Carrie reports that over the fourteen years that she
has taken care of the children in her community, there are many more
sick kids today than ever before. "It seems that every kid that comes
in here [to her day care center] has a runny nose, or a cough—and
they didn't used to be like this." Carrie also reports seeing new problems like eczema, red cheeks and red ears on many of her children.
Gastrointestinal problems also seem to be on the rise in her center.
"We get quite a bit of frequent loose stools and diarrhea—more so now
than ever."

Carrie admits that it is easy to dismiss these subtle changes in children, as they are so mild, but she expressed concern about other, more
troubling, changes she has seen in her population of children. "We are
getting a lot more kids that we think may be autistic. We have had quite
a few kids in the last few years that will lie on the floor, watching

wheels—wheels on the strollers, wheels on toys—just go round and round. They line up toys. There are some that don't look you in the eye or talk to you—they just aren't there." When Carrie started working in the day care center, there was one child that displayed this sort of abnormal behavior (this child was later diagnosed with autism), and many accommodations were made for this child. Now, Carrie says, she currently has at least four children in her day care center who display these types of behaviors, yet no one talks about it or provides any information about how to interact with or best care for these children. She also sees a variety of other new behaviors such as head banging, sensitivity to sounds, and significant anxiety. "We had a little girl who would scream when she heard the vacuum cleaner; she would just panic when she heard that. She didn't even like the sound of a broom sweeping."

The chronic childhood conditions plaguing our country today are many. Some are subtle and underdiagnosed (such as food sensitivities/allergies) while others are quite observable (such as autism/pervasive developmental disorders). Among the most common and growing chronic conditions are autism spectrum disorders (ASD), ADHD (attention deficit hyperactivity disorder), allergies, and asthma—what integrative physician and author Dr. Kenneth Bock calls the Four-A Disorders.[4] But many more chronic conditions are hitting new highs in children, including depression, bipolar disorder, obsessive-compulsive disorder, type-II diabetes, multiple sclerosis, and even new disorders that have recently been discovered or labeled, such as sensory processing or sensory integration disorder. Sensory processing disorder is a relatively new diagnosis that includes children who have difficulties processing external stimuli such as noise, sights, smells, touch, and motion. Children with this disorder cannot tolerate the most ordinary of sensations, such as a hug, the feel of sand, or the sound of a vacuum cleaner. Interestingly, many children with autism also struggle with sensory disorders. This diagnosis has become so common in recent years that a pediatrician in New Canaan, Connecticut, calls it the latest "fad" diagnosis. Should the unprecedented numbers of children being diagnosed with sensory disorders be interpreted as a cultural fad, or is there something more biologically and environmentally complex that is causing so many children to experience this type of disorder?

Recent studies and surveys indicate that not only are chronic childhood illnesses on the rise, they are reaching epidemic proportions. The prevalence of inflammatory illnesses such as asthma and allergies, and disorders classically viewed as neurological such as autism and ADHD, have skyrocketed over the past few decades. There is much debate over whether reported prevalence rates are perceived (attributable to improved diagnostic techniques and other technical mechanisms) or actual, but as new epidemiological studies emerge and the data mounts, it becomes clear that these astonishing rates are real and indicative of a serious health crisis in our country.

Classic inflammatory disorders comprise the bulk of childhood chronic illness today. Asthma, characterized by inflammation of the airways of the lungs that results in wheezing, coughing, difficulty breathing as well as acute respiratory attacks, affects over 9 million children in America and is the most commonly diagnosed chronic disease among children.[5] According to a National Center for Health Statistics (CDC) report, the prevalence of childhood asthma nearly tripled from 1980 to 2006.[6] According to the Summary Health Statistics for Children from 2006, African American children are affected disproportionately with 17 percent of African American children under 18 years reporting that they had asthma. This is nearly one in five African America children in America. Of the children surveyed for the CDC report, over 40 percent were classified as being in "fair" or "poor" health. These are sick children with a chronic and often debilitating condition. Minority children who live in inner cities are reported to have even higher rates of asthma. One study reported in the *Annals of Allergy, Asthma & Immunology* found that 27 percent of African American children in Little Rock, Arkansas had asthma, and other studies report similar findings.[7]

The prevalence of allergies among children is difficult to nail down because diagnosed cases of allergic disease are believed to represent only a small portion of the total burden of atopic (allergic) disease in America. The term *allergy* itself is a controversial one because many allergists use a fairly narrow definition of allergy and only define true allergy as immediate-onset, IgE-mediated reactions to environmental triggers (see chapter two for more on the types of allergies). These types of allergies are diagnosable in an in-patient setting with diagnostic techniques specifically designed to test for immediate-onset allergies. However, a growing body of physicians and research scientists argue that the classic allergies that the allergy/immunology community acknowledges as true allergy may represent only one way in which the human body adversely reacts to environmental antigens or immunogens (e.g., foods, dust, insects, molds, etc.).

Although the concept has been around for decades, increasingly, allergists and integrative clinicians are beginning to recognize the relevance of other types of allergic or immune-related reactions to environmental antigens. These reactions include IgG, IgA, or IgM-mediated allergies and are often called sensitivity reactions, hypersensitivities, or delayed-onset allergies. Practitioners who look for physiological symptoms caused by these types of adverse reactions to food, chemicals, or other substances tend to use the term *allergy* quite liberally, and apply it to any immunologically based adverse reaction to external stimuli in the body. Most allergists would call IgG and delayed-onset allergies *sensitivities* or *intolerances,* which are acceptable working definitions, except that they tend to connote symptoms that are a nuisance and not a serious clinical problem. Many clinicians who treat allergies, particularly in the integrative or holistic community, would disagree, believing instead that delayed-onset allergies are responsible for precipitating a whole host of symptoms that range from severe eczema and migraine headaches to manic behavior, chronic fatigue, and even clinical depression. Thus, evaluating the prevalence of allergies from an epidemiological perspective is complicated.

Allergic disease (atopy) is a broad category that covers a variety of symptoms, including hay fever/allergic rhinitis (itchy/watery eyes, sneezing, congestion), urticaria (hives), atopic dermatitis (eczema/scaling), contact dermatitis (skin rashes), asthma, food and chemical allergies (including allergies to pharmaceuticals like penicillin) and insect sting allergies. According to the American Academy of Allergy, Asthma and Immunology (AAAI) the prevalence of diagnosed allergic disease is as follows:

- Allergic rhinitis affects over 40 percent of children
- True (severe) food allergy is estimated to affect approximately three million children (roughly 4 percent of American children under eighteen)[8]
- The prevalence of undiagnosed food sensitivities is unknown; however, they are believed to account for the vast majority of all food allergy (in the broad sense), thus the number of children likely affected by this type of allergy is considerable[9]
- Children under four years of age have the highest prevalence of true food allergy at 6-8 percent[10]
- Atopic dermatitis affects between 10-20 percent of children[11]

While the debate continues over what exactly constitutes allergy, the prevalence of easily diagnosable allergic disease continues to rise in the U.S. Results from the Third National Health and Nutrition Examination Survey (NHANES, conducted by the CDC) reveal that for six hay-fever-associated allergens common to both NHANES II (1976-1980) and NHANES III (1988-1994) prevalences were 2.1 to 5.5 times higher in NHANES III. NHANES IV has not yet been completed, so the degree that hay fever has increased since 1994 is uncertain. The NHANES III revealed that nearly 55 percent of the U.S. population tested positive on a skin prick test (IgE allergy test) for at least one of ten common allergens known to cause symptoms of hay fever. Children are, of course, among those who are increasingly developing hay fever. Hay fever, considered "an exceedingly rare occurrence" in the early nineteenth century, has become a household term and an everyday experience for many Americans. [12]

In addition to respiratory allergies, atopic skin disease has increased substantially in recent years. The American Academy of Pediatrics reports that atopic dermatitis has increased threefold over the last decade. Reported food allergies in children are also on the rise, increasing 18 percent from 1997 to 2007.[13] Some early studies indicate that peanut allergy is among the fastest growing food allergy and may have tripled since the late 1980s.[14] No population-based studies have been done to assess the likely prevalence of food hypersensitivities or intolerances in children in the U.S.; however, most governmental health organizations and professional medical organizations tend to agree that food sensitivities seem to be increasing, but it is difficult to ascertain to what degree.

The American Academy of Allergy, Asthma, and Immunology has stated that up to 25 percent of the US population has reported adverse reactions to foods and the highest prevalence of this is among infants and young children. Other sources cite as many as 35 percent of people self-reporting adverse reactions to foods. Dr. William Walsh, allergist and author of *Food Allergies: The Complete Guide to Understanding Your Food Allergies,* noted in an interview that despite earlier ideas about food intolerances, they are an exceedingly common and serious problem. "It is widely thought by many people, including many allergists, that food intolerance is not much of a problem. I believe that the opposite is true—for every patient who has a food allergy, there are perhaps ten with food intolerances that cause real problems—there's just a huge number of people affected." Most of those affected by food intolerances are undiagnosed, and thus continue to suffer from symptoms of "unknown etiology."[15]

Perhaps the most troubling statistics emerging regarding chronic childhood illness in America are those that pertain to what have classically been defined as neurological, psychiatric or behavioral disorders. The rates of children now being diagnosed with autism, ADHD, depression, and bipolar disorder, among others, are at unprecedented levels. The current statistics are as follows:

- 1 in 6 children have a learning disability, developmental delay or behavioral disability.[16]
- The Centers for Disease Control (CDC) reports that 1 in 150 children have been diagnosed with autism. Studies have shown that the rates vary significantly by geography with rates

as high as 1 in 80 in some parts of the US and UK. New Jersey
is among the states with the highest prevalence of autism, reporting that 1 in 94 children, and 1 in 60 boys, have been diagnosed with autism.[17] A more recent unpublished study
conducted by the Cambridge University Autism Research
Center found that 1 in 60 British students had autism.[18] The
National Children's Health Survey released new data in October of 2009 revealing that 1 in 91 children (or 1 percent of
children) have an autism spectrum disorder.[19] This translates
to 1 in 57 American boys.[20]

- Estimates of the number of children who have ADHD range
  from 2-9 percent of children; The National Institute of Mental
  Health (NIMH) estimates approximately 5 percent of American children have ADHD, but recent CDC reports put the
  number closer to 8 percent.[21]

- The estimated number of children with severe mood dysregulation or pediatric bipolar disorder ranges from 3 to 7 percent.[22]

- Estimates for the prevalence of oppositional defiance disorder
  range from 1 to 16 percent of children.[23]

- According to physician and author of *Gut and Psychology Syndrome,* Dr. Natasha Campbell McBride: 10 percent of all children are dyspraxic (unable to coordinate motor function
  effectively), 1 in 100 children have been diagnosed with obsessive compulsive disorder, and 1 child in every classroom
  has depression.[24]

- According to a December 2008 report in the *Archives of General Psychiatry,* nearly 50 percent of college-age individuals
  have a psychiatric disorder. This study found that approximately 18 percent of college-age students met the criteria for
  personality disorders.[25]

Many of these conditions or diagnoses are rising at astonishing rates.
Although much debate surrounds the recent studies demonstrating
rates of autism are skyrocketing, a consensus is slowly emerging

around the idea that the prevalence of autism is indeed increasing, and the rising numbers cannot be attributed solely to improved or changing diagnostic techniques. Autism or Autism Spectrum Disorder (ASD) is a label given to children who exhibit symptoms of a syndrome that is characterized by abnormal development of social, behavioral and communicative functions. The American Academy of Pediatrics and most physicians describe ASDs as "brain-based" disorders, but an increasing body of literature supports the notion that ASDs are, in fact, the physical manifestation of systemic biological (not brain-specific) dysfunctions related to imbalances in inflammatory, detoxification, and oxidative mechanisms within the body.

Dozens of studies report a rising prevalence of autism in the United States (in addition to other western countries). For example, from 1995 to 2007, the prevalence of autism in children aged three to five years in California (those receiving state intervention services) increased from 0.6 per 1,000 to 4.1 per 1,000. This is a *sevenfold* increase in just twelve years! From 1994 to 2003, in an aggregate of all U.S. states (excluding Massachusetts and Iowa), the prevalence of autism for children in special education programs increased from 0.6 per 1,000 to 3.1 per 1,000. The prevalence has been shown to vary from state to state, with New Jersey showing the highest prevalence of 1.06 children per 100 as of 2002. It is estimated that the number of children diagnosed with autism has grown anywhere from three times to ten times in the past twenty years.[26]

Like ASDs, ADHD appears to be a relatively new epidemic, affecting children born in the late twentieth and early twenty-first century. Today, *at least* 5 percent of American children are classified as having ADHD, ADD or some variation of that diagnosis, but estimates range as high as 9 percent or even 12 percent of American children.[27] Researchers at the University of Cincinnati College of Medicine have argued that fewer than half of children with ADHD actually have a formal diagnosis. Thus, it is considered a condition that is grossly underdiagnosed. In the late 1960s, a disorder known as hyperkinesis or hyperkinetic reaction of childhood, characterized by hyperactivity, inattention and impulsivity was entered into the DSM-II (a mental health diagnostic manual). At the time, however, the occurrence of this disorder was considered relatively rare. According to the CDC, the annual increase in ADHD diagnoses in children averages about 3 percent annually. Some who are skeptical of the recent epidemic of ADHD argue that perhaps the increase is due to the American penchant for pathologizing behaviors that fall slightly outside the range of normal. This phenomenon, exacerbated by anxious parents and over-prescribing pediatricians, certainly accounts for some ADHD diagnoses. Many physicians who treat large numbers of children with ADHD will tell you that a majority of these children exhibit symptoms that go far beyond misbehavior or ineffective parenting.

Speak to the parent of a child with ADHD and they will assure you that ADHD is a very real condition that is both challenging and confounding. Furthermore, and perhaps most convincingly, studies in brain imaging and biochemistry confirm that ADHD does, in fact, have a biological basis. Regardless of the skeptic's view of ADHD, it is a health condition that is putting tremendous strain on our nation's health and education systems. ADHD, the top mental health problem affecting children today, is typically the most common diagnosis in special education settings, and is the main behavioral problem that classroom teachers encounter.[28]

The new epidemics of chronic childhood illnesses go beyond the Four-A Disorders. Mounting evidence indicates that other chronic childhood illnesses and disorders are on the rise. Many autoimmune disorders seem to be increasing, including: juvenile diabetes (increasing at 6 percent per year in children under four[29]), Crohn's disease, and ulcerative colitis. Recent studies in Denmark and Scotland have confirmed existing beliefs that the prevalence of pediatric Crohn's, colitis and inflammatory bowel disease has increased over the last decade in industrialized nations.[30] Celiac disease, an autoimmune disease where an individual cannot tolerate eating wheat or gluten, was once thought to be a rare childhood disease. It is now estimated that as many as one in eighty children has celiac, and for every diagnosed case, there are thirty undiagnosed cases.[31] Recent reports indicate that the prevalence of celiac has quadrupled since the 1950s.[32] Celiac disease has become so common that most supermarkets are now clearing their shelves to make way for gluten-free products. Even Starbucks just rolled out their new gluten-free Valencia Orange cake. The marketplace doesn't lie—if the supply is there, it reflects demand.

There is no doubt that we are experiencing an unnatural increase in chronic illnesses classically labeled as inflammatory, neurobehavioral, psychiatric and autoimmune. Author Donna Jackson Nakazawa made headlines in 2008 with the publication of her book *The Autoimmune Epidemic*, which brought national attention to the "escalating tsunami" of epidemiological evidence pointing to an American epidemic of autoimmune disease, affecting adults and children alike.[33] However, the autoimmune epidemic is only one small piece of the chronic illness epidemic that is sweeping the industrialized world. Our children are the canaries in the coalmine, warning of an epidemic of much greater proportions on its way. What does this epidemic mean for America?

THE ECONOMIC IMPACT OF CHRONIC DISEASE IN CHILDREN

A look at chronic childhood illness through the lens of economics is an effective way to gauge the total impact of this epidemic. It is a somewhat cold, yet sobering, exercise. Many studies have been done to estimate the cumulative costs associated with chronic disease. In 1999, the CDC estimated that the costs associated with special education for ADHD students totaled $3.5 to $4 billion annually. More recently, Pelham *et al.* estimated that based on a 2005 prevalence of ADHD (5 percent of sixty million children), the aggregate annual cost for health and mental health care alone was $7.9 billion. When costs associated with special education, as well as crime and delinquency, are added to this estimate, the total aggregate cost associated with societal management of ADHD is estimated to be $42.5 billion annually, with a per capita cost of $14,576 per child.[34] It is important to take into consideration that these estimates were done on a prevalence rate of 5 percent of sixty million children. Estimates in 2009 have been as high as 9 percent of seventy-three million American children, which adds up to a price tag of approximately $95 billion annually. The costs associated with ADHD continue to spiral out of control.

The costs associated with autism are equally devastating. Dr. Michael Ganz, an Adjunct Assistant Professor at the Harvard School of Public Health, estimates that the "the lifetime *per capita* incremental societal cost of autism is $3.2 million," with adult care and lost productivity accounting for the largest percentage of the cost. Dr. Ganz developed a model to estimate the total cost of one year's birth cohort of children with autism to determine the total societal economic impact of autism. His model, which uses a hypothetical birth cohort (based on prevalence data) from the year 2000, places the total lifetime cost associated with one year's birth cohort at $35 billion. This means that for all the children born in 2000 who have autism, society will absorb $35 billion in cost associated with their care (direct and indirect costs) by the time these children are sixty-five years old.[35] Extrapolating from this model, by 2065 American society will have incurred (conservatively estimated) over $1.15 trillion in costs associated with individuals with autism born in 2000 and thereafter.[36] Other estimates of the financial burden of autism place the U.S. annual economic cost at nearly $9 billion.[37] This is considered a conservative estimate. The Autism Society of America predicts that by 2013 the cost of autism will run at $200-400 billion a year.[38] With an estimated cost of $35,000 of direct medical costs per year up until age 5, it is unlikely that many families of individuals with autism will be able to carry the financial burden of caring for their children, thus it becomes America's financial burden. According to the National Autistic Society, only 6 percent of adults with autism are able to hold full-time employment and many individuals with autism require full time day care.[39] The epidemic of autism in America represents an economic crisis as well as a human crisis.

The skyrocketing costs associated with ADHD and autism are only one piece of the economic crisis our nation faces in coming years. According to the AAAI, the annual economic cost of asthma in America is $19.7 billion. Direct costs make up about $14.7 billion of that total, and indirect costs, such as lost productivity, add another $5 billion. Over $6 billion of the direct cost of asthma is attributable to the cost of prescription medication used to manage asthma. According to a 2005 publication in the *American Journal of Public Health*, Foster *et al.* estimated that the cost to society of youths diagnosed with conduct disorder are estimated at $70,000 per child over a seven-year period (ages seven to thirteen). "In one longitudinal study in London, by age 28, children with childhood conduct problems had cost society 3.5 to 10 times more than a comparison group, mainly costs associated with crime and education."[40] All in, the societal cost associated with children suffering from chronic illness is billions upon billions of dollars annually. The time will come when our nation will break under the financial burden of chronic illness, and the generation of chronically ill children growing up in America today threatens our social and economic stability. Something must be done to stem the tide of illness in America.

IS THE EPIDEMIC OF CHRONIC CHILDHOOD ILLNESS REAL?

Is this gloomy picture of childhood illness and America's uncertain future real, or are we experiencing health hysteria created by a media-frenzied, anxiety-ridden population of parents and physicians erroneously labeling children who are poorly parented and over-indulged as sick? It is difficult to dispute the diagnoses of true allergy and asthma, as these diagnoses can be made fairly objectively using diagnostic criteria that is reproducible, controlled, and fairly accurate. However, the diagnosis of neurological, behavioral, and psychiatric disorders becomes somewhat more complicated because more subjective criteria are incorporated into the diagnosis. It is for this reason that many people question the existence of these types of illnesses and wonder if we are not pathologizing certain types of human behavior that used to be more acceptable. The question remains: are the epidemiological numbers regarding chronic childhood illnesses like autism and ADHD real? Let us first examine the epidemiological evidence.

The CDC and NIH (National Institutes of Health), the main governmental bodies that track the health and wellness of America's children, seem to be hedging themselves on the question of rising chronic childhood illnesses. Although the CDC confirms that the prevalence of autism is indeed 1 in 150 (as compared to estimates from the 1970s that ranged from <1 in 2000 to 1 in 10,000), they have not yet definitively conceded that the change in the number of children diagnosed with ASD is due to an increase in actual cases. The CDC concludes: "It is clear that more children than ever before are being classified as having autism spectrum disorders (ASDs). But, it is unclear how much this increase is due to changes in how we identify and classify ASDs in people, and how much is due to a true increase in prevalence."[41] Similarly, in a 2008 policy statement on autism, the American Academy of Pediatrics (AAP) concluded that "the [increased] prevalence of autism and, more recently, ASDs, is more closely linked to a history of changing criteria and diagnostic categories."[42] Thus, both the CDC and AAP acknowledge the increased prevalence of ASDs in America, but tend to attribute the increase to changing diagnostic and classification techniques.

The main evidence the CDC and AAP use to support these conclusions comes from a study authored by P.T. Shattuck and published in *Pediatrics* in 2006.[43] Shattuck argues that the increase in prevalence of autism is due to a concurrent decrease in mental retardation diagnoses. Therefore, the perceived increase in prevalence of autism was due to substitution of the label *mental retardation* with the label *autism*. Yet, additional studies have disproven this hypothesis, and subsequent studies have all together discredited the notion that increased prevalence can be attributed to changing diagnostic criteria.[44] Although changes in diagnostic procedures in conjunction with better tracking and "capture" of patients with autism in the primary care setting may account for some part of the increase in prevalence, the number of new cases of autism cannot be explained away by this overly simplistic analysis.

In a 2004 study published in *Public Health Reports* (official journal of the U.S. Public Health Service) Mark Blaxill reviewed over fifty-four available public health survey publications to determine whether the reported increased prevalence of autism was perceived (e.g., because of factors such as changes in diagnostic criteria) or real (actual number of cases of autism increasing as time advances). The report concludes that the large increases in prevalence of autism in both the U.S. and U.K. cannot be explained by diagnostic changes alone. Blaxill concludes: "A comparison of U.K. and U.S. surveys, taking into consideration changing definitions, ascertainment bias, and case-finding methods, provides strong support for a conclusion of rising disease frequency," and there is "little evidence that systematic changes in survey methods can explain these increases, although better ascertainment may still account for part of the observed change."[45] In a subsequent study, Mark Blaxill and Dan Hollenbeck challenged some of the conclusions drawn by Shattuck in his 2006 study. Again, Shattuck's study argued that increased numbers of autism diagnoses coincided with decreased numbers of children being diagnosed as mentally retarded beginning in the late 1980s. However, as Blaxill and Hollenbeck point out, Shattuck did not take into account the introduction of the diagnostic label *developmental delay*, which was increasingly used in lieu of mental retardation as a diagnostic label in the late 1980s. (See Graph 1.)

A study published in the January 2009 issue of *Epidemiology* concluded that the increasing prevalence of autism could not be explained away by diagnosis, awareness or other factors related to tracking or counting individuals with autism. The study, conducted by researchers at the UC Davis M.I.N.D. Institute, concluded that no more than 56 percent of the 600 to 700 percent increase in reported cases of autism could be attributed to the inclusion of milder cases of autism, such as PDD-NOS (pervasive developmental disorder — not otherwise specified). Furthermore, only 24 percent of the increase

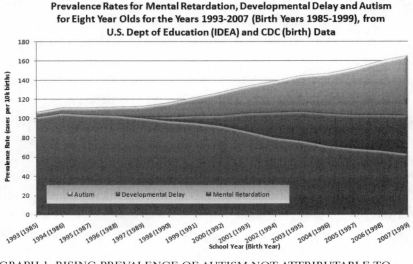

GRAPH 1. RISING PREVALENCE OF AUTISM NOT ATTRIBUTABLE TO
DIAGNOSTIC CHANGES

Permission to reprint: www.thoughtfulhouse.org.[46]

could be attributed to earlier age at diagnosis. The study found that
the increase in the number of children born in California with autism
since 1990 was likely to be a result of an increase in actual disease frequency, despite their best efforts to uncover other factors that contributed to increased numbers of diagnosed children.[47] Although the
rise in prevalence of reported cases of autism is still the subject of controversy, the evidence is beginning to mount behind the fact that
autism is indeed an epidemic in this country.

In the case of ADHD, the Centers for Disease Control and the
American Academy of Pediatrics take a stance similar to that of
autism: "The number of children who are being treated for ADHD
has risen. It is not clear whether more children have ADHD or more
children are being diagnosed with ADHD."[48] Although these organizations persist in taking a neutral stance on whether or not the prevalence of ADHD is actually increasing, most veteran teachers can
substantiate the trend by describing the changes they see in the class-

room. The hyperactivity, inattention, and impulsivity are only one part of the changes that these teachers see. The CDC's prevalence data suggest that one in twelve children in America is *diagnosed* with ADHD or a learning disability. Extrapolating from a 2007 study that indicated the gross underdiagnosis of ADHD, the prevalence of ADHD and learning disorders is one in six children. This means that every classroom has five or more children with ADHD and learning disabilities. This estimate does not even address the other mental health issues, such as bipolar disorder or depression, that affect learning and performance in school.

Even without diagnoses like ADHD, autism, or asthma, children today are just plain sicker than they were thirty years ago. Less severe illnesses like otitis media (ear infections), sinus infections, acid reflux, or chronic colds (runny noses, coughs) are extremely common today. These types of illnesses often fly under the radar screen of epidemiologists because they are not necessarily diagnosed or treated so they may not be tracked or logged in health records the way other illnesses would be. Children are getting ear infections earlier and with greater frequency than ever before in history. Ten years ago, the peak incidence of otitis media occurred between two and six years of age, and by six years of age, 75 percent of children had at least one episode.[49] Today, it is estimated that nearly 100 percent of children will have two episodes of otitis media by the time they are two years old (with the peak incidence being between six and twelve months of age). Moreover, children are routinely getting illnesses, such as sinus infections, that used to be found mainly in older populations.[50]

One more type of illness is nearly impossible to track because the symptoms are often mild, and it is not something that is frequently diagnosed in the doctor's office. Nonetheless, these subtle symptoms are indicative of a physiological dysfunction that could be critical to the health and wellness of the children that exhibit them. This type of illness is ubiquitous among American children today, and is perhaps the greatest warning signal that something is not right with our children. This illness could be called generalized gastrointestinal dysfunction or GI syndrome, but it is marked by an increasing number of children who have mild to severe gastrointestinal symptoms, such as reflux, vomiting after eating, colic, eosinophilic esophagitis, chronic diarrhea, abnormal stooling (stools that are yellow, foamy, excessively stinky, explosive or that float or contain large amounts of undigested food), chronic constipation, abdominal pain ("tummy aches"), or even hernias. Drop in on a playgroup for babies or young children, or visit an early childcare center or daycare center and ask how many of the children in the room exhibit these symptoms on a frequent basis. The answer will astound you. Despite what pediatricians might tell you, these symptoms are *not* a normal part of childhood, not if they are occurring on a frequent or everyday basis. Occasional diarrhea or constipation or vomiting happens with children. But children today are living with these symptoms *every day*. It is *not normal*.

WHAT IS MAKING OUR CHILDREN SICK?

Although not all governmental and professional organizations are willing to embrace the label of *epidemic* regarding chronic childhood illnesses today, they are beginning to look with concerted effort into what is causing the development of chronic illnesses like autism and ADHD in children. Despite intensive research efforts, no one has been able to explain why children today are affected so profoundly with illnesses that were relatively rare in children just thirty years ago. The explanation for each illness varies but there are some common ideas that many researchers and physicians cite as possible explanations for the increases in chronic illness in kids today.

The Hygiene Hypothesis and Related Theories

Perhaps the most honest answer given by physicians when asked what is causing so many children to become chronically ill is, "we don't know." However, there does seem to be a consensus emerging around the theory of the *hygiene hypothesis* as a possible contributor to the epidemic of chronic childhood illnesses. This theory is often cited by physicians who treat children suffering from allergies, asthma, and autoimmune disorders as a possible, although not fully developed, explanation for atopic and autoimmune disease. The hygiene hypothesis is not typically cited when discussing neurological, behavioral or psychiatric illnesses.

The hygiene hypothesis, as described by the American Society for Microbiology, "suggests that allergies and autoimmune diseases are caused or aggravated by depriving the immune system of microbial stimulation during its development."[51] The theory essentially argues that the human being's exposure to microbes early in life has been reduced substantially in the modern (industrialized) era. Humans were once exposed to a myriad of microbiota in everyday life, through contaminated water, soil, raw foods and contact with other people and animals. As many of these microbes have been removed from our experience through sanitation, sterilization, chlorination, etc., our immune systems are no longer effectively "primed" when we are children, and therefore do not function properly. Jessica Snyder Sachs, author of *Good Germs, Bad Germs*, uses the hygiene hypothesis to speculate on the importance of microbes to our very existence. "Could it be that the human immune system evolved in such a way that it came to rely on constant exposure to bacteria and other 'germs' to function properly? If so, what happens when over one or two centuries, an evolutionary blink of an eye, we separate ourselves from this continual exposure by sanitizing our water, processing our food, dousing our bodies with germ-killing drugs and soaps, and distancing ourselves from the natural landscape?"[52]

The hypothesis was developed by epidemiologist David Strachan in the late 1980s when he was researching atopic disease in British families. In trying to determine a rationale for the increased prevalence of atopic disease in Britain (in the 1980s, it was estimated that one in eight British children suffered from some form of atopy), Strachan found that families with more children generally had a lower incidence of atopic disease. "The modern epidemic of allergies and asthma, Strachan concluded, stemmed directly from a decrease in the usual viral infections of childhood, from the common cold to measles, mumps, and rubella." Essentially, Strachan argued that a lack of exposure to "germs" in early childhood robbed their immune systems of the practice needed to become fully developed, mature and effective immune systems. The consequence was immune systems that were hypersensitive and that would respond to benign substances such as pollen and dust. Strachan titled his study, "Hay Fever, Hygiene, and Household Size" which was later transformed into "The Hygiene Hypothesis" as it made its way through the mainstream media and into the medical community.[53] Subsequent researchers have reinforced his finding by looking at other factors that contribute to the development of more hardy immune systems (e.g., older brothers or pets in the home).

After Strachan and others proposed the mechanism behind the hygiene hypothesis, immunologists began to look for further evidence to prove or disprove this theory. Many studies have emerged to support this theory, yet an equal number refute this initial hypothesis. Recently, researchers have begun to develop modified versions of the hygiene hypothesis where the focus has begun to move away from the importance of microbes that cause infection (pathogens) and toward the importance of exposure to *any* microbes. Initial studies seem to indicate that early and frequent exposure to all sorts of microbes (through farm animals, fecal exposure, day care/other children) has a sort of immune-strengthening or protective benefit, especially with regard to the development of atopic and autoimmune disorders. A modified hygiene hypothesis now proposes that the lack of exposure to microbes in early childhood can lead to immune disorders (especially in those individuals who might have a genetic predisposition toward atopy or autoimmunity). It is not exposure to infection, per se, but exposure to microbes in general that offers some sort of protection.[54]

This theory was further developed by Graham Rook of University College in London in what has become known as the Old Friends hypothesis. The theory proposes that reduced exposure to microorganisms that have long lived symbiotically with human beings, such as intestinal parasites and other bacteria ("old friends"), may hinder the ability of our immune system to regulate appropriate responses. In other words, the human immune system is trained to regulate itself (against attacking its own cells and against hyper-reactivity to benign antigens) by early and frequent exposure to microscopic old friends. Although the hygiene hypothesis is widely known among physicians treating patients with atopic and autoimmune diseases, Rook's old friends hypothesis is less well known, but is beginning to gain traction. Nonetheless, these early theories as to the etiology of chronic disease are not fully developed and have yet to make an impact in terms of treating or preventing chronic atopic and autoimmune disease.

Etiology of ADHD, ASDs and other "Neurobehavioral" and "Psychological" Illnesses

For the most part, physicians and many scientists are still attributing ADHD, ASDs, and illnesses such as depression and bipolar disorder to genetics and neurobiology. The conventional wisdom on the etiology of ADHD, as expressed by the NIMH (National Institute of Mental Health) is as follows: "Most substantiated causes appear to fall in the realm of neurobiology and genetics. This is not to say that environmental factors may not influence the severity of the disorder, and especially the degree of impairment and suffering the child may experience, but that such factors do not seem to give rise to the condition by themselves."[55] Much of the research in ADHD has focused on abnormalities in the brain of individuals with ADHD (such as brain volume, reduced "white matter," etc.). However, few of these many and well-funded studies have looked elsewhere in the body to determine if any other systemic or physiological disruptions in the body might contribute to particular abnormalities in brain structure and function.

Similarly, researchers looking to explain mental illnesses such as bipolar disorder, schizophrenia or depression tend to operate within the construct of neurobiology. The vast majority of research focuses on studying and manipulating levels of brain chemicals known as neurotransmitters, such as dopamine, norepinephrine, and serotonin, in an effort to regulate mood and behavior. Yet, in looking for answers regarding mental illness, few researchers seem to focus on the parts of the human body where many neurotransmitters are manufactured, namely, the gastrointestinal system. As Michael Gershon's groundbreaking research on the enteric nervous system (*The Second Brain*, 1999) revealed, neurotransmitters manufactured in the gut can impact the function and health of both the gut *and* the brain. Unfortunately, because so many researchers are still fixated on the mechanics of the brain, neurologists and psychiatrists are left with an arsenal of medications that can manipulate and alter the brain chemistry of individuals with mental illness, but they are still unable to explain why these brain chemical imbalances occur in the first place.

Despite recent growth in funding for autism research, the etiology of ASDs is unknown. Researchers use the same genetics and neurobiology paradigm as ADHD and other "psychological" illnesses to explain what causes autism. Most theories as to the etiology of ASDs rely heavily on genetics as an explanation. Increasingly, researchers are looking at the interplay between genes and environment to explain autism, but even these preliminary investigations tend to operate with the assumption that genetics is the predominate force in etiology. There is such a strong belief that ASDs are genetically rooted that even epidemiological studies work off of this paradigm. One study, conducted by Rogers *et al.* in 2008, proposed that the increased prevalence of autism was due to more women taking folate supplements prenatally, which results in greater survival of fetuses with "a genetic polymorphism that does not maintain normal folate levels which, in turn, resulted in an increase in children at risk for diminished methylation and consequently, abnormal neurodevelopment resulting in autism/ASD."[56] Essentially, this hypothesis speculates that all children with autism are destined to be autistic because of their genetic makeup, but spontaneous miscarriage that would normally occur (through natural selection) does not happen because of the mother's increased folate intake during pregnancy. Although this theory is novel, it does not address many of the biological dysfunctions that are present in children with ASD, and it also relies heavily on genetics as a sole explanation for ASDs. Theories abound, from the plausible to the absurd, but there is still no consensus as to the likely etiology of autism.[57]

The most widely circulated, and certainly most controversial, theory among laypersons explains the increase in autism as somehow related to childhood vaccination. The theory proposes that autism is caused by brain damage affected by the MMR (measles, mumps and rubella) vaccine, or thimerosal, a vaccine stabilizer. This theory was first introduced in a study conducted by Dr. Andrew Wakefield in 1998. Wakefield's study found evidence that measles vaccination had been associated with intestinal abnormalities, which precipitated a cascade of events ultimately resulting in the development of ASD in twelve patients. Subsequently, critics of Wakefield's study have been vitriolic in their attacks on Wakefield and his research. According to most sources, Wakefield and his 1998 study have been fully discredited. Moving beyond the controversy and flaws of his 1998 MMR study, Andrew Wakefield continues to publish studies examining the role of the gastrointestinal system in the development of ASDs. Despite the larger medical community's apparent antipathy for Dr. Wakefield, many researchers, integrative physicians, and holistic practitioners continue to follow Wakefield's work in hopes of a breakthrough regarding the etiology of autism.

Other research has used Wakefield's study as a platform for further examination. A 2008 study conducted by Young *et al.* found that "significantly increased rates of autism, ASD, attention deficit disorder, attention deficit hyperactivity disorder, learning disorders, emotional disorders and tics [were] associated with increased mercury exposure from thimerosal-containing vaccines during the period from 1990 to

1996."[58] Thimerosal, (sodium ethylmercurithiosalicylate) which contains ethylmercury, a known neurotoxin, has been the focus of intense and emotional debate since the late 1990s. Many parents of children with autism claim that thimerosal is responsible for triggering autism in their children, and battles between parents and vaccine manufacturers continue to play out in the court system. A number of studies demonstrate a link between thimerosal and autism, but there are even more studies that *disprove* a link between thimerosal and autism. For instance, a 2008 study conducted by Schecter and Grether reported that "the prevalence of autism in California increased after thimerosal was eliminated from vaccines."[59] More studies continue to emerge that only intensify the debate.

Despite the best efforts of the CDC, the AAP, and other public health organizations to try to bury the vaccine-autism link because of its impact on rates of vaccination (which may lead to increased prevalence of dangerous infectious diseases in the general population), the debate simply will not go away. The jury is still out among many clinicians and researchers regarding the vaccine-autism theory. Most of the American medical community continues to begrudge Wakefield for generating what they view to be "vaccine hysteria" responsible for a reduced rate of childhood vaccinations. Should the emerging science uncover a link between vaccines and autism, Wakefield and subsequent researchers who claim a link will experience the greatest of all vindications. As previously stated, much of the debate concerning the vaccine-autism link centers on the role of thimerosal. Increasingly, however, researchers are beginning to look beyond thimerosal, and instead look at what impact routine childhood immunizations may have on the immune system. This research stems, in part, from clinical observations made by physicians using a functional or integrative medical approach to treat and heal children with autism.

To date, there do not seem to be any explanations for autism that the American medical community wants to embrace outside of genetics. However, a small but growing numbers of physicians (particularly alternative or integrative), research scientists, and other clinicians are beginning to outline a complex theory as to the etiology of autism, where genetics play only one small part. Within this theory may also lie the answers to etiology of other chronic childhood illnesses, such as ADHD, allergies, asthma and many autoimmune disorders.

The Alternative Theory

Increasingly, scientists are documenting biochemical imbalances as well as physiological dysfunctions in the body that help to explain the existence of clinical symptoms associated with neurobehavioral or psychiatric diagnoses. These imbalances or dysfunctions could include anything from hormone imbalances or inflammation in the brain to heavy metal toxicity. For example, when a child demonstrates "abnormal behavior" with symptoms that resemble the diagnosis of ADHD, we can find physiological imbalances or abnormalities in this child (as compared to his neurotypical, or "normal" peers) that provide a biological rationale for the behavior.

In 2002, researchers in the NIMH Child Psychiatry Branch studied 152 boys and girls with ADHD, matched with 139 age- and gender-matched controls without ADHD. Researchers determined after scanning the children's brains multiple times that, "the ADHD children showed 3-4 percent smaller brain volumes in all regions—the frontal lobes, temporal gray matter, caudate nucleus, and cerebellum."[60] Many researchers take this information regarding the smaller brain size of children with ADHD and immediately begin looking for clues to etiology of "small brain" in the genes. These researchers are seeking the "ah ha!" moment when they can isolate the particular gene or gene sequence that regulates brain growth and development.

In contrast, researchers and physicians operating under a different paradigm regarding human health and wellness believe that chronic illnesses like ADHD have complex etiologies that are particular to each individual, and genetics alone cannot explain the origin. Instead, they speculate that chronic childhood illnesses develop from a perfect storm of toxic overload, improper nutrition, dysregulated immune function, and unhealthful lifestyles, among other contributing factors. In other words, there are no *simple* explanations for the epidemic of chronic childhood illnesses in America in the twenty-first century, but there are explanations. These explanations are elaborated upon in chapter two.

Importantly, the explanations presented by this group of individuals offer hope for prevention, treatment and cure of children's chronic illnesses. This new way of understanding the etiology of chronic childhood illness in America is complicated, yet logical, and even intuitive, once you move beyond Western medicine's disease- and organ-based medical paradigm. Unfortunately, the modern medical establishment is reluctant to embrace these theories because the preventative and therapeutic protocols that can save our children question existing immunization and pharmaceutical practices, as well as environmental and cultural influences.

Nonetheless, it is time for America to wake up to the epidemic of chronic illness burdening our pediatric population. By ignoring the problem or denying that it exists, we are unwittingly creating a grim future for our children and ourselves. Children of today are overmedicated, poorly nourished, and exposed to a tremendous toxic burden on a daily basis. What's more, many children suffer from immune dysregulation, a condition that makes them more susceptible to all of the toxic influences in their lives. It is entirely possible that we are raising the first generation of children that does not outlive its parents. The consequences of doing nothing are not only tremendous in terms of human cost, but the economic cost associated with an entire generation of children saddled with chronic illness is a burden that this country does not want to encounter, and cannot afford.

chapter 2

The Etiology of Chronic Illness in American Children

🌱

One of the reasons skeptics question the validity of the emerging epidemiological evidence regarding the epidemic of chronic childhood illness is that it just seems *too* unbelievable. Can there possibly be *that many* ill children in this country? Why is it that all these diseases that seem to be relatively unrelated (like autism and juvenile diabetes) are rising concurrently? It would be logical, for instance, if it were *only* neurological disorders that were on the rise. A rise in just neurological disorders would tell us to look at what affects neurobiology to try to ascertain what might be causing more children to become sick.

However, the diseases that are striking our children today affect the brain, the pancreas, the lungs, and the skin among other organs. The diseases are psychiatric, inflammatory, autoimmune, behavioral, gastroenterological, and immunological. What could possibly be affecting all of these seemingly disparate parts of, and functions within, our children's bodies?

The answer is first that these parts of our body are *not* distinct entities; rather they are all interconnected parts of the same biological systems, and if one organ appears to be dysfunctional, then it is likely that underlying biochemical dysfunctions or imbalances are affecting all organs, systems, and mechanisms in the body. Therefore, these diseases (which are not really diseases at all) are just names that we give to symptoms of underlying biological dysfunctions that are as unique and varied as the individuals who suffer from them. To an untrained eye, a child who presents with a disease like asthma seems to have a problem in the lungs, but the "diseased" lungs are merely one outward physical manifestation of other serious systemic dysfunctions occurring within the body.

One of the fundamental flaws of our existing medical paradigm is the tendency to approach health and sickness only through a disease-based, or organ-focused, lens. Most branches of medical specialties are almost exclusively dedicated to specific organs, organ groups or diseases. The exceptions are those specialties that focus on a particular patient population (e.g., pediatrics or geriatrics) or skill (e.g., surgery or radiology), or particular settings (e.g., emergency medicine, or intensive care medicine). (See table 1.) Physicians are some of the most intelligent, hard working, and highly trained professionals in our society, but few are trained to use a "systems biology" approach to manage the health of their patients.

When an asthmatic patient presents at a pediatrician's office, the pediatrician is trained to diagnose and manage the asthma ("name it, blame it, tame it"). It is not always possible for a physician to figure out why the patient developed asthma in the first place. Certainly, the physician can help a patient to determine that the household cat

TABLE 1: REPRESENTATIVE AMERICAN CLINICAL MEDICAL SPECIALTIES

Medical Specialty	Organ/Disease/System Focus	Setting Focus	Patient Population Focus	"Systems Biology" Focus	Generalized Skill
Anesthesiology	Pain/Anesthetics				
Orthopedic/Ofthopedic Surgery	Skeletal system				
Otolaryngology/ENT/Surgery	Ear, nose, neck, face, throat				
Pediatrics/Pediatric Surgery			Children		
Plastic Surgery	Skin, muscle, nerve etc.				
Oncology/Hematology	Cancer				
Surgical Oncology					Surgery
Urology/Urological Surgery	Urogenital system				
Vascular surgery	Vascular system and peripheral vessels				
Transplant surgery	Organs				
Thoracic surgery	Chest organs				
General Surgery					Surgery
Cardiology	Heart/Cardiovascular system				
Cardiovascular surgery	Cardiovascular system/heart surgery				Surgery
Trauma Surgery					Surgery
Maxillofacial surgery	Face/jawith neck				Surgery
Dermatology	Skin and its appendages				
Emergency Medicine		ER			
Intensive Care Medicine		ICU			
Endocrinology	Endocrine system				
Gastroenterology	GI system				
Hepatology	Liver/biliary tract				
Infectious diseases	Infectious diseases				
Nephrology	Kidney disease				
Proctology	Rectum, anus, colon				
Pulmonology	Lungs/respiratory tract				
Rheumatology	Joints/inflammatory disease				
Neurology	Brain				
Geriatrics			Elderly		
Obstetrics/Gynecology	Reproductive system				
Psychiatry	Psychiatric disorders ("diseases" believed to affect the brain)				
Integrative Medicine				Systems Approach	
Functional Medicine				Systems Approach	
Environmental Medicine				Systems Approach	

triggers episodes of asthma, but he or she cannot provide an explanation as to why that particular patient's immune system is intolerant of cat dander. The doctor knows that the patient's immune system is hyper-reactive to ordinarily innocuous substances, and may know every minute detail of the cascade of biological events that lead to wheezing when a cat enters the room, but he or she can provide only theories (such as genetics or the hygiene hypothesis) to explain why this occurs in a particular patient. The patient can be referred on to another medical subspecialist, such as a pulmonologist or an allergist, but even here, the specialist mainly focuses on a particular system or biological mechanism, which may not provide any insight into etiology.

Western medicine tends to be fairly silo-ed, particularly in the United States. This institutional organization has benefits. If an organ needs to be removed, you want the surgeon removing it to be highly trained in the care and management of that particular organ. The problem with this structure is that the etiology of disease is almost never to be found by looking at one particular organ or system in the body. Thus, silo-ed medicine is not optimal for understanding etiology of disease.

What causes chronic illness? The truth is, as most honest physicians will tell you, we do not know precisely what causes these illnesses, although we do know about things that are correlated with the development of the diseases. If causes are not known then it is virtually impossible to prevent or cure these illnesses. Our existing medical paradigm is not bringing us any closer to prevention, treatment or cure of these chronic illnesses, but medical research and developing branches of medicine such as functional medicine and environmental medicine are getting closer every day.

Preliminary Medical Research and Functional Medicine Shed Light on Chronic Disease Etiology

Although earlier, less developed versions of functional medicine have been around for a long time, functional medicine, as a new medical paradigm, has really been operating only for the latter part of the twentieth century. Essentially, functional medicine uses systems biology (or "body ecology") to understand and correct imbalances in the human body that impede health and wellness. Practitioners believe that disease is something that develops because fundamental life-giving mechanisms in the body (most often found in places other than the "diseased" organ) break down. A properly functioning body is one that effectively assimilates vitamins, minerals and nutrients, digests food properly, and eliminates wastes and toxins properly. When a body is not properly functioning, because of any number of physiological or biochemical imbalances, the body can manifest disease-like symptoms in any organ or system. This is why disease labels are not helpful in providing any insight into etiology of disease. The "diseased" organ is usually only one outwardly manifested symptom of a whole host of underlying imbalances. Thus, it is of critical importance to look for underlying imbalances in a "diseased" patient, for this will point to etiology of disease, and it can provide a prescription for treatment and cure.

Functional medicine applies a new paradigm to health management in patients.

For instance, recent medical research has discovered that one of the primary mechanisms behind cardiovascular disease is inflammation.[1] In fact, physicians can now assess a particular patient's risk for cardiovascular disease by looking for particular biological markers of inflammation such as c-reactive protein (a substance that can be found in the blood). But where does the inflammation come from? Conventional medicine might use a drug to try to block inflammatory processes from affecting the heart and vascular system. This is like putting a bucket under a leaky roof. Functional medicine, on the other hand, aims to find the root cause of the inflammation and turn it off—or fix the hole in the roof to stop the leak. For each individual patient, functional medical practitioners look for and test for particular imbalances or stressors known to be associated with disease, and treat the disease by correcting the imbalances and eliminating the stressors.

The most basic example of applied functional medicine is what was done in the eighteenth century on ships where crewmembers were suffering from scurvy. Scurvy, an illness that was particularly common among seafarers, is caused by vitamin C deficiency. A Scottish surgeon in the British Royal Navy by the name of James Lind treated and prevented scurvy in sailors by making them eat citrus fruits. Although this approach is technically known as "orthomolecular medicine," the two disciplines overlap and share common principles. Orthomolecular medicine tends to focus on the role of nutrients and vitamins in the body, and functional medicine incorporates a wider spectrum of analysis of bodily processes and factors, including but not limited to: nutrients, neurotransmitters, hormones, proteins, microorganisms, immunological cells, energy and of course, genes. Classic functional medicine uses a fairly simple concept: evaluate the individuality of a patient, then find and correct their particular imbalances/deficiencies/stressors. The twenty-first century version of functional medicine is quite complicated, and it does not fit into the existing western medical paradigm. Functional medicine requires extensive laboratory testing and often does not result in the prescription of pharmaceutical agents. It requires a highly individualized approach to patient management, which is an approach that has been widely replaced by the "one-size-fits-all" approach preferred in the age of managed care. Many American physicians today are under so much pressure to meet the demands of their patients and practices that they barely have enough time to write a prescription for their patients, let alone discuss metabolic testing.

Practitioners who apply functional medicine to their patient population have experienced remarkable results with regard to treatment, prevention, and cure of disease. While functional medicine cannot be easily assimilated into the existing American healthcare system, it is the future of healthcare. Practitioners who use the latest scientific research to apply the functional medicine paradigm to the care of their patients are at the cutting edge of medical treatment and health management. It is a remarkable and awe-inspiring field that may usher in a new age of human health and wellness. It is in the cutting-edge scientific and medical research, and in the offices of functional medicine practitioners that the etiology of chronic illness in children is coming to light.

THE ETIOLOGY OF CHRONIC CHILDHOOD ILLNESS

There are many names for today's chronic childhood illnesses. These names are autism, ADHD, allergies, asthma, multiple sclerosis, depression, bipolar disorder and many other labels that can be found in the DSM-IV (standard diagnostic manual). From a pharmaceutical and clinical management perspective these are meaningful terms because certain pharmacological and behavior modification techniques for each of these illnesses can help improve some symptoms. However, these labels become somewhat inadequate when considering how to prevent and cure such illness in children. No one seems to know what causes any of these illnesses outside of some correlations to genetics, but these findings are not fully developed. Chronic illnesses like autism and ADHD are a real problem for all conventional medical clinicians. Typically, they can offer their patients little outside of symptom management.

To practitioners of functional medicine, autism, asthma, multiple sclerosis and many other illnesses are not so much diseases as they are observable manifestations of human bodies with fundamental biochemical and physiological imbalances. Conventional western medicine describes ADHD as a genetically based brain dysfunction that results in inattention, hyperactivity, and impulsivity. This way of understanding ADHD tells us to look in the brain or at a genetic profile for answers as to what causes ADHD. The functional medicine approach is different.

Through established scientific research and laboratory testing, functional medicine recognizes that ADHD is associated with imbalances in the levels of micronutrients (or vitamins and minerals used by the body for basic functions), neurotransmitters (necessary brain chemicals), and excesses of heavy metals in the body, among other dysregulated processes. Through diagnostic laboratory testing, clinicians can evaluate a particular patient's imbalances and look for what might have contributed to these imbalances. For instance, deficiencies in micronutrients in the body (such as zinc, selenium, magnesium) can be explained by looking at the diet and how effectively or ineffectively the body assimilates these nutrients into the gastrointestinal tract.

Similarly, mood and behavior problems can be assessed by looking at the levels of neurotransmitters (such as dopamine or serotonin) circulating in the blood. Disorders associated with a deficiency in serotonin, a critical brain chemical required for mood stability, can be explained by looking at how effectively the body produces serotonin, which, interestingly, is produced in the gastrointestinal tract. In fact, 95 percent of your body's serotonin is manufactured in the duodenum (part of the small intestines)![2] For a patient with depression or ADHD (both conditions marked by altered levels of neurotransmitters or brain chemicals), one cannot begin to understand the origin of these "diseases" without first looking at the health of the gastrointestinal tract. Many of the imbalances in the body's brain chemicals actually originate in the "gut."

The *gut*, or gastrointestinal tract, simply refers to the long hollow tube that stretches from the tip of your tongue to your anus. Since the bulk of neurotransmitters are produced in the gut, it would seem logical that a physician would examine the gut health of a patient with a mood disorder. Yet few physicians, and even fewer psychiatrists, examine gut health when diagnosing and treating this sort of illness. This completely ignores a biological system that is likely to play a critical role in the onset of illness.

What functional medicine offers that conventional western medicine does not is the ability and the potential to determine etiology of illnesses that were previously understood only as chronic, incurable, or worse, genetic. If you understand the root cause(s) of illness, then the chances of treating, curing and preventing illness increase exponentially. For example, millions upon millions of dollars have been spent on, and hundreds of thousands of research hours have been invested into, the search for the cause of autism. Most of this time and money has been spent looking at the brain and genetics. Is there no greater puzzle in the medical world today than the etiology of autism? Functional medicine is beginning to uncover some of the root causes of autism (and there are many). Applied functional medicine has reversed autism in *thousands* of patients across the country. Many of these children have completely lost their autism diagnoses and are now considered neurotypical, indistinguishable from their "normal" peers. These same protocols have been applied to children suffering from ADHD, allergies and asthma, and they have also recovered from their illnesses.

What, then, causes autism? What causes asthma, ADHD, allergies, juvenile diabetes, bipolar disorder, depression, and the many other chronic illnesses plaguing our children today? The answers to these questions are complicated and vary significantly from patient to patient, but some underlying mechanisms and environmental factors are present in various combinations in virtually all chronic illnesses in children. Particular changes in American life over the last century have precipitated an increased likelihood of children developing chronic illness, but the changes that have been seen over the last few decades are accelerating this likelihood at an unprecedented rate.

ROOT CAUSES: THE PERFECT STORM

The epidemic of chronic childhood illness in America is the product of "a perfect storm" of environmental factors, including the overuse of medications, poor diet and nutrition, excessive hygiene, indoor sedentary lifestyles, excessive or improperly administered vaccination, and continuous exposure to a panoply of environmental toxins. To a degree, genetics play a role in the development of illness for particular children, but genetically based explanations do not explain the unprecedented and widespread biological dysfunctions among children today. There are no epidemics of genetic illnesses, only environmentally derived illnesses. There are simply too many sick children today to substantiate the theory that genetics cause their illnesses.

Note to Readers: The following content is rich in scientific evidence and medical detail. The science may be complicated or overwhelming for those who are not scientifically oriented, but it is a necessary part of the explanation of why children become chronically ill. I have tried to simplify some of the medical concepts and I have also placed some of the more rigorous medical detail in the endnotes. Taking the time to understand the science is well worth the effort. If you are ready to learn the root cause of chronic illness in children, in all of its fascinating scientific detail, read on. If you find yourself becoming overwhelmed, move on to chapter three and come back to chapter two when you feel ready to digest the science.

An Explanation of Common Biological Dysfunctions at the Root of Chronic Illness

Instead of looking at chronic childhood illnesses as distinct entities, let us look at common underlying biological and physiological imbalances that are present in most of these illnesses. One of the first clues that points to common underlying biological dysfunctions in all of these illnesses is that most children present with a primary diagnosis (such as asthma), but they also present with a variety of comorbidities. *Comorbidity* is a term used to describe the presence of a secondary, and often less severe, chronic disease in a patient. Many children with ADHD, for instance, are saddled with other conditions, such as seasonal allergies, eczema, or obsessive-compulsive disorder. It is very common for children with asthma to also have food allergies and eczema. Children with autism typically carry the worst comorbidity load, suffering from gastrointestinal illnesses such as colitis, reflux, and chronic diarrhea, but they also tend to have allergies (food and respiratory), and other neurological comorbidities such as anxiety or ADHD. The fact that many of the symptoms of chronic illness in children overlap leads us to ask if there are common underlying biological dysfunctions.

In kids with chronic illnesses some of the most basic biological systems and functions are "broken" or operate improperly. One of the common underlying biological dysfunctions found in virtually all children with chronic illnesses is something known as *immune dysregulation*. This simply means that their immune systems are not functioning properly. This phenomenon has been observed in the clinical setting, but it has also been demonstrated through laboratory analysis.

It is well known that the etiology of allergies and asthma is tied to immune dysregulation. However, what is less well known, at least outside the medical community, is that almost all of the chronic illnesses in children today are in some way related to immune dysregulation. In recent years, medical researchers have established immune dysregulation as one of the principle suspects in the etiology of autism.[3] Other illnesses are also believed to be rooted in immune dysregulation. Juvenile diabetes, long believed to be a genetic disorder, is now understood as an autoimmune disorder.[4] Autoimmunity (when the immune system attacks a body's own cells/tissues) is no longer an obscure term used to discuss illnesses such as multiple sclerosis or lupus, but rather a vast umbrella that covers hundreds of illnesses as seemingly distant as rheumatoid arthritis and celiac disease.

Immune dysregulation is ubiquitous in American children today, and it goes beyond just those who are "sick." Many children who might be considered healthy by an untrained eye have more subtle signs of immune dysregulation like chronic constipation, moderate behavioral problems, reflux, chronic sinusitis, recurrent ear infections, or a particular susceptibility to colds and flu. America is experiencing a historic epidemic of immune dysregulation in its children and researchers are finally beginning to figure out why.

Despite the medical establishment's most desperate desires to find the holy grail of disease in our genes, there is no one "autism gene" or "ADHD gene." Genetic information is important for understanding the etiology of these chronic illnesses, as it can provide us with information on an individual's degree of susceptibility to particular environmental factors. But the genetic susceptibilities may not be meaningful if we do not understand how these susceptibilities work in concert with environmental triggers and influences. It is an extraordinarily complicated web of specific environmental factors that have precipitated this recent trend of chronic illness in American children. Simply put, every day we send our children out into a world that is saturated with toxins and immunological challenges, but many of our children are what could only be described as immunocompromised. In other words, the immune systems of many children have been altered and made dysfunctional by an assortment of environmental factors. The origin, as well as the clinical consequence, of each child's immune dysregulation varies. This is why it is so difficult to pin down the etiology of chronic childhood illnesses: the specific root causes of each child's illness vary according to his or her particular environmental exposures and unique genetic make up.

Immune Dysregulation and Chronic Childhood Illness

Although many environmental factors contribute to chronic illness in children, one of the most important outcomes of all these environmental influences is a dysregulated immune system. A dysregulated immune system can overreact to innocuous stimulus; it can attack its host's own cells and tissues; it does not have the ability to eliminate harmful substances that enter the body, and it cannot effectively combat pathogenic (disease-causing) microbes that invade the body. The most common environmental factors that can contribute to a dysregulated immune system include:

- Disruptions to existing healthy colonies of bacteria in the body (most often caused by antibiotics or other pharmaceuticals)
- Diet and nutrition
- Lifestyle factors (such as indoor, sedentary lives)
- Exposure to environmental toxins and electrical pollution
- Modern forms of immunization

Many of these factors create a vicious cycle in the body that, once begun, is difficult to reverse. For instance, environmental toxins can dysregulate an immune system and once an immune system is dysregulated, it becomes increasingly difficult for a body to effectively process new environmental toxins, thus leading to a vicious cycle.

Immune dysregulation occurs when human immunological cells no longer respond to immune stimuli in natural and benign ways. The immune system is an extraordinarily complex system in our bodies, and for as much as scientists know about it, new information is being generated all the time. By looking at the development of infants' immune systems, much can be learned about how and why the immune system can become dysfunctional. When babies are born, their immune systems are immature and inexperienced. As they come in contact with environmental stimuli such as microbes, food particles, and other antigens, their immune systems learn how to differentiate "friend" from "foe." They also learn how to effectively eliminate harmful substances (pathogens, toxins, etc.) from the body.

Most of this learning occurs in the gastrointestinal tract. Oral tolerance (the immune system's tolerance of benign antigens such as food), tolerance of beneficial bacteria, and immunological responses to pathogenic bacteria occur mostly in the gastrointestinal tract. Since approximately 90 percent of known pathogens enter the body through the gastrointestinal tract, it makes sense that the vast majority of the immune system would be located here.[5] Within the first few months of an infant's life, the gastrointestinal tract goes from being completely sterile (in the womb) to becoming colonized by hundreds of different types of microorganisms. These colonies of microorganisms are critical to immune system development, and to fundamental biological processes such as digestion, nutrient assimilation, as well as detoxification.[6] When there is an imbalance between the number of "good germs" (commensal or beneficial microorganisms) and "bad germs" (pathogenic yeasts, bacteria, viruses, etc.) in the gut, a condition known as "gut dysbiosis" occurs. This simply means that the good germs that live in the gut have been overrun by bad germs.

When populations of commensal microorganisms ("good germs") are disrupted or overtaken by pathogenic microorganisms ("bad germs"), the effects can be devastating. The immune system becomes compromised, the body is not able to efficiently assimilate nutrients or produce energy, and a whole cascade of physiological disasters can occur. Although gut dysbiosis can occur anywhere along the gastrointestinal tract, it is of particular concern when this occurs in the small intestine, as this is where the bulk of food and nutrients are assimilated into the body. Gut dysbiosis can lead to intestinal permeability (when certain contents of the intestine "leak" out into the body), which is directly linked to the development of allergic disease. Gut dysbiosis contributes to the total inflammatory burden in the body, which can have wide-reaching consequences. Gut dysbiosis can also impede a person's ability to detoxify harmful substances that pass through the gastrointestinal system, since friendly gut bacteria help to make toxic substances less toxic to the body. Figure 1 illustrates some of the possible consequences of gut dysbiosis.

Normal interface between microorganisms ("friends" and "foes") and an infant's immune system is a critical part of the development of a mature and properly functioning immune system. Normal interface means that microorganisms come into contact with an infant's mucosal surfaces (the "wet surfaces" in the eyes, mouth, nose, gastrointestinal tract, etc.) where the immune system is designed to handle these immunological challenges. It is unknown exactly the impact of bypassing these mucosal surfaces via direct antigen presentation into the muscle, or under the skin (as is the case with vaccination). However, there is speculation that such an interface between antigen and the immune system can lead to immune dysregulation.

Relatively recently, scientists have discovered that disruptions to the development of the critical colonies of microbiota (microorganisms) in the gut can lead to a variety of immune system dysfunctions.[7] Although the science is still evolving, a substantial amount of evidence indicates that particular strains of commensal bacteria in the gut play a critical role in biochemical processes such as dendritic cell maturation, epithelial cell (lining of the gut) signaling to immune cells, and modulation of systemic cytokine (immune signaling molecules) pro-

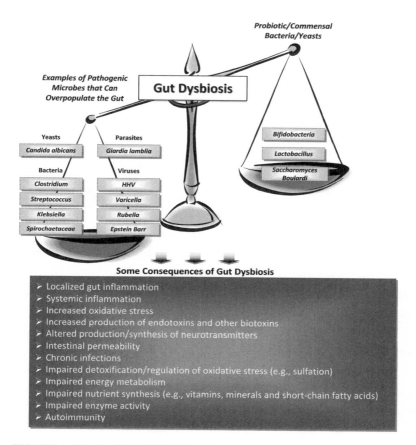

Probiotic/Commensal
Bacteria/Yeasts

Examples of Pathogenic
Microbes that Can
Overpopulate the Gut

Gut Dysbiosis

Yeasts	Parasites
Candida albicans	Giardia lamblia

Bacteria	Viruses
Clostridium	HHV
Streptococcus	Varicella
Klebsiella	Rubella
Spirochaetaceae	Epstein Barr

Bifidobacteria

Lactobacillus

Saccharomyces
Boulardi

Some Consequences of Gut Dysbiosis

➤ Localized gut inflammation
➤ Systemic inflammation
➤ Increased oxidative stress
➤ Increased production of endotoxins and other biotoxins
➤ Altered production/synthesis of neurotransmitters
➤ Intestinal permeability
➤ Chronic infections
➤ Impaired detoxification/regulation of oxidative stress (e.g., sulfation)
➤ Impaired energy metabolism
➤ Impaired nutrient synthesis (e.g., vitamins, minerals and short-chain fatty acids)
➤ Impaired enzyme activity
➤ Autoimmunity

FIGURE 1: SOME CONSEQUENCES OF GUT DYSBIOSIS.

duction.[8] In other words, friendly microbiota in the gut are known to provide essential building blocks for the human immune system, especially with regard to regulatory functions (the parts that keep the immune system in check). A lack of these essential building blocks can result in an immune system that cannot shut itself off, and will treat benign substances as invaders.

Germ-free animal models, where animals are raised with sterile guts, have demonstrated that absence of commensal bacteria in their guts results in defective gut-associated lymphoid tissue (GALT), the tissue directly beneath the epithelial (surface) cells that is considered the headquarters of immune function in our bodies.[9] In other words, animals raised without gut flora develop immune systems that do not work properly, and thus, they can become very sick.

Although multiple factors contribute to immune dysregulation, it is commonly seen in conjunction with (and often as a result of) gut dysbiosis. Gut dysbiosis can affect many mechanisms within the gastrointestinal tract, thus it is important to first understand the many roles of microorganisms in the gut. Some have called the microorganisms in the gut the "organ within an organ."[10] If you compare the number of human cells versus bacterial cells that each of us contains, we are more bacterial than we are human. Of all the cells in our body, about 10 percent are human and 90 percent bacterial. If you compare the number of human genes in our body to bacterial genes, we are 1 percent human and 99 percent bacterial. All of these bacteria that we carry around weigh an average of two to five pounds.[11] Other microbiota (microorganisms) that can inhabit the gut include yeasts, parasites, viruses, and protozoans. Approximately 99 percent of the human body's microbiota inhabit the digestive tract.[12] The primary roles of healthy intestinal microbiota include metabolism, defense, and immunomodulation (regulation of the immune system). The metabolic functions of commensal microbiota include (but are not limited to) vitamin synthesis, fermentation of carbohydrates, and energy production. Commensal microbiota are also necessary to protect the gastrointestinal tract from pathogenic invaders by producing bacteriocidins (highly specific antibiotics) and by competing with pathogenic organisms for food and space.[13]

To summarize their many complex roles, good germs in the gut help us to:

- Break down and effectively digest food
- Draw nutrients out of food so that they can be used by our cells
- Make immune cells
- Turn certain immune cells on

- Turn other immune cells off
- Break down toxins like mercury or carcinogens so they are less harmful as they travel through our bodies
- Keep large molecules of food from passing through the intestines into the blood (which would lead to allergic reactions) by creating a "bacteria barrier"
- Keep bad germs from colonizing our gut by producing powerful and highly specific chemicals (a "bug spray" of sorts)
- Make the precursors to neurotransmitters and other important biological chemicals.

If an individual has gut dysbiosis, or an overgrowth of bad germs in the gut, his or her ability to do any of the aforementioned functions can be seriously impeded. If he or she cannot perform these basic functions, physical signs and symptoms of illness begin to appear. Without a healthy population of good bacteria, we cannot make critical brain chemicals like serotonin or dopamine; we cannot effectively protect ourselves from infectious agents like viruses or disease-causing bacteria; we cannot nourish our cells, because we are unable to extract nutrients from the food that we eat; we cannot protect ourselves from damaging toxins like aluminum, mercury, or pesticides.

A lack of good germs, or an overgrowth of bad germs in the gut, can result in many different physical symptoms, including:

- Diarrhea
- Constipation
- Depression
- Anxiety
- Obsessive behaviors
- Hyperactivity
- Symptoms of food allergies/sensitivities such as red ears or cheeks, hives, wheezing, headaches, eczema, wetting accidents in young but potty-trained children, etc.
- Fatigue, low energy

- Mood swings and irritability
- Pain
- And many other symptoms

When colonies of friendly bacteria are unable to populate the gut (because of gut dysbiosis), a whole host of physiological problems can arise. One of the more common consequences of gut dysbiosis is a phenomenon known colloquially as leaky gut syndrome, or intestinal hyperpermeability. *Intestinal hyperpermeability* simply means that the normal barrier function of the intestinal mucosa (the surface layer of cells in the intestines and the microorganisms that populate it) is compromised by the presence of microscopic "holes." The holes permit substances normally contained within the intestines to leak into the circulatory system. Consequently, under-digested food antigens and microbes leak into the immune cells and circulatory system beneath the mucosal layer. The immune system views these food particles as foreign invaders rather than molecules of nourishment. The result is an immune response to everyday foods (food allergies).

Furthermore, pathogens that normally pass through the intestinal barrier via immune system gatekeepers, are instead able to bypass the protective gatekeepers and proceed directly into the rest of the body. A normally functioning barrier is able to effectively prevent certain substances (such as viruses, pathogenic bacteria, and improperly digested food molecules) from entering the blood stream without first interacting with appropriate immune cells, while allowing the appropriate substances (properly digested food molecules) through to the bloodstream. When the barrier is dysfunctional, the body develops unnatural responses to the presence of these substances in the lymph and circulatory systems.

Intestinal hyperpermeability and gut dysbiosis can have the effect of making toxins more toxic to our bodies. The role of commensal bacteria in host detoxification is well established. Friendly bacteria help to metabolize, or break down, substances that might otherwise be toxic to the body:

> They [microflora] participate in the metabolism of drugs, hormones and carcinogens, including digoxin (Lindenbaum et al., 1981), sulphasalazine, and estrogens (Gorbach, 1982). By demethylating methylmercury, gut flora protect mice from mercury toxicity (Rowland et al., 1984).[14]

Hyperpermeability allows toxins that would normally be metabolized by commensal bacteria and eliminated through the bowel, to make their way into the epithelial layer (surface cells in the intestines) and into the bloodstream. The liver, which may not be able to process these toxins, is forced to store these toxins in fatty tissues in the body, including the brain. "Increased tissue toxicity is thought to be a major trigger for mitochondrial dysfunction" which has been implicated in the development of autism.[15]

Intestinal hyperpermeability has been implicated as one of the critical physiological dysfunctions that precedes (or runs parallel with) both immune dysregulation and the development of chronic illness.

> Breaching this single layer of cells [the epithelial layer], which encompasses a huge surface area that can be exposed to approximately 1×10^{13} microorganisms along with a myriad of food antigens at any one time, can lead to pathologic stimulation of the highly immunoreactive subepithelium. Breakdown of this barrier is implicated in the pathogenesis of acute illnesses such as bacterial translocation leading to sepsis and multiple organ system failure. It also has been implicated in several diseases having their origins during infancy that manifest in later life. These include atopic disease such as eczema, food allergies, celiac enteropathy, type 1 diabetes, asthma and inflammatory bowel disease.[16]

The authors of this review article published in the highly respected, peer reviewed journal *Acta Paediatrica* also indicate that intestinal hyperpermeability is likely to play a significant role in the pathophysiology of autism.

Intestinal hyperpermeability affects children with food allergies, eczema, asthma and many other chronic illnesses, but it also affects many children who are seemingly healthy. Some signs of food allergy and intestinal permeability are not readily recognized as such. Parents and physicians may not connect symptoms such as frequent loose stools, depression, or excessive tantruming in young children to intestinal hyperpermeability, but if they occur persistently, this is a likely culprit. The largest proportion of children affected by immune dysregulation and gut dysbiosis may actually be children who have not been diagnosed with a chronic illness—children deemed healthy by most standards. It seems incredible that so many children could be suffering from gut dysbiosis, leaky gut syndrome, and associated immune dysfunction. However, once the causes of these physiological dysfunctions are examined, it does not seem so incredible at all. In fact, it makes perfect sense, given the modern American lifestyle.

The Origins of Gut Dysbiosis and Leaky Guts

Because a properly functioning intestinal barrier is a complex system of human cells and enteric (intestinal) microbes (such as bacteria), there are multiple ways in which the barrier can break down. Specific environmental factors common in many children's lives contribute to gut dysbiosis and intestinal permeability.

Gut dysbiosis occurs when pathogenic microbes such as yeasts and bacteria edge out friendly bacteria. Once friendly bacteria are already compromised, further assaults on the gut occur. Yeasts and pathogenic bacteria affect the integrity of the intestinal lining physically but also biochemically through the secretion of toxins (such as mycotoxins).[17] In addition, overexposure to particular pharmacological or chemical agents, such antibiotics, NSAIDS (ibuprofen, naproxen etc.) or industrial emulsifiers, can result in increased intestinal hyperpermeability.[18] Stress is another factor that is believed to contribute to intestinal hyperpermeability. Gut dysbiosis, intestinal hyperpermeability and immune dysregulation are a vicious cycle. Once a gut is dysbiotic, it leads to intestinal hyperpermeability, which leads to immune dysregulation, which can lead to autoimmunity, and aberrant immune re-

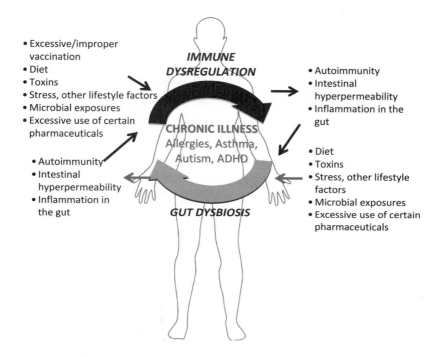

FIGURE 2: ILLUSTRATION OF FACTORS CONTRIBUTING TO GUT
DYSBIOSIS, IMMUNE DYSREGULATION AND CHRONIC ILLNESS.

sponses where the immune system attacks and destroys epithelial cells
and commensal bacteria, which perpetuates gut dysbiosis and intestinal permeability. The cycle is unrelenting. (See figure 2.) To understand how this vicious cycle begins, it is important to look for the roots
of gut dysbiosis.

The Beginnings of Gut Dysbiosis

As mentioned previously, an infant is born into the world with a sterile
gut, but colonization with bacteria begins immediately as the baby
passes through the mother's birth canal. Here, the infant acquires the
same bacteria that are present in the mother's body via vaginal and
fecal exposure. Bacteria that are present in the mother's body are also
transferred to her baby through breastfeeding. In a mother who has a
healthy body ecology herself, she will transfer two particular types of

bacteria in great quantities: *Bifidobacteria* and *Lactobacilli*. These two types of bacteria are considered among the most important bacteria for homeostasis (stable health) in the gut. Studies in neonates in intensive care units have shown that delayed colonization with *Bifidobacteria* can result in the overgrowth of potentially pathogenic strains of bacteria such as those of the *Clostridia, Streptococcus* and *Enterobacteriaceae* genus.[19] If a mother's gut or vagina is dysbiotic, with overgrowth of pathogenic bacteria such as certain strains of *Clostridia, Klebsiella, Staphylococcus,* or yeasts such as *Candida albicans,* then she may transfer these same pathogenic microbes onto her child.[20] These pathogenic microbes often exist in our guts in small quantities (relative to the friendly bacteria) without any problems, but when their populations overtake the friendly bacteria, the seeds of illness are sewn. Thus, it is important that both mother and child maintain healthy gut ecology.

In everyday terms, if a pregnant woman has vaginal yeast infections, or persistent diarrhea or constipation, excessive flatulence or bloating, gastroesophageal reflux, or other GI symptoms, she may have gut dysbiosis or dysbiosis in her vagina. The imbalance of microorganisms in her body will be passed along to her baby if the baby is delivered vaginally. This may not present a problem for the baby, as the baby's body may be able to restore balance on its own (especially through breastfeeding). If, however, this baby is exposed to additional environmental challenges, such as antibiotics, environmental toxins, and in some cases vaccinations, the baby may not be able to restore balance and may begin to show signs of ill gastrointestinal health and immune dysregulation. It is speculated that colic may be one such symptom.[21]

Yeasts in particular can be problematic for the host. Although many forms of innocuous yeast inhabit the human body, skin, tissues, mucous membranes and gastrointestinal tract, *Candida albicans* is the most common, and can proliferate to become an infection or overgrowth with significant consequences. Any woman who has had a vaginal yeast infection has likely experienced an overgrowth of a *Candida* yeast in her vagina. If the yeast proliferates and colonizes a portion of the gastrointestinal tract, the fungus can produce rhizoids (mycelia), which produce toxins that can be quite damaging to the human body.

> [Rhizoids] are very long root-like structures, which can penetrate the mucosa. . . . Penetration of the gastrointestinal mucosa can break down the boundary between the intestinal tract and the rest of the circulation and allow introduction into the bloodstream of many substances that may be antigenic. Both incompletely digested dietary proteins and *Candida* organisms are reported to enter the blood stream in this way, with specific consequences.[22]

Like all living organisms, yeasts and bacteria produce wastes or byproducts. The wastes produced by the microbiota in the gut can be beneficial or harmful to the human host. In the case of *Candida albicans*, many harmful toxins are produced. The toxins released by these yeasts can interfere with the production and synthesis of neurotransmitters such as serotonin and dopamine, brain chemicals essential for normal and healthy neurological function.[23] Yeasts (and some bacteria) are particularly sensitive to the effects of diet. Yeasts such as *C. albicans* thrive on high sugar, high carbohydrate foods, which are mainstays of the American diet. The typical American today consumes over 140 pounds of sugar per year, up from 114 pounds in 1967 and 10 pounds in 1821.[24] Alcohol consumption can also contribute to the development of intestinal and vaginal yeast overgrowth.

One of the environmental factors that can have a profound effect on the health of commensal bacteria colonies in the gut is the use of certain pharmacological agents, such as antibiotics, steroids, NSAIDS and oral contraceptives.[25] Some of the newer broad-spectrum antibiotics are particularly damaging to commensal bacteria. When an antibiotic disrupts the bacterial ecology of the gut by killing a portion of the resident bacteria, spaces are left along the GI tract for opportunistic or pathogenic bacteria and yeasts to flourish. Antibiotics can destroy entire colonies of beneficial bacteria in the gut, but other pharmacological agents can alter gut flora, especially when used chronically.

Approximately 80 percent of American women have used oral contraceptives at some point in their lives, and these are drugs that are taken
chronically.[26] Interestingly, indomethacin, a nonsteroidal anti-inflammatory drug (NSAID) that is one of the most commonly used drugs
in the neonatal intensive care unit, has been shown in several studies
to increase intestinal permeability in this fragile population.[27]

Of all drugs used in this country, the ones with the most devastating
effects on gut ecology are the ones prescribed the most. "Ninety percent of the sore throats we Americans experience each year are viral
in nature and immune to antibiotics, but medical statistics indicate
that 73 percent of the estimated 6.7 million visits by adults to physicians complaining of a sore throat between 1989 and 1999 resulted
in a prescription for antibiotics."[28] Exposure to antibiotics is not limited to the ten-day course of oral antibiotics taken by a mom with a
sore throat, or a child with an ear or sinus infection. Antibiotic exposure occurs subtly through our food and water. Antibiotics have long
been used as animal feed additives in an effort to promote growth and
optimal health among factory farm animals. Recent reports are now
alerting consumers to the fact that pharmaceutical agents, including
antibiotics, have been found in public water supplies. Thus, even if
you have never taken antibiotics personally, you may have experienced exposure through diet and environment.

Further Stresses on the Gut

Once gut dysbiosis is present, additional assaults on the integrity of
the intestinal mucosa can occur. Within the epithelial barrier there
are intercellular junctions called tight junctions, or desmosomes.
These are regulated (purposeful) spaces between the cells (enterocytes). These tight junctions can be disrupted in a variety of ways, but
when this delicate layer is disrupted, hyperpermeability, or leaky gut,
results. Some preliminary research has been done in vitro and in animal models that demonstrate that certain chemicals and foods additives may degrade the tight junctions between cells. These food
additives may include emulsifiers such as carrageenan or sugar esters,

which are often used as dispersing agents in dry powdered foods, or as whipping agents in dairy foods.[29] For every food additive that has been studied in relationship to gastrointestinal impact, thousands more simply have not been studied for their effect on the gut. While information about the effect of food additives on gut health slowly emerges from research labs, Americans continue to consume massive quantities of food additives every year, with unknown consequences.

Also, recent research has revealed that certain microbes, such as *Clostridium difficile* and overgrowth of *Enterococcus* and *Streptococcus* strains, can affect the permeability of the intestine not only by squeezing out the more protective probiotic ("friendly") bacteria, but also by releasing toxins that work to degrade the tight junctions between epithelial cells in the gut.[30] Other studies have shown certain bacteria have the same effect by altering gene expression in epithelial cells. Viruses are also known to increase intestinal permeability.[31] Thus, there are multiple mechanisms through which pathogenic microbes contribute to enhanced intestinal permeability. Typically, when a host is infected with a microbe such as rotavirus, the rotavirus degrades enterocytes of villi (surface cells) as well as the tight junctions, but once the immune system removes the pathogen, these features will begin to repair. However, children whose immune systems are not able to effectively eliminate these pathogens may experience chronic infection in the gut (or elsewhere), ensuing inflammation, and pervasive intestinal permeability. For instance, many children with autism are found to have chronic infections with *Borrelia burgdorferi* (the spirochete that causes Lyme disease) or other tick-transmitted microorganisms that prevent the gut (and other tissues) from ever fully healing.[32]

THE PATHWAY TO DISEASE: FROM PHYSIOLOGICAL DYSFUNCTION TO SYMPTOM PRESENTATION

A small group of integrative physicians and researchers are leading a national movement for the promotion of functional medicine in an effort to change America's broken medical paradigm. These well-published and highly regarded physicians and scientists include Dr. Mark Hyman, Dr. Jeffrey Bland, Dr. Woodson Merrell, among many other opinion leaders. These professionals are working tirelessly to raise American awareness of the connection between fundamental physiological dysfunctions (e.g., biochemical imbalances) and the development of chronic illness. The scientific research supporting their assertions is dense, and the library of publications demonstrating that chronic illnesses can be cured through personalized medical interventions is growing every day. Dr. Hyman, who recently published a book on mental health titled *The UltraMind Solution*, urges Americans to pay attention to underlying physiological dysfunctions as they hold the key to curing mental illness.

> What is emerging is a model that incorporates understanding the role of nutritional deficiencies, hormonal imbalances, inflammation, altered immunity, toxins, oxidative stress, mitochondrial dysfunction, altered cell bioenergetics, and digestive dysfunction in altered behavior, mood, and brain function. It is only by teasing apart how each of these fundamental physiological processes alters brain function and studying how correcting them can restore normal function that a new model of psychiatry, neurology, and clinical neuroscience can emerge that provides more satisfactory answers than only partially effective pharmacological treatments.[33]

Dr. Hyman asks us to consider the question, is mental illness really "all in the head?"

These opinion leaders are also drawing detailed outlines of how physiological dysfunctions lead to chronic illness, and what must be done to correct them. Thus, we are learning that each chronic childhood illness can be treated by searching for these underlying dysfunctions (which are highly specific to each individual child) and by correcting the implicated imbalances. Let us take a look at some representative illnesses to see how this paradigm can be applied clinically.

Allergies and Asthma: The Root Causes

It is important to understand the history of allergic disease as a "modern malady" because it demonstrates how allergies are an environmentally derived illness and not simply caused by genetics. (Although, as Dr. Sudhir Gupta of UC Irvine has noted, genetics clearly "load the gun," while environment "pulls the trigger.") Although the rare occurrence of allergy exists in the historical record at least as early as Hippocrates, allergy as a widespread human disease really emerges during the industrial era. In the nineteenth century, hay fever, the earliest form of modern allergies, began to emerge among the upper and middle classes in America and Great Britain, but largely spared the poor. The first cases of this new industrial hay fever were recorded as early as 1819, but the vast majority of hay fever cases emerged during the late nineteenth century. The fact that poor people, often living in unhygienic conditions, were spared from allergic afflictions helped to give rise to the hygiene hypothesis. Too much hygiene and germ avoidance seemed to correlate with the development of atopic disease. In *Allergy: The History of a Modern Malady*, Mark Jackson explores how hay fever became somewhat of a badge of social rank, and those of the upper classes were content to suffer with it, as it served as a marker of social privilege. During the interwar years (between the first and second world wars), it was estimated that one in thirty people suffered from allergies. That number has now grown to one in three, or even one in two by some estimates.[34] There is no question that the development of widespread allergies evolved in tandem with industrialization, but the specific reasons for this are still somewhat uncertain.

Today, a wide array of symptoms are considered allergic, including but not limited to urticaria (hives), erythema (skin rash/reddening), angiodema (swelling of the skin), vomiting, anaphylaxis, itchy/watery eyes, atopic dermatitis (eczema) and wheezing (airway and lung inflammation) associated with asthma.[35] Symptoms believed to be associated with food allergies are somewhat controversial. As author, allergist, and food allergy expert Dr. William Walsh has said, "Describing the illnesses caused by food allergy is like trying to gift-wrap an elephant—there's not enough paper to do it. What's more, even if you had enough paper, where would you start?"[36] Often times, food allergy symptoms present specifically in the gastrointestinal tract with manifestations such as esophagitis, gastritis, and gastroenterocolitis, colitis and proctitis, celiac disease, gastroesophageal reflux (GERD), colic, diarrhea, and constipation, but can also include more generalized symptoms, including tachycardia (racing pulse), poor growth or failure to thrive, edema, lethargy or muscle weakness, aching joints, nausea, and "brain fog."

With such a long list of associated symptoms, it is exceedingly difficult to diagnose allergy, let alone find the root cause. As is the case with all chronic illnesses, not *all* of the biological mechanisms behind the disease are fully understood, but medical science has established a fairly comprehensive understanding of the cascade of physiological events that precede an acute allergic response. Simplified, an allergic reaction occurs when the body produces excess white blood cells in response to environmental stimuli. These white blood cells produce certain antibodies whose job it is to recognize the offending antigens (food particles, molds, etc.) and alert other white blood cells (mast cells and basophils) to their presence.

Once mast cells and basophils are "activated," they release histamines and other substances into the circulatory system that cause inflammation, mucus secretion, smooth muscle contraction (bladder, respiratory tract), and vasodilation (which accounts for redness, swelling).[37] This is why *anti*histamines such as Benadryl are effective at mitigating allergic symptoms; these drugs block the release of histamine and thus reduce symptoms. (Again, like most conventional drugs, this is like putting a bucket under a leaky roof, but it does not address the cause of the leak.) The antibodies that are known to stimulate mast cell and basophil activation in an acute allergic reaction are called IgE (immunoglobulin E) antibodies. In fact, clinical diagnosis of allergy typically relies on serum (blood) IgE levels or IgE skin-prick testing which indicate that an allergic response has occurred.

Other immune factors besides IgE antibodies play a role in acute or even delayed immune responses, including IgG, IgA and IgM. However, the role of these antibodies is not as well studied as IgE. Studies have been done where patients suffering from allergic or other inflammatory disorders have removed foods or chemicals that correlated with raised IgG levels and improved their symptoms. Many people have gone to allergists to be tested for allergies because of acute or delayed responses to particular foods, chemicals or airborne substances, only to be told that they do not have an allergy because their IgE-levels were not elevated. However, the patient still believes that they experience some kind of immunological reaction to food or another substance. This is most likely because they *are* experiencing an allergy (conventional medicine might call this an intolerance), but it is not IgE-mediated. This does not make it any less real or clinically relevant. Typically, the patient is sent out of the physician's office frustrated because he or she knows on an intrinsic level that the symptoms are caused by some sort of allergic reaction, yet the physician insists that there is no allergy because their IgE tests came up negative.

The reasons why many physicians do not accept the possibility of non-IgE-mediated allergic responses are complex. It is partly because the science behind the other immune factors is still underdeveloped. It is also partly a function of the fact that the professional organizations within the field of allergy and immunology have not officially validated anything other than IgE-mediated responses as clinically meaningful. However, it does not obviate the need to understand what is causing the immunological responses (IgE-mediated or not) to innocuous stimuli in the environment. Eliminating exposure to allergens is one way to manage allergies, but this approach offers no hope of cure. There is no universal root cause of atopic disease in children, but as previously mentioned, underlying physiological commonalities can serve as a jumping off point for understanding the pathogenesis of allergy in children.

Food allergies are often the simplest to explain because the physiological mechanisms are better understood compared to other chronic illnesses. Food allergies are directly linked to the presence of intestinal hyperpermeability caused by gut dysbiosis. To be sure, more complicated mechanisms can be involved (as with the case of gluten sensitivity and celiac disease, where autoimmunity plays a significant role). However, when trying to understand what is causing food allergies in a particular child, it is best to look at what is going on in the gut.

When food allergy occurs, mucosal adaptive immunity (what normally enables the GI mucosal layer to differentiate between pathogens and benign friendly bacteria and ingested foods) is dysfunctional. Numerous studies have demonstrated a link between dysbiotic microbes in the gut and the presence of allergic disease.

> The altered composition of intestinal microbiota appears to precede the development of atopy: Infants who develop atopy have more *Clostridia* and fewer *Bifidobacteria* and *Enterococci* in their stools as compared with infants who remain healthy (Bjorksten et al., 2001, Kalliomaki et al., 2001a). Furthermore, recent observations indicate that infants who suffer from atopic disease harbour a distinct pattern of *bifidobacteria* comprising mostly of adult-like strains, as compared to healthy infants with a typical infant pattern consisting mainly of *Bifidobacterium bifidum* (Ouwehand et al., 2001).[38]

A study published in *BMC Pulmonary Medicine* in 2008 revealed that altered gut flora (as determined by a gut colonized by *Bacteroides fragilis*) in infants three weeks of age was correlated with increased incidence of asthma predictive factors in the first three years of their life.[39] As previously discussed, gut dysbiosis is one of the precursors to intestinal permeability and the development of allergic and inflammatory illness. When food particles leak through the mucosal layer in the intestine, the body stimulates an immune response, which unleashes a cascade of events, including inflammation, excessive production of mucosal secretions, vasodilatation, and many other physiological occurrences.

Multiple environmental and genetic factors contribute to the development of allergic disease. Many studies have been done to try to establish or disprove a link between early antibiotic use and allergic disease, including asthma. Antibiotic use may be a significant factor contributing to the development of gut dysbiosis, but it is unlikely that it is the sole causative factor in the development of atopy. The results of studies looking for a causal relationship are often conflicting. Some conclude a meaningful link between antibiotic use and atopy, and some conclude that the link is not substantive. A close examination of antibiotic-allergy studies reveals design flaws in many of them, both those that support a link and those that do not. The studies that use only serum IgE (a type of immunoglobulin or immune cell) and skin prick as measures of atopic disease or allergy tend to show that there is no correlation. However, studies that use different parameters for measuring allergy (such as clinical history) tend to show a stronger correlation.

As previously discussed, IgE-mediated response is not the only way to evaluate the presence of atopy. The lack of an IgE-mediated response to environmental stimuli does not mean that atopy does not exist. In fact, we now know that there are many ways in which the immune system responds to antigens, and not all of them are mediated by IgE. Likewise, few human studies have been done that examine the relationship between food allergies/intolerances and antibiotic use. To exclude food allergies and intolerances is to use a fairly narrow definition of atopy, which sets up an automatic bias in the studies. Following is a chart summarizing several studies done in this area and their outcomes (table 2). Notice the studies that used only IgE serum levels or skin prick tend to show a negative relationship and studies that use other modalities to evaluate atopy show a positive relationship.

Thus, it is unclear whether there is a causal link between the use of antibiotics and the development of atopic disease because many of the studies in this area are flawed in methodology. Other clinical scenarios have not been examined extensively, such as maternal antibiotic use during or prior to a child's birth and the subsequent risk of developing atopy. A common procedure today is the administration of IV or oral antibiotics for laboring women who are Strep B positive or who have

TABLE 2: EXAMINATION OF STUDIES LOOKING FOR CORRELATIONS BETWEEN ANTIBIOTICS AND ATOPY/ASTHMA.

Study [Author, publication, date.]	Correlation b/t early antibiotics and atopy demonstrated?	Type of measurements used to assess atopy	Comments/Design Flaws
P. Cullinan *et al.* *Thorax*, 2004.	**Mixed Results** • Association between antibiotics and asthma shown in self-reported cases. • No association shown for general atopy (when skin prick was used as measurement).	• Skin prick tests (IgE); Atopy = one or more positive skin tests to cat fur, grass pollen, and dust mites. • The study also looked for correlations between atopy and self-reported hay fever and asthma.	• Study was done in adults. • Authors conclude that the relationship is reverse; that respiratory infections (for which antibiotics were prescribed) are more likely to be the causal factor of asthma, rather than antibiotics causing asthma. • Narrow parameters for definition of atopy used. Skin prick test (IgE) was used as a determination of atopy; Food allergy was not examined, thus the full spectrum of atopy was not evaluated.
Noverr, MC *et al.* *Infection and Immunity*, 2005.	**Positive Correlation** • Association between dysbiotic microflora (caused by antibiotics and yeast inoculation) correlated with allergic disease. • Mouse models treated with antibiotics and inoculated with *C .albicans* (yeast) developed allergic-type responses to mold, where as control mice exposed to mold did not.	• Presence of immune factors, including: IgE AND levels of eosinophils, mast cells, IL-5, IL-13 and gamma interferon.	• Wide parameters for definition of allergic response used. • Addition of *C. albicans* does not allow for pure examination of the role of antibiotic. • Mouse model—results in humans may not correlate exactly.
Cohet, C. *et al.* *Journal of Epidemiology and Community Health*, 2004.	**Positive Correlation** • Association between use of antibiotic and/or paracetamol in first year of life (or in month prior to study) and increased risk of asthma.	• Used surveys to determine presence of asthma and atopy.	• Inherent problems with subjective nature of surveys to determine presence of asthma and atopy. • Inclusion of paracetamol obscures role of antibiotics.
Kusel, MM *et al.* *Clinical and Experimental Allergy*, 2008.	**Negative Correlation** • Use of antibiotics used early in life not correlated with development of atopy, allergy, eczema.	• Skin prick (IgE)	• Narrow parameters for definition of atopy used. • Food allergy was not examined, thus the full spectrum of atopy was not evaluated.
Celedon *et al.* *American Journal of Respiratory and Critical Care Medicine*, 2002.	**Negative Correlation** • Use of antibiotics used early in life not correlated with development of atopy, allergy, eczema.	• Used skin prick test at two years (IgE) and physician's diagnosis of atopy or allergy.	• These studies, like many others looked only for atopy as defined by skin prick OR hay fever, eczema diagnosed by a physician. • Allergies (especially food allergies) are underdiagnosed and thus the actual incidence of allergy was likely underestimated. • As authors of study admit, early diagnosis of asthma (<5yrs) is not always accurate, and asthma often develops later in life. Children were evaluated for asthma at age 5.

certain health conditions, such as mitral valve prolapse. Administration of oral or IV antibiotics to a laboring mother would likely alter the gut flora of the mother at a time when homeostasis of her gut flora is most critical for her newborn's immune development. In short, more studies need to be done to examine the impact of antibiotics on gut flora and subsequent impact on developing immune systems.

It is naïve to assume that a single causative factor, like antibiotics, is responsible for the development of atopy. There are too many other variables with antibiotic use to clearly define it as a sole causative agent. For instance, a patient who takes antibiotics but is on a low sugar diet that is rich in probiotic bacteria (e.g., fermented foods such as yogurts, kefir, raw cultured vegetables etc.) may not experience gut dysbiosis (the causal mechanism) because levels of gut microflora would be rapidly restored to homeostasis in this situation. On the other hand, a pregnant mother who consumed a high quantity of sugar and processed foods prior to labor would likely be setting herself up for gut dysbiosis, as these types of foods feed pathogenic microbes, especially yeasts like *Candida*. Excessive consumption of glucose (sugar) in an already dysbiotic gut can lead to the overgrowth of certain strains of lactic acid producing bacteria, such as *Streptococcus* and *Enterococcus*, which can cause a condition where the gut cannot support the necessary balance of beneficial microflora, perpetuating further gut dysbiosis.[40]

Other factors, such as diet or exposure to environmental stimuli like viruses, mold, urban pollution, or cigarette smoke, should be considered among the other ingredients that contribute to the development of allergies and asthma. For instance, many children experience asthma when exposed to a virus. Furthermore, a recent study in Saudi Arabia demonstrated that western diets were correlated with the development of asthma.[41] Neither antibiotics, nor diet, nor other environmental factors are likely to act as sole causative agents in the development of atopic disease; however, each may play a very important role in disease etiology. It is still critically important to look at the role that antibiotics (as well as other medications) and all other environmental factors play in the perfect storm that leads to atopic disease. What is certain, however, is that regardless of the types of environmental variables present in a particular child's life, gut dysbiosis is an important, and perhaps even central, feature in the development of chronic illness.

Autism, ADHD, and other Mental Health and Developmental Disorders: The Root Causes

It is very difficult for most people to understand that autism, ADHD, depression and other disorders formerly labeled as psychiatric may actually have a systemic biological basis. We have been trained to think of these disorders as "all in the head." Recent scientific discoveries are slowly unraveling these old ideas. The latest research reveals that the root cause of these disorders may actually be found in other areas of the body—areas that have become dysfunctional because of environmental stressors.

Although autism spectrum disorders, ADHD and other disorders of developmental and mental health are all very different from one another both in etiology and presentation of symptoms, they share enough of the same underlying physiological and biochemical dysfunctions that it is worthwhile to examine these disorders in tandem. Most children with these disorders suffer from gut dysbiosis and immune dysregulation. As discussed in relation to the development of allergies and asthma, the immune systems of these children are skewed, either responding too aggressively to immune stimulus (as with food allergies), or responding inappropriately so that normal immune pathways become altered or destructive. Often, the neurological symptoms of these children are manifestations of brain function that has been affected by problems elsewhere in the body, such as a chronic infection in the gut or cellular damage in the liver caused by toxin exposure.[42]

Presently, a small, but growing, group of clinicians are treating these sorts of illnesses by addressing quantifiable biochemical and physiological imbalances found in the bodies of their patients. For example, a patient that has symptoms such as hyperactivity or inattention may also show high levels of heavy metals in laboratory testing or clinical evidence of severe gastrointestinal dysfunction, in addition to any number of other biological imbalances. These clinicians use clinical exams, medical history, and laboratory testing to try to understand the root cause of their patients' symptoms so that they can then develop individualized treatment protocols to stop or even reverse biological damage. Thousands of children have recovered from illnesses like autism, ADHD, and depression using this clinical methodology.

The Etiology of Neurological and Developmental Disorders Through the Prism of Autism

Autism is a term that is commonly used to describe what is actually a spectrum of disorders, characterized by abnormalities in the development of communication, socialization, and behavior. More precisely, one is said to be "on the autism spectrum," or diagnosed with an "autism-related disorder," which leads to a rather heterogeneous group of individuals that share some of the same neurological and behavioral symptoms. The condition of autism was first described in 1943, by Leo Kanner, a psychiatrist and physician, considered by many to be the father of modern child psychiatry. At the time, it was characterized by withdrawal from social interaction, repetitive behaviors and impaired communication. Today, autism is understood as a much more complex and dynamic group of disorders and dysfunctions. A child with an Autism Spectrum Disorder (ASD) can be considered severely disabled, or "high functioning," and capable of assimilating quite normally into society, as is seen with the label of Asperger's Disorder.

Increasingly, ADHD (and ADD) is now being considered by many to be a spectrum disorder. Often times, children with Asperger's and ADHD are highly intelligent individuals (exceeding their peers) who struggle with some social and behavioral issues. There are many variations in symptoms and onset of symptoms; consequently, individuals are categorized differently according to these and other variables. It is believed that some children are born with autism, while another subset of children may have what is known as regressive autism, where a child develops according to normal standards for a period during their infancy, only for their communicative, social, and behavioral skills to disintegrate, either rapidly or overtime.

Because ASDs are a heterogeneous group of disorders, a wide variety of different attributes are associated with each diagnosis, and the symptoms vary from child to child. Some of the symptoms displayed by children with ASD may include:

- Limited/impaired/no speech/communication capabilities
- Social impairment
- Lack of eye contact
- Sleep difficulties
- Gastrointestinal symptoms/conditions such as chronic diarrhea, constipation, reflux, abdominal pain
- Repetitive motions (spinning, rocking, flapping)
- Seizures, tics
- Sensory integration/processing disorders (sensitivity to stimuli such as light, noise, touch, taste)
- Aggressive/defiant or other problematic behaviors
- Dyspraxia, apraxia (impaired motor skills)
- A variety of comorbidities, including allergies (food and respiratory), asthma, ADHD, anxiety, depression, etc.[43]

For many years, when autism was still an extremely rare disorder, it was believed to be a psychiatric or behavioral disorder that originated from cold and inattentive parenting, particularly by the mother. In fact, in the 1960s, the official literature and psychiatric textbooks at the time advocated that both mother and child receive psychotherapy, so that the mother could "acknowledge her guilt and disclose why she hated the child and wished it had never been born." The child was "provided with a paper or clay image of a women (his mother) and was encouraged to tear it to bits, thus expressing his hostility toward his mother, whom the psychotherapists were positive had caused his autism." The "refrigerator mother" (the cold and inattentive mother) was the predominate explanation for the etiology of autism well into the 1980s.[44] It was in the 1980s when new ideas about the etiology of autism began to emerge. Most researchers and physicians began to understand autism as a disorder stemming from neurobiology or "nature" (an inherent disorder), rather than from learned behavior ("nurture"). A smaller group of physicians and researchers interested in understanding the etiology of autism began to investigate the underlying dysfunctions in the body that might be affecting the brain.

Although autism is perhaps the most complex of all neurological and developmental disorders, an examination into the underlying systemic and biological dysfunctions in autism provides insight into how dysfunction in the body can result in dysfunction in the brain. As Dr. Mark Hyman describes it, "Autism is a hologram for chronic disease. In it is reflected all the causes and cures for chronic disease." This is true because so many of the most basic physiological functions of the human body are profoundly altered in a child with autism. Thoughtful House, an internationally known and somewhat controversial treatment center in Texas, lists just some of the "biological impairments" present in children with autism:

- Chronic diarrhea/constipation
- Yeast/bacterial overgrowth of bowels
- Inability to clear heavy metals
- Impaired sulfation
- Leaky gut syndrome
- Imbalanced immune system
- Mineral deficiencies (zinc, magnesium, selenium)
- Malabsorption/malnutrition
- Impaired neuronal development
- Disrupted hippocampus/amygdala
- Gluten/casein sensitivity
- Impaired detoxification

- Impaired antioxidation
- Omega-3 fatty acid deficiency
- Significant food allergies
- Impaired pancreatic function
- Frequent viral and bacterial infections
- Vitamin deficiencies
- Autoimmunity
- Neurotransmitter imbalance/dysfunction
- Seizures
- Impaired methylation[45]

Children with autism may have all or some of the above impairments. While a child with depression, asthma, or even diabetes may have some of the same imbalances and dysfunctions as a child with autism, the child with autism seems to aggregate many of the possible biological dysfunctions into one struggling body. These irregularities are well documented by the autism community and in the scientific literature because determined parents of children with autism have gone to great lengths to fully understand the root cause of their children's disorder. This means that many more children with autism have undergone extensive blood work, endoscopies, as well as stool, urine, hair and genetic analysis, than their neurotypical peers. There is a vast body of literature regarding the particular systemic biological dysfunctions in children with autism. This is less the case with children who suffer from "milder" disease forms such as asthma or depression because the available medical treatments are satisfactory enough that many parents do not continue to look for answers to etiology of disease. It goes without saying that these children could benefit greatly from this type of biomedical analysis.

Mounting evidence supports the fact that children with autism have profound systemic biological dysfunctions. These dysfunctions correlate with neurological and behavioral symptoms, yet, the mainstream medical community and the vast majority of autism treatment and research programs treat autism as if it were a purely genetic disorder (without acknowledging the systemic biological components of the disorder) or a disorder stemming from idiopathic brain dysfunction. In an article published in *Neuropsychology Review* in December 2008, author Lynn Waterhouse surveyed the landscape of autism etiology theories and research to see whether the scientific and medical community had reached any kind of preliminary consensus as to the etiology of autism. Waterhouse concludes: "Despite the overwhelming flood of causal theories for autism, the field has not made progress in creating a synthesized, standard predictive causal theory of autism, and it may well be time to abandon the effort to find a unifying causal deficit model for autism."[46] Waterhouse addresses the fact that so many researchers have devoted their lives to locating the singular cause of autism, a fruitless effort given the multiplicity of variables that are likely to play a role in the etiology of autism today. The search for a singular "autism gene" continues despite the discouraging results of decades of research in this area.

Part of the reason that genetics are a primary focus in autism is that some autism-related disorders, such as Fragile-X and Rett syndrome, have been associated with a single gene, and twin studies in autism have demonstrated a high heritability trend among children with autism—indicating that genetics are likely to play a role.[47] Thus, the focus remains squarely fixed on genetics. According to Waterhouse, researchers in the field of autism agree only on the following four "truths":

1) That autism exists (as defined in the DSM-IV TR)
2) That there are variants in the disorder (hence ASD) and it includes subsets of diagnostic groups (e.g., Asperger's, Rett, etc.)
3) That there is wide variability in diagnostic traits and in associated impairments in ASD individuals
4) That the majority of autism cases result from gene effects.[48]

It seems that few within the mainstream medical community (e.g., American Academy of Pediatrics, the Society for Developmental and

Behavioral Pediatrics) are interested in understanding what role systemic biological impairments might play in the development of neurological and behavioral disorders. According to most neurobehavioral physicians treating children with autism, the only treatments believed to be effective for these conditions are psychotropic drugs, or ABA, Applied Behavioral Analysis. ABA is a difficult and arduous method of training children with autism to modify their behaviors. Although psychotropic drugs may alleviate some symptoms, and ABA is effective for many children (often helping them to improve daily functioning and interaction), both of these modalities completely ignore the relationship between the symptoms of autism and the underlying biological imbalances that interfere with the most basic everyday functions that a body performs, such as digestion, metabolism, and detoxification.

However, some autism researchers and clinicians fundamentally believe that most ASDs (possibly excluding disorders such as Rett's and Fragile-X) are the result of a perfect storm of environmental and genetic factors that result in a breakdown in some of the most basic biological processes in human function. Although this is a heterogeneous group of researchers and clinicians, most believe that ASDs can be treated, reversed, and perhaps even prevented with the appropriate biomedical interventions. Today hundreds of clinicians in this country are treating ASDs and other chronic illnesses, such as asthma, allergies, depression and many others, by applying biomedical intervention strategies to their patient population.

The origins of this "discovery" and the subsequent development of treatment protocols truly began in the 1960s, under a research psychologist by the name of Dr. Bernard Rimland. Dr. Rimland, himself the father of a son with autism, established the Autism Society of America in 1965 and the Autism Research Institute in 1967, in an effort to further research and discovery in the field of autism. Rimland's early work on the neurological impairments of individuals with autism helped to eventually discredit the refrigerator mother hypothesis. Rimland's work then began to focus on biomedical interventions that could improve symptoms of children with autism. By the 1990s, Rimland and the Autism Research Institute had raised enough awareness and enough money that they were able to make significant strides in uncovering some of the key biological dysfunctions common in children with ASDs.

In 1995, the Autism Research Institute convened its first Defeat Autism Now! Conference, a think tank initiative sponsored by autism scientists and physicians aimed at utilizing the latest research and clinical experiences to expedite the development of effective treatment protocols. The outcome of this first meeting was the creation of a resource book (the autism bible) of biomedical intervention research and guidelines, written by Dr. Sydney Baker and Dr. Jon Pangborn. This book was published and disseminated to clinicians and parents across the country in hope that the paradigm of autism could be changed so that children could receive effective treatments. Defeat Autism Now! has since become a worldwide network of clinicians and researchers who are actively engaged in treating and recovering children with autism. Perhaps the best known figure associated with Defeat Autism Now! outside the autism community is Jenny McCarthy, celebrity, author, and mother of a son with autism. Jenny McCarthy wrote several books about her experiences with Defeat Autism Now! and the recovery of her son. Physicians trained using the Autism Research Institute and Defeat Autism Now! approach are known colloquially as "DAN! doctors," and although they are not recovering every one of their patients with autism, they are recovering some, and are making dramatic quality of life improvements in others.

The approach that these clinicians use to heal their patients stems from the belief that ASDs are not so much diseases as they are the manifestation of an extraordinarily complex web of physiological and biochemical dysfunctions of environmental and genetic etiology. The Autism Research Institute describes their philosophy regarding biomedical intervention in these terms:

> The biomedical approach is not 'alternative' medicine; it's a science-based, molecular-biological approach to treatment. Everyone agrees that psychotropic drugs do not treat the problem—they simply reduce or eliminate some of the symptoms. Our aim, in contrast, is to

> address the underlying health problems. The guiding principle is
> simple: remove what is causing harm, and add what is missing.[49]

Essentially, this is the same approach used by practitioners of functional medicine who treat every chronic illness from cardiovascular disease to juvenile diabetes. Also, other associations of clinicians and researchers, such as Thoughtful House in Austin, Texas, the Homeopathy Center of Houston, the Rhinebeck Health Center in Rhinebeck, New York, and others, have rallied around the systems biology approach to treating and learning about autism. It is through research and the treatment approaches used by practitioners of functional medicine and systems biology that the etiology of autism is beginning to emerge. Although these practitioners are unlikely to claim that they know what causes autism, many have a solid understanding of the major contributing factors. A consensus statement regarding the etiology of autism has not yet emerged out of this community, but it's something to look out for in the very near future.

The Etiology of Autism Spectrum Disorders

Most causal theories advanced for autism emphasize neurobiology and genes. Very few look at the body as a system where dysfunctions in one remote area of the body can impact other areas of the body. Autism is viewed as either: "a genetically determined fixed brain-based disorder" or "a reversible systemic disorder that is influenced by genetics and that affects the brain."[50] In order to understand how systemic dysfunctions can affect the brain, it is necessary to examine the root causes of dysfunctions that occur in ASDs. Interestingly, many of the root causes of the biological impairments associated with ASDs are related to a diseased and dysfunctional gastrointestinal system. Yet, rarely is this observation made by conventional physicians who treat children with autism. Following is a table that demonstrates the number of biological impairments in autism that have origins in gastrointestinal dysfunction, or are directly related to gastrointestinal functions. Many dysfunctions associated with autism are linked, either directly or indirectly, to the gastrointestinal system.

TABLE 3. BIOLOGICAL IMPAIRMENTS IN AUTISM: RELATIONSHIP TO GASTROINTESTINAL SYSTEM.

Biological Impairment	Gastrointestinal System Implicated?	Comment
Chronic diarrhea/constipation	√	
Yeast/bacterial overgrowth of bowels	√	Gut dysbiosis
Inability to clear heavy metals	√	Microflora in the gut are involved in detoxification of heavy metals.
Impaired sulfation	√	Microflora may play a role in enabling sulfation (gene expression)[51].
Leaky gut syndrome	√	
Imbalanced immune system	√	70 percent of the immune system is located in the gut— gut dysbiosis leads to immune irregularities.
Mineral deficiencies (zinc, magnesium, selenium)	√	An impaired gut cannot properly assimilate minerals and nutrients.
Malabsorption/malnutrition	√	An impaired gut cannot properly assimilate minerals and nutrients.
Impaired neuronal development		
Disrupted hippocampus/amygdala		
Gluten/casein sensitivity	√	Stems in part from intestinal permeability.
Impaired secretin signaling	√	Pancreatic function compromised.
Impaired detoxification	√	Again, microflora play a significant role here; impaired glutathione results in impaired detoxification.
Impaired antioxidation	√	Related to glutathione deficiency. Amino acids necessary for glutathione may be impeded by impaired protein digestion.
Omega-3 fatty acid deficiency	√	Although diet plays an important role, impaired assimilation of nutrients due to a diseased gut may be in play also.
Significant food allergies	√	Intestinal permeability, autoimmunity (immune dysregulation).
Impaired pancreatic function	√	
Frequent viral and bacterial infections	√	Impaired immunity due to compromised gastrointestinal system. Impaired gut-associated lymphoid tissue.
Vitamin deficiencies	√	An impaired gut cannot properly assimilate minerals and nutrients.
Autoimmunity	√	A function of immune dysregulation; may be related to gastrointestinal immune system.
Neurotransmitter imbalance/dysfunction	√	Most are produced in the gastrointestinal system.
Sensitivity to vaccinations	√	Impaired immune system (because of gut damage) cannot effectively respond to vaccinations.
Seizures		
Impaired methylation		

According to many Defeat Autism Now! physicians and researchers, autism is a treatable, environmentally driven illness (with noted genetic susceptibilities) much like other inflammatory illnesses, such as cardiovascular disease or diabetes, where gut and immune health play a leading role in etiology. Since so many chronic illnesses are finally being recognized as the end product of inflammatory processes in the body, researchers and physicians are desperately looking for the causes of the inflammation, so that appropriate treatments may be developed. Defeat Autism Now! pioneer Dr. Sydney Baker has argued that autism is similar to every other inflammatory illness in that once the root cause of the inflammation is understood and fixed, healing can begin. Many Defeat Autism Now! clinicians believe that the source of most inflammation is the gut, thus, the first biomedical interventions typically applied to a new patient with autism are aimed at healing a dysfunctional gut.

Much of this treatment protocol evolved out of these clinicians' experiences treating an overwhelming number of patients with autism who also had gastrointestinal (GI) symptoms and disorders. Although many children with autism have outward signs of gastrointestinal dysfunction, such as chronic diarrhea or constipation, vomiting, or reflux, many GI disorders go undiagnosed, either because the children are nonverbal and cannot describe certain symptoms (such as abdominal pain), or because a child's particular gastrointestinal dysfunction is not always linked to the GI by parents and doctors. For instance, many children with autism have food allergies, eczema, or hyperactive behavior, and unfortunately, most parents and many physicians do not associate these symptoms with gut dysfunction. It has been established that these symptoms can be the result of intestinal hyperpermeability (in combination with a dysregulated immune system and the ingestion of certain foods/substances). Intestinal hyperpermeability is a gastrointestinal malfunction. Yet, few would look at a child's allergies, eczema or hyperactivity and link them to the gut. Many children are asymptomatic and do not show any outwards signs of GI dysfunction, but this does not mean they are not there.

A common phenomenon that is widely observed among children with autism is what is known as posturing. When nonverbal children experience abdominal pain, they can be observed seeking abdominal pressure. Children will lie on their bellies and press their abdomens against tables, chairs or other pieces of furniture in an effort to relieve their pain.[52] This type of posturing behavior has also been misdiagnosed as a tic disorder, as some children will contort their bodies in particular shapes in an effort to curb their discomfort.[53] Many GI disorders (such as lymphonodular hyperplasia or eosinophilic esophagitis) are made apparent only through the use of endoscopy, and most children with autism will never receive an endoscopy in their life. Thus, it is quite common for children with autism to live silently (often painfully) with GI disorders, simply because parents and doctors are not aware of the high prevalence of GI disorders in this population of children.

Although it is not definitively known what percentage of children with autism have gastrointestinal disease or dysfunction, estimates range anywhere from 20 percent to 77 percent.[54] It is difficult to assess how many children with autism truly have gastrointestinal disorders because many children will never present with symptoms associated with GI disease, even if disease is present. GI studies done in children with autism involving endoscopy tend to find very high rates of gastrointestinal disease, but these studies may be biased due to the nature of patient sampling (e.g., children tend to receive endoscopies because of apparent GI complaints). One well-designed study aimed at evaluating intestinal permeability of children with autism found that 43 percent of tested children showed evidence of intestinal hyperpermeability as compared to 0 percent of controls (normally developing children). A second study of the same type found that 76 percent of children with autism demonstrated intestinal hyperpermeability.[55]

Multiple studies examining gut dysbiosis in children have found significantly higher rates of pathogenic bacteria in the guts of children with autism. A study by Finegold *et al* in 2002 assessed thirteen children with autism and eight neurotypical children for gut dysbiosis.

The researchers found nine species of *Clostridium*, known pathogens, in the children with autism that were not present in the neurotypical children. Many other studies have consistently found significantly higher rates of diarrhea, constipation, and abdominal pain in children with autism as compared to their neurotypical peers or siblings. To date, no known studies have used endoscopy and pill camera (a technology used to evaluate the small bowel) to examine either autistic or neurotypical children that have no GI history or GI complaint for evidence of underlying gastrointestinal disease or dysfunction. It is difficult to understand the true prevalence of gastrointestinal disease, in the clinical sense, among children with autism because the epidemiological research and data are in their infancy.

Some researchers and physicians, including the controversial pediatric gastroenterologist Andrew Wakefield, [56] have given the GI dysfunctions associated with autism their own diagnostic term, autistic enterocolitis. Wakefield and colleagues argue that regressive autism, in particular, is a function of "primary inflammatory bowel disease." In other words, the symptoms of autism come from inflammation and dysfunction in the gastrointestinal tract. Dr. Wakefield explains the full landscape of GI dysfunction in children with autism that he calls autistic enterocolitis:

> There appears to be an autoimmune attack against the lining of the intestine. In association with this we get a compromise of the barrier function of the intestine. Digestive enzymes on the surface of the villi are essential for the normal digestion of food and the maintenance of intestinal health. When these enzymes are not working properly—as in children with various infectious enteropathies (following a rotavirus infection, for example)—then the consequence may well be malabsorption and diarrhea. The presence of undigested food in the stool is something that we commonly see in these children. This has been demonstrated in children with autism both by Dr. Tim Buie at Harvard and by Karoly Horvath. We also see ulceration—the breakdown of the lining of the intestine. There is dys-

biosis, which is an overgrowth of potentially pathogenic aerobic and anaerobic bacteria in the colon and in the small bowel. This reportedly leads to the proliferation of Paneth cells as a source of antibacterial peptides. This is the constellation of pathology in the intestine that forms the disease we now call autistic enterocolitis.[57]

It is becoming increasingly clear that many children with autism (particularly those with regressive-type autism) suffer from some gastrointestinal disorders (both diagnosed and undiagnosed). However, the cause of these gastrointestinal disorders is still the subject of much debate.

As part of his research examining the nature of inflammatory bowel disease in patients with autism, Dr. Wakefield has studied the near ubiquity of immune dysregulation in these children. Although gastrointestinal dysfunction can cause immune dysregulation itself, Wakefield is particularly interested in the role that viruses play in the development of immune dysregulation and inflammatory bowel disease. Dr. Wakefield has hypothesized that infection with certain viruses (the measles virus in particular) may be linked to the development of immune dysregulation, gastrointestinal dysfunction and subsequent regressive autism. Dr. Wakefield has become a controversial figure because his studies imply (but do not assert) a possible link between the MMR vaccine (measles, mumps, and rubella) and the development of regressive autism. A study that Wakefield published in 1998 was a lightning rod for controversy, as public health officials were concerned about the impact that Wakefield's study might have on national immunization program compliance, and subsequent infectious disease outbreaks. Although this particular controversy still rages, Wakefield continues to pursue the virus-etiology theory and has published a considerable amount of research examining the role that viruses and gastrointestinal dysfunction play in the pathophysiology of autism.[58]

Much of the mainstream medical community has dismissed Dr. Wakefield's research (for complex reasons, including the publication of studies that refute the findings of Wakefield's 1998 study[59]); however, he is not the only physician and researcher to pursue the virus-etiology theory of autism. Other researchers are testing the hypothesis that viral infection may precipitate some forms of autism in some children.[60] To date, no definitive studies have proven a link. This is partly why Dr. Wakefield has been so villainized by the medical establishment; many believe that his hypotheses regarding viruses are unproven, yet they have created a vaccine scare among the public. Although Dr. Wakefield's particular studies do not provide definitive evidence of a link among viruses, gut inflammation, and the development of autism, this does not mean that they are not part of the etiological picture.

"It's the Flora, Stupid."

The gastrointestinal problems in children with autism are many, and each child displays unique GI symptoms and physiology. However, it is becoming increasingly clear that the one factor common to all children with autism is gut dysbiosis. Frustrated with the apparent slow uptake of these facts by mainstream medical professionals, Dr. Sydney Baker urges us all to seriously examine the role of our most inner environment: the human microbiome. The microbiome is a fancy word for the ecological domain of thousands of species of microorganisms, most of which inhabit our gastrointestinal tract. Dr. Baker elaborates:

> The most dazzling experience I have had observing the healing of problems in cognition, language and human interaction in autistic children over the past 30 years have come from steps aimed at modifying gut flora. If we can believe what we see rather than seeing what we believe to be true, we should expand our concept of the ways in which the metabalome [metabolites, signaling molecules, etc.] of the gut flora drives its host's agenda. If those of us who have been on the front lines trying to do every biomedical thing we can think of for children in the autism spectrum were to have just one plea to make to our academic colleagues and others charged with public policy it would be, "It's the flora, stupid."[61]

Simplified, Baker means to say, so many of the biological impairments of autism (and any chronic disease, for that matter) can be linked back to the health and balance of microbiota in the gastrointestinal system.

Dr. Baker refers not just to the role of the microorganisms themselves, but to the *metabalome*, which is a term used to describe the thousands of different types of molecules (many produced by microorganisms) inside our bodies. The metabolites, hormones, and signaling molecules produced by microorganisms are involved in a myriad of physiological processes, including human gene regulation, detoxification, metabolism, immune cell signaling and production, and many, many more complex and poorly understood functions.[62] The functions performed by microorganisms in our bodies are critical to our very health and survival. If we had sterile guts, we could not live. The "bugs" in our gut are perhaps the most underestimated and underappreciated organisms in all of medical science. It is time for us to wake up and smell the *Clostridia*!

How Does Gut Dysbiosis or Gut Dysfunction Affect the Brain?

A gut that is over-populated with pathogenic microbes often degenerates into a diseased state. The type and degree of disease vary according to a large number of environmental factors (such as diet, microbial exposure, toxin exposure, vaccination history, genetic history, etc.). As discussed in the context of allergies and asthma, altered gut flora can contribute to the development of immune dysregulation, as the gut flora play a critical role in the immune system. It is possible that gut flora are only one part of the total immune dysregulation picture in autism, but it is certain that healthy gut flora are a prerequisite for a properly functioning immune system.[63]

It is well documented that children with autism have severely dysregulated immune systems. [64] This may result in symptoms associated with compromised immunity, such as chronic viral and bacterial infections. Chronic ear infections and rhinoviruses are commonly seen among autistic children.[65] In addition, a subset of individuals with

autism is classified as having PANDAS (Pediatric Autoimmune Neuropsychiatric Disorders Associated with Streptococcal infections),
which is a neuropsychiatric disorder associated with a particular type
of strep infection. Children without an autism diagnosis may also be
diagnosed with this disorder. Children may be susceptible to this disorder because of dysregulated immune function.[66] Some children
with autism are known to have hyperresponsive immune systems,
meaning that their immune systems overreact to stimuli, often resulting in autoimmunity. Children with autism are not typically diagnosed
with primary immunodeficiency (like AIDS patients), yet serious immunological dysfunctions are present in their bodies, which are believed to impact neurological function. This is especially true for
children with the regressive type of autism.[67] A review study published
in the *Journal of Leukocyte Biology* in 2006 examined the link between
immune dysregulation and neurological dysfunction in individuals
with autism:

> There is emerging evidence and growing concern that a dysregu-
> lated or abnormal immune response may be involved in some forms
> of ASD. In general, the links between the immune and neurological
> systems are becoming increasingly well known. Cytokines and other
> products of immune activation have widespread effects on neuronal
> pathways and can alter behaviors such as mood and sleep. Aberrant
> immune activity during critical periods of brain and neuronal de-
> velopment could potentially play a role in neural dysfunction, typical
> of autism. Various hypotheses have attempted to link dysfunctional
> immune activity and autism, such as maternal immune abnormali-
> ties during early pregnancy, increased incidence of familial autoim-
> munity, and childhood vaccinations. Several lines of research have
> shown abnormalities in the nature, extent, and regulation of the im-
> mune response in autism, including a skewed generation of antibod-
> ies, cytokines, and immune cells.[68]

Any doubts about the link between the immune system and neurological function can be allayed by looking at historical examples of

infectious diseases that have caused neurological symptoms, such as the neurological syndrome associated with typhoid fever. Typhoid fever was a condition caused by infection with a bacterium (*in the gastrointestinal system*) that was characterized by encephalitis (brain inflammation), delirium, hallucinations, light-sensitivity, seizures, and apraxia. Many other infectious diseases are known to cause neurological impairment and damage (both temporary and permanent), including toxoplasmosis, rubella, herpes, gonorrhea, syphilis, group B streptococcus, meningitis, varicella, polio, malaria, *Borrelia burgdorferi*, and HIV. In fact, our children are currently vaccinated against many of these pathogens precisely because of the concern of neurological complications associated with infection. Often, the immune system can clear the pathogen from the body and normal neurological function can return. However, many of these infections can cause lifelong neurological impairment when an immune system is not able to kick the pathogen out.

Perhaps one of the best known examples of such an infection is what is known as encephalitis lethargica. A pandemic of encephalitis lethargica swept the western world in the 1920s and left some victims in a permanent catatonic state. Many who did not recover from the acute infection were left severely disabled, with impairments in speech, communication, behavior, and movement. The story of patients left in such a catatonic state was popularized by the 1973 book *Awakenings* by Oliver Sacks, which was made into a film starring Robin Williams in 1990.[69] Recent studies have examined the possibility that the neurological impairment following encephalitis lethargica may in fact be a "post-infectious autoimmune CNS [central nervous system] disorder." Essentially, researchers demonstrated that in this particular disorder, the immune system attacks "deep grey matter neurons" in the brain.[70] This is not unlike the autoimmunity that has been discovered in autism.

Much recent research has focused on the role of autoimmunity in the etiology of autism. One hypothesis proposes that the immune system may actually be "attacking" cells in the brain, thereby creating inflammation and neurological damage. In a 1999 study published in

The Journal of Pediatrics, Anne Connolly *et al.* found serum antibodies to brain epithelial cells in patients with autism, signifying a type of autoimmune destruction of particular brain cells.[71] No definitive conclusions have been drawn yet about the origin of autoimmune responses, but a variety of autoimmunity triggers have been proposed, including viral infection, bacterial infection or overgrowth, yeast overgrowth, genetic and environmental (e.g., toxins) interaction, and of course, vaccines.

Literally hundreds of studies over the last few decades have examined the role of autoimmunity and immune dysregulation in the pathophysiology of autism. More specifically, researchers are uncovering the fact that inflammation in the bowel (often of autoimmune origin) is directly related to inflammation in the brain. A study conducted by Diane Vargas, and published in the *Annals of Neurology* in 2005, demonstrated that inflammation in the brains of children with autism is *secondary*, meaning that inflammation originating elsewhere in the body (such as the gastrointestinal tract) can ultimately lead to inflammation in the brain. Vargas and colleagues hypothesized that this "active and chronic neuroinflammatory process in patients with autism" holds important keys to understanding the pathophysiology of autism, yet, much more work on immune dysregulation in this population needs to be done.[72]

This takes us back to Wakefield's and others' research in the area of gastrointestinal inflammation.

> Is it possible that what we are observing is a systemic inflammatory response from the intestine leading to secondary immune activation in the brain, and cell damage? We've seen this before, in celiac disease—a primary immunopathology of the intestinal mucosa associated with an allergic sensitivity to gluten. Celiac disease [an autoimmune disorder] is associated with a wide variety of secondary neurological complications, including autistic behavior, dementia, peripheral neuritis, focal and generalized seizures, and cerebral calcification. Celiac disease provides a perfect example of a primary gut

disease leading to secondary brain damage. Placing patients on a gluten-free diet may lead to some amelioration of these neurological features.[73]

Evidence continues to mount behind the "gut-brain" hypothesis, or the idea that acute and chronic events in the gut (inflammatory, infectious, etc.) have a direct impact on neurology and neurobehavior.

Thus far, we have established that individuals with autism often suffer from gastrointestinal dysfunction (sometimes asymptomatic) and immune dysregulation. These physiological dysfunctions involve both inflammation and autoimmunity that may impact neurological function. Yet, there is no consensus on the origin of the inflammation, other than that it is *secondary* with a possible origin in the gut. Theories abound as to the origin of inflammation in the gut, ranging from viral infection to genetic polymorphisms (genetic variation) that predispose an individual to autoimmune activation on gastrointestinal tissues. Dr. Natasha Campbell-McBride, a British physician specializing in neurology, who is also a nutritionist, and the mother of a son recovered from autism, believes that the origin of inflammation is a dysbiotic gut. When the gut flora are improperly balanced (because of a variety of environmental factors) the immune system becomes dysregulated. Dysregulated immune systems often produce excessive inflammation, as they are unable to self-regulate. Dr. Campbell-McBride published a book entitled *Gut and Psychology Syndrome* in 2004, where she details the connection between gut dysbiosis and neurological disorders such as autism, ADHD, depression and schizophrenia. The common symptom in all these neurological disorders, according to Dr. Campbell-McBride, is inflammation—inflammation originating in the gut.

How gut dysbiosis leads to inflammation is a complex process and varies according to each individual. The following is a simplified synopsis of some of the ways in which disruption to colonies of beneficial microflora in the gut can lead to inflammation, according to Dr. Campbell-McBride:

- Beneficial flora (commensal/friendly) provide a physical barrier against pathogenic or opportunistic flora (such as *Candida*). When beneficial bacteria are reduced or absent, opportunistic flora thrive, which can stimulate an immune response that leads to inflammation. "Studies with microscopic examination of a biopsy of the gut wall show that in healthy individuals there is a thick bacterial band attached to gut mucosa, keeping it intact and healthy. In inflammatory bowel disease different pathogenic bacteria are found in the mucosa, even inside the gut cells, which means that the protective bacterial band has been broken and allowed the pathogens to reach the sacred gut wall."[74]

- Beneficial gut flora are also involved in digestion of foods. Insufficient beneficial gut flora result in food that is insufficiently digested. The gut wall also becomes more permeable without the protection of the beneficial flora. Combine these two factors, and food allergy (an inflammatory process) develops, as under-digested food molecules leak through the intestine into the circulatory system, which stimulates an immune response. This immune response results in inflammation that is experienced throughout the entire body.[75]

- Beneficial bacteria are critical to immune function. "For example, in the cell wall of *Bifidobacteria* (the good bacteria largely populating the human colon) there is a substance called Muramil Dipeptide which activates synthesis of one of the most important groups of immune system cells—lymphocytes. . . . Scientific research shows that in people with damaged gut flora, there are far fewer lymphocytes in the gut wall." Beneficial flora are also necessary for the proper functioning of other immune cells such as neutrophils, macrophages, as well as immune molecules like cytokines and interferons. A person with compromised gut flora can become "immunocompromised" because the production of these important immune molecules is hindered. Consequently, other immune responses [humoral immunity] replace "cell-mediated immunity." These "back up" immune responses are responsible for excessive inflammation in the body.[76]

The entire cascade of events that links gut dysbiosis and inflammation is complex, and researchers continue to learn more about the relationships every day. Nonetheless, there is clear evidence that healthy gut flora are a critical part of gastrointestinal function, immune function, inflammation modulation, and ultimately, neurological function. This is why Dr. Campbell-McBride, Dr. Mark Hyman, Dr. Sydney Baker and so many other physicians and researchers are urging us to pay attention to the guts of those who suffer from neurological or psychiatric disorders.

Although gut dysbiosis (and associated gastrointestinal dysfunction) and immune dysregulation may be at the core of the etiology of autism, they are certainly not the only factors that contribute to autism. There is no question that other factors such as genetic polymorphisms (genetic variables) and toxic exposures (particularly to heavy metals) play an incredibly important part in the pathophysiology of autism. Environmental toxins have long been suspected of contributing to the development of autism. The current generation of American children is exposed to more neurotoxins than any previous generation, and many children do not have effective detoxification equipment to survive in this environment. Neurotoxins are simply substances (metals, chemicals, venom, etc) that are destructive to nerves and nerve cells. Neurotoxins are proven to impact intelligence (IQ), and cognitive, motor, speech, and behavioral functions. Key detoxification capabilities in children become compromised when the gut is dysbiotic. The toxic burden of children with autism is often quite high, and their gastrointestinal dysfunction (which may have been caused in part by toxic exposure) only compounds their total toxic load.

As previously mentioned, gut flora play a critical role in the detoxification of a variety of compounds. Research scientists have demonstrated that microorganisms in the gut such as *Lactobacillus* readily detoxify ingested environmental substances so that we can excrete them from our bodies with minimal harm. It is well known that different individuals metabolize drugs differently. This variation in metabolism is partly due to variations in gut flora in any given individual. The gut flora metabolize many compounds and, depending on the particular strain of flora, may either make compounds inert, or increase their toxicity to the body. It has been demonstrated that certain pathogenic microorganisms not only produce their own metabolites that can be toxic to the body, but they may also enhance the toxicity of other compounds through metabolism. It is critically important to have the correct balance of microflora in the gut because not only do beneficial bacteria effectively lessen the impact of ingested toxins, their colonization also edges out other pathogenic microorganisms that tend to produce more toxic substances in the body.[77]

Mercury, a potent neurotoxin, is of particular interest in autism. Associations have been drawn between mercury poisoning and autism, as the symptoms of the two are similar. Mercury is also ubiquitous in the environment, and can be found everywhere from dental amalgams, to our food and water supply, to vaccines. Under normal conditions, the gut flora are able to demethylate (degrade) mercury, making it less toxic to the body. A study performed by Rowland *et al.* in 1984 demonstrated that mice fed methylmercury demethylated and excreted mercury at different rates depending on the type of diet they were fed. Furthermore, when the mice were fed antibiotics (to disrupt the intestinal flora) their fecal excretion of mercury was reduced, while their retention of mercury in tissues increased substantially.[78] What this study illustrates is that gut dysbiosis can disable this critical detoxifying capability, making an individual susceptible to the neurotoxic effects of mercury. Mercury and other toxins are also known to negatively impact commensal bacteria, possibly reducing their numbers and thus protective benefits to their host.

There is no debate about the neurotoxicity of mercury. It is a neurotoxin and can cause neurological damage in children at even very low levels of exposure. The Environmental Protection Agency (EPA), the Food and Drug Administration (FDA), and the US Agency for Toxic Substances and Disease Registry (ATSDR) have all established safety guidelines as to the upper limit of methylmercury exposure. The EPA's "safe" limit of methylmercury exposure is 0.1g/kg/day, and the FDA's "action level" is 0.4g/kg/day.[79] The most common sources of exposure to mercury (including methylmercury, and its close relative, ethylmercury) include dental amalgams, consumption of certain fish (especially large, deep water, fatty fish like tuna and swordfish), soil, air, and water contamination (often the result of coal-fired power plant emissions, or other industrial byproducts), vaccines containing the additive thimerosal, and now evidence supports that mercury can be found in certain processed foods.[80]

Many studies link prenatal and childhood exposure to heavy metals like mercury to developmental delays, intelligence deficits, and neurological disorders. One study examined the levels of mercury in the baby teeth of children with autism and neurotypical children and found higher levels of mercury in the baby teeth of the autistic set of children.[81] Baby teeth are known to be a good indicator of stored toxins in the body. Baby hair, on the other hand, can be a good indicator of how effectively an individual excretes heavy metals. Detectable levels of mercury in a hair sample indicate that the body is effectively eliminating toxins. A study by James B. Adams *et al.* found higher levels (7 times!) of mercury excreted in the hair of neurotypical children as compared to autistic children, an indication that the neurotypical children were appropriately detoxifying and excreting mercury from their bodies, while the autistic children had retained the mercury in their bodies. There was also a reverse association between the amount of mercury in the hair and degree of severity of autism. Those children with the *least* mercury in their hair had the most severe forms of autism. The body retained the mercury in these children, compounding the neurotoxic effects. [82]

Other studies have tried to assess the impact of heavy metals epidemiologically: A 2006 study conducted by Windham *et al.* in the San Francisco Bay area found an epidemiological association between autism and concentrations of hazardous air pollutants (HAPs) such as heavy metals and chlorinated solvents. Windham's study looked at 284 children with autism and 657 control children and found that exposure to higher ambient levels of HAPs, especially mercury, during pregnancy and early childhood correlated with an increased risk for autism.[83] Another epidemiological study out of Texas found a slight but positive correlation between the amount of mercury released into the environment from industrial sources (e.g., coal-burning power plants) and rates of autism in surrounding school districts.[84]

Mercury is, by no means, the only toxic substance in our environment that may be adversely affecting children. The list of toxins under investigation for links to autism, ADHD and other neurodevelopmental disorders is long and includes: fluoride, lead, arsenic, aluminum, perchlorate, bisphenol A, and many, many other household, commercial, and industrial chemicals and toxins.[85] Over four hundred chemicals commonly used in industrial countries are identified as neurotoxins. Children with autism who also tend to have dysregulated immune systems (e.g. autoimmune responses to brain tissue), intestinal hyperpermeability, gut dysbiosis and other biochemical imbalances (such as impaired sulfation, a necessary process for detoxification) are going to experience the effects of neurotoxins in a much more dramatic way than children who have fully developed immune systems, and are biochemically balanced. It is important to remember that autism is a spectrum of disorders, so children along the spectrum (and even *off* the spectrum) will experience the effects of neurotoxins differently. Some children will have greater susceptibility, while others will prove to be more resilient. This susceptibility is both genetic and environmental.

The debate surrounding the role of environmental toxins in the development of autism is fierce, primarily because this hypothesis naturally leads to the indictment of childhood vaccines, which up until 2000, were a significant source of ethylmercury exposure for infants.[86] Studies have been done to try to disprove a link between autism and mercury exposure from vaccines, but most of these studies have been done in healthy children. No studies have looked specifically at the impact of ethylmercury exposure on infants and children with significant gut dysbiosis or other impaired detoxification pathways. If a study were to examine the impact of ethylmercury on children by using a comprehensive stool analysis (or other type of biomedical diagnostic tool for evaluating gut dysbiosis), and compare the impact of ethylmercury exposure on children with balanced gut flora versus imbalanced gut flora, the results might be different. Children with significant gut dysbiosis are more likely to be affected by ethylmercury exposure than those with healthy gut flora.

Many argue that thimerosal cannot be implicated in the development of autism because autism rates have continued to climb even after thimerosal was removed from most vaccines. This is true. However, a few details need to be considered before thimerosal can be completely vindicated. First, thimerosal was not removed from all vaccines. In fact, most states now mandate that babies as young as six months old receive a yearly influenza vaccination (which may contain up to 25mcg/dose of thimerosal). Pregnant women are also advised to receive a thimerosal-containing flu vaccine. In addition, other vaccines still contain thimerosal, including some tetanus boosters, and a vaccine used for meningitis. Second, other toxins are present in vaccines, including aluminum, MSG, and formaldehyde. Children with strong, regulated immune systems may have no problem processing any of these toxins. Most children do absolutely fine with vaccinations. However, some children are just not equipped to handle toxic assaults, no matter the form.

Children with autism (and perhaps many more children that we do not know about) have a decreased ability to protect themselves from toxic and other immunological assaults because of the presence of very specific metabolic imbalances. Dr. Jill James, director of the Metabolic Genomics Laboratory at the Arkansas Children's Hospital and Research Institute, has published groundbreaking research demonstrating that children with autism have impairments in the most basic detoxification pathways in the body. Dr. James has found that children with autism have chronic metabolic imbalances that prevent them from effectively "neutralizing" the oxidative stress that their bodies encounter.[87] In other words, when we encounter oxidative stress (a process that damages cells and cellular functions) in the form of toxins, radiation, immunological assaults, an inflammatory diet, or other forms, healthy bodies regulate and reduce this oxidative stress through a complex metabolic detoxification pathway. What Dr. James and colleagues found is that children with autism have reduced levels of certain metabolites that serve as markers of properly functioning detoxification pathways.[88] One of the biomarkers that they found in children with autism is a reduced level of glutathione. Glutathione is the most important naturally formed antioxidant in the body that is used to reduce the impact of oxidative stress. A child with reduced levels of glutathione will not be able to effectively handle toxic assaults, such as exposure to mercury.

Dr. James' work raises the question, do these children have inborn errors of metabolism that make them more vulnerable to the impact of oxidative stress (pollution, infections, heavy metals, junk food diets, etc.), or is there something in their environment that is impacting and altering their metabolic detoxification pathways? This science is still evolving; however, enough evidence indicates that children with autism (and perhaps many others, including those with ADHD and other spectrum disorders) are simply more vulnerable and sensitive to environmental toxic assaults. This has implications for everything from vaccinations to the use of chemical household products and technological gadgets that emit strong radio frequencies. If nothing else, Dr. James' research warns us that we cannot assume that all children have intact detoxification capabilities, so we need to be vigilant about keeping toxic exposures to a minimum, for all children. Thimerosal or other environmental mercury exposures may be effectively metabolized and detoxified in the bodies of some children, but we now know that at least a subset of children simply cannot safely handle exposure. Without knowing if your child has this particular metabolic impairment, is it safe to risk exposure to mercury or other toxins?

Journalist Arthur Allen wrote a well-researched and detailed history of vaccination in a book entitled *Vaccine: The Controversial Story of Medicine's Greatest Lifesaver*. In his book, Allen provides a strong defense for America's current vaccination protocols, and offers a compelling critique of the thimerosal-autism hypothesis. Allen argues that mercury toxicity requires much greater exposure to organic mercury than the trace amounts found in vaccines. He provides a nostalgic anecdote to illustrate his point: ". . . many a baby boomer could recall breaking one [a mercury thermometer] open to roll the gleaming silvery puddle around in the palm of one's hand—inhaling its toxic fumes all the while."[89]

Allen is referring to the fact that many of us—before the autism epidemic—can remember literally holding beads of mercury in the palm of our hands, absorbing its toxic effects, with little or no health consequences. Allen is right—baby boomers were able to expose themselves to high levels of mercury with little clinical impact because most baby boomers had immune systems that were strong and could effectively absorb and excrete toxins. Baby boomers did not usually have five, six or seven courses of antibiotics in the first two years of their lives. Baby boomers' mothers did not take chronic cycles of birth-control pills, NSAIDs, steroids, and other pharmaceuticals known to disrupt the gut flora, which would then be passed on to their children. Baby boomers might have received a handful of vaccinations in their early childhood, as opposed to the dozens received in the first year of life by children today (which may contribute to immune dysregulation). Baby boomers were not exposed as children to one-tenth of the amount of toxins absorbed by children today. As children, baby boomers were not suffering from gut dysbiosis and immune dysregulation. The children of today do suffer from these conditions, and it places them at an incredible disadvantage in an increasingly toxic world. Is thimerosal the sole causative agent behind the epidemic of autism? Probably not. Could it be the straw that broke the camel's back in a few susceptible children? Maybe. What is more likely, is that the mercury from thimerosal is (to use Doris Rapp's and Donna

Jackson Nakazawa's metaphor[90]) one more drop of water in a barrel that is already overflowing with toxic, immune-disrupting, and gut dysregulating influences. The children of today need to minimize exposure to *any* substances that might "tip the barrel," and send them in a downward spiral into disease and biological dysfunction.

Autism is an extraordinarily complex disorder. There are numerous etiological variables in each case of autism. The degree to which each variable plays a role in etiology varies by individual. Following is a graphic illustration of the some of the variables believed to contribute to the development of autism. The first graphic (figure 3) shows a simplified illustration of causal factors that lead to the development of autism. Not all of these factors are present for each individual. For instance, although vaccination is shown as one of the predisposing factors, it is possible for a child who has never been vaccinated to develop autism as a result of the presence of any number of the other variables believed to contribute to autism. The second graphic (figure 4) is a more complex illustration of the etiology of the symptoms of autism by looking in detail at some of the wide reaching biological and physiological consequences of gut dysbiosis, immune dysregulation and certain environmental variables. These graphics are meant to illustrate the incredible complexity of autism, and are not meant to represent a complete illustration of the etiology and pathogenesis of autism. They are meant to illustrate that autism results from the confluence of multiple environmental and genetic variables.

The Etiology of ADHD and Other Neurological Disorders

Although the etiology of autism is complex, it is a prism through which other neurological disorders can be understood. Many have argued that ADHD is a disorder that ought to be placed upon the autism spectrum. In the opinion of some physicians and researchers, all neurological disorders could be placed on the same, albeit more complex, spectrum, as the etiology of many neurological disorders is the same: gut dysfunction and immune dysregulation.

Since much of the etiology of autism is environmental (with perhaps genetic predispositions that "load the gun"), it is likely that many

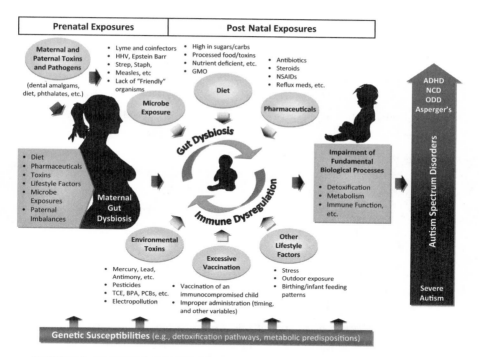

FIGURE 3: FACTORS CONTRIBUTING TO ETIOLOGY AND PATHOGENESIS OF AUTISM SPECTRUM DISORDERS.

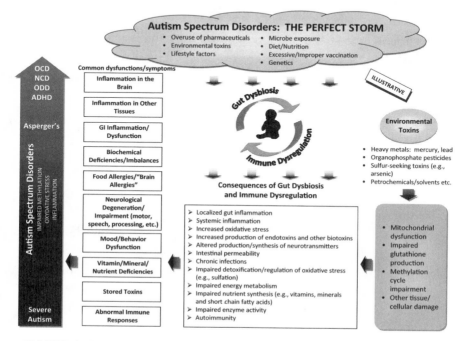

FIGURE 4. FACTORS CONTRIBUTING TO ETIOLOGY AND PATHOGENESIS OF AUTISM SPECTRUM DISORDERS (DETAILED).

more children are adversely affected by these same environmental assaults. The physiological and biochemical dysfunctions that affect
children with autism also affect children diagnosed with specific neurological disorders (such as ADHD, depression, bipolar disorder, etc.)
and it is probable that they are also affecting neurotypical children as
well. Children that are neurotypical but suffer from sensory processing
disorder or oppositional and defiant behavior, or excessive rage,
tantrums, or other atypical behavior may be exhibiting symptoms of
biological imbalances.

ADHD is the most common of all diagnosable neurological disorders in children today. It is a diagnosis that has evolved over time. Like
autism, allergies, and asthma, it is a modern diagnosis; comparable behavioral and clinical characteristics were rarely seen in the preindustrial age. This is not to say that it did not exist preindustrially, but like
the other "modern maladies," it was a rare occurrence. For the earliest
description of modern ADHD, many historians point to nineteenth
century physician and author Heinrich Hoffman, who described
among his own children ("fidgety Philip") a boy who might today be
classified as ADHD. A physician named Sir George Still also described
a disorder with characteristics similar to ADHD around the turn of the
century. By the 1960s, the diagnosis of hyperkinesis was increasingly
common, but nowhere near the proportions seen today. Some estimates place the prevalence of ADHD as high as 10 percent or more of
American children. Like autism, ADHD is believed to be of genetic
origin. Like autism, epidemiological studies continue to throw a
wrench in the genetic-etiology theory. The question that is asked about
autism is also asked about ADHD: how is it possible that we are seeing
an epidemic of a genetic brain disorder? It just does not add up.

Nonetheless, most researchers continue to point to genetics as the
main etiology of ADHD. In fact, one recent review of ADHD noted
that twin studies indicated that 75-90 percent of the etiology of ADHD
is genetic.[91] Twin studies (looking at the rates of a particular disorder
among identical twins) provide compelling evidence of genetic origin.
If 75-90 percent of identical twins both have ADHD, it would seem

that this were dictated by their shared genes. Yet, what about the other 10-25 percent of twins, where one does not have ADHD? And for those twin sets who both have ADHD, is it possible that both twins developed ADHD simply because they received the same gut flora from their mother, ate the same diet, breathed the same air, drank the same water, and received the same immunological assaults as infants? As more clinicians who use a biomedical or functional approach begin to treat children with ADHD, new ideas about etiology emerge. Environmental factors are suddenly a new focus for etiological research.

Interestingly, children diagnosed with ADHD often carry other co-morbidities, such as allergies, asthma, obsessive-compulsive disorder, anxiety disorder (33.5 percent prevalence[92]), oppositional defiant disorder, depression, conduct disorder, bipolar disorder and other diagnosable disorders. Has the pediatric psychiatric community gone on a diagnosis spree, wildly stamping labels on children that are simply misbehaving? Or is there something more complicated going on? Perhaps the fact that individual children are often diagnosed with multiple psychiatric disorders could provide a clue about the etiology of these neurobehavioral disorders. Children do not fit neatly into diagnostic boxes because they are individuals, each experiencing unique biochemical and physiological dysfunctions that impact neurobehavior. Diagnosis with a disease or a disorder is medical science's way of ordering what is otherwise a completely confounding phenomenon. Children are struggling; children are misbehaving; children are out of control, but we do not understand why.

Applying the model of autism to ADHD and other neurological disorders allows us to see why diagnosis is so difficult. Each child has a different genetic makeup and a variety of environmental variables that affect the pathophysiology of their neurobehavioral disorders. The same variables that affect the development of allergies, asthma and autism (genetic/diet/vaccine/medication-induced gut dysbiosis and immune dysregulation, compounded by environmental toxins) also affect the development of ADHD, depression, bipolar disorder, and other disorders. Among the environmental variables most commonly

linked to the etiology of ADHD are diet/allergies, disruptions to neurotransmitter systems (which is related to gut dysbiosis and immune
dysregulation), and chemical/toxic exposure.

Parents of children with ADHD have long considered diet to be
among the factors most influential on symptoms and severity of their
children's disorder. In the early1970s, a psychiatrist by the name of
Richard Mackarness argued that diet was a critical component of
many of his patients' neurological disorders, including those with hyperactivity.[93] Mackarness was not the only physician in the 1970s to
concern himself with dietary management of ADHD. Perhaps one of
the best known medical figures in the ADHD community is Dr. Ben
Feingold, who developed the infamous Feingold Diet, a dietary plan
that calls for the elimination of certain food additives and substances
believed to exacerbate symptoms of ADHD.

Orthomolecular psychiatry is another domain where physicians understand ADHD as the manifestation of underlying physiological and
biochemical imbalances. In this field, physicians examine a particular
patient's diet and vitamin/nutrient/biochemical imbalances in an effort to understand how certain psycho-nutrients (e.g., foods that trigger
abnormal psychological and behavioral symptoms) can lead to neurobehavioral abnormalities.

Dr. William Philpott, an orthomolecular physician, published a
book entitled *Brain Allergies* in 1980, which details his clinical experiences treating neurobehavioral and psychiatric disorders through
diet and nutrient management. Dr. Philpott provides many examples
of patients whose symptoms improved with individualized dietary and
nutrient management. Following are two case studies he relates in
Brain Allergies:

> A twelve-year-old boy diagnosed as hyperkinetic had the following
> symptoms on testing for spinach: he became overtalkative and phys-
> ically violent, had excessive saliva, was very hot, developed a severe
> stomachache, and cried for a long time. Watermelon made him ir-
> ritable and depressed; cantaloupe made him aggressively tease other
> patients. Once he avoided the incriminating substances in his diet,

> his hyperkinesis symptoms diminished dramatically. . . . A four-year-old boy diagnosed as hyperkinetic had a variety of reactions. String beans made him hyperactive, and he wanted to fight with everyone. Celery gave him a severe stomachache, after which he cried and became grouchy. Strawberries made him angry and hyperactive and caused a great deal of coughing. Unrefined sugar caused him to be irritable, after which he coughed and developed a stuffy nose.[94]

These hyperkinetic symptoms, Dr. Philpott argues, are actually the result of food allergies or sensitivities. The functional medicine approach would examine the guts of these boys to look for intestinal hyperpermeability (leaky gut). Essentially, brain allergies are simply food allergies/intolerances that result in an inflammatory response that impacts the brain. This is not unlike the inflammatory processes seen in autism. Preliminary studies are examining the possibility that obsessive-compulsive disorder and schizophrenia (often accompanied by ADHD) may be of autoimmune etiology.[95]

While diet may be of critical importance in the pathophysiology of ADHD, it does not provide the complete etiological picture.

As with autism, understanding the etiology of ADHD and other neurological disorders requires putting together many disparate pieces of a genetic and environmental puzzle. Environmental toxins are another factor likely to play a role in the etiology of ADHD and other neurobehavioral disorders, either by directly disrupting the gut flora (critical for detoxification, immune regulation, etc.) or by directly impacting brain or nerve cells. Multiple studies have linked ADHD to environmental toxins. Lead, in particular, is implicated in the etiology and pathophysiology of ADHD. A 2008 study of over twelve hundred children in China demonstrated that children with ADHD had much higher levels of lead in their blood than neurotypical children. These results were found to be consistent with previous studies correlating blood lead level to neurological disorders.[96] Similarly, another study demonstrated that children exposed prenatally to tobacco smoke were 2.5 times more likely to develop ADHD than unexposed children.[97]

An inability to effectively detoxify may be genetic, but it may also be related to the health of our first line of defense against environmental toxins, our gut flora. As food allergies would indicate, children with ADHD likely suffer from some form of gut dysbiosis and immune dysregulation. As with children with autism, children with ADHD and associated behavioral disorders often struggle with gastrointestinal issues ranging from chronic constipation and encopresis (soiling problems) to abdominal pain and diarrhea. Studies have demonstrated a clear link between constipation/soiling problems and psychological and behavioral problems. One study conducted in the UK found that children with emotional and behavioral disorders had a significantly higher incidence of daily and weekly soiling incidents than normal peers.[98] In general, children with defecation disorders are known to have more behavioral problems than children without defecation disorders.[99]

If these studies are not compelling enough to demonstrate a link between neurobehavioral disorders and gastrointestinal dysfunction, speak with special education teachers or social workers that care for children with mental health diagnoses. One former social worker with the Department of Children and Families (a child welfare agency in Massachusetts) recounted her experiences with children with neurobehavioral disorders:

> I had a caseload of about 22-24 kids with mental illness. Examples of primary diagnoses were Bipolar Disorder, Mood Disorder, Reactive Attachment Disorder, ADHD, Autism, Asperger's, and also kids who had autistic or Asperger's traits. These kids usually have multiple diagnoses. I have noticed that most of my kids have trouble with their digestive systems. They often have constipation, pain, are fearful of going to the bathroom and will hold it until the last minute possible. These kids also tend to have accidents and bowel leakage and require a change of underwear throughout their school day. I also remember some previous co-workers agreeing that they have experienced the same thing with the kids on their caseloads.[100]

It is commonly believed that the *discomfort* of constipation contributes to abnormal behavior, or that psychological issues cause children to hold their feces and thus experience constipation. Conventional western medicine wants to believe that the aforementioned disorders are brain-based, or begin in the head, and every other symptom is downstream of the brain. There seems to be very little focus on the role of environmental factors such as diet and antibiotics in the development of gastrointestinal dysfunction, and there is even less consideration of the notion that gastrointestinal issues might provide clues with regard to etiology of behavioral disorders.

As with autism, dysfunction in the gut leads to dysfunction in the brain. One of the most promising recent developments in the field of ADHD research is the finding that children with ADHD suffer from deficits of dopamine, an important neurotransmitter that promotes calm and feelings of well-being.[101] This discovery was made in part by the observation that stimulant medications (such as methylphenidate/ Ritalin), which increase available dopamine levels, help mitigate symptoms of ADHD. Impaired dopamine systems can impair cognitive function, but can also impact motor control and regulation of kinesis. While research involving impaired dopamine systems continues, the vast majority of published studies look at the synthesis of dopamine as it occurs in the brain (in nerve terminals). Again, we see the brain-first approach to understanding neurobiological disorders.

However, studies demonstrate that the critical biochemical precursors to dopamine are not produced in the brain. In order for the body to produce dopamine in the brain, a cascade of biochemical reactions needs to occur first. The following is the cascade of events that lead up to the production of dopamine: The amino acid L-phenylalanine is converted to L-tyrosine, which is then converted to L-DOPA, which is required for the production of neurotransmitters such as dopamine, norepinephrine, and epinephrine. Interestingly, L-phenylalanine is made available through food we ingest and is then converted into L-tyrosine by an enzyme known as tyrosine hydroxylase. Tyrosine hydroxylase is coded on the TH gene, which requires induction by butyrate—a short-chain fatty acid that is produced by *microorganisms in our gut.*[102] Whew. This is a rather involved process to explain, but the key takeaway is that without good gut flora, we cannot effectively make the neurotransmitters that we need to regulate our behavior and moods.

> Circulating short-chain fatty acids (SCFAs) are primarily derived from bacterial fermentation of carbohydrates in the colon where they function as physiologic modulators of epithelial cell maturation. Butyrate [one of these short-chain fatty acids] has been shown to induce tyrosine hydroxylase, the rate-limiting enzyme of catecholamine synthesis.[103]

In simplified language, butyrate (which is produced by the good gut flora) induces the production of tyrosine hydroxylase, which is necessary for the production of dopamine.

Our bodies cannot effectively manufacture dopamine if we do not have butyrate readily available in our guts. Children with gut dysbiosis have low levels of butyrate. Children with neurobehavioral disorders also have low levels of butyrate. To summarize, in some children: low levels of good gut flora=>low levels of butyrate=>low levels of dopamine=> mood and behavioral problems.

The production of neurotransmitters such as serotonin, dopamine, norepinephrine and epinephrine, which are so important to neurological function in human beings, is critically dependent upon a healthy and balanced gastrointestinal system. As Hippocrates stated in the fifth century B.C., "All diseases begin in the gut." Perhaps now is the time that we as a society begin to listen to our gut, and examine the truth behind this statement.

A significant amount of compelling evidence points to the fact that the gastrointestinal system is of utmost importance in human health and wellness. Yet, it is of equal importance to understand that the pathophysiology of chronic illness is a complex and highly individual phenomenon. No two people are likely to develop disease in the same way. However, there are lessons to be learned by looking closely at how individuals become chronically ill, as common environmental variables (many of them cultural) contribute to etiology of disease. Americans, the same people who theoretically have many health advantages over other people on this planet, are much sicker than they ought to be, and it is high time we pay attention to the environmental (that is to say, cultural) factors that make this so. Particular parts of American culture (e.g., diet, industrial capitalism, lifestyle etc.) predispose us to chronic illness. Unfortunately, it is our children that must serve as the canaries in the coal mine, alerting us to the fact that our ways of living are self-destructive.

chapter 3

Why Our Children? Why Now?

ᘏ

AMERICA'S PROBLEM

Illness in children is not a new phenomenon. But until fairly recently, infectious diseases were the main cause of serious illness in children. Historically speaking, chronic illnesses affected older people or those who had survived an infectious disease earlier in life, which might lead to postinfection complications (e.g., paralysis from polio). It would seem that the demise of deadly infectious childhood diseases in America would usher in an era of tremendous health and wellness for our youth. Unfortunately, this is not the case. Today, American children are largely spared from deadly infectious diseases, but they carry a heavy burden of disease, nonetheless. As a society, we have transitioned out of the age of deadly infectious disease, and into the age of chronic disease.

In the early 1970s, a UNC epidemiologist by the name of Abdel Omran wrote a paper on the subject of human population change that helped to frame our current understanding of health and disease in the modern world. In his paper, "The Epidemiology of Transition," Omran describes how human societies can be grouped according to mortality patterns, or how people in a society typically die. Omran used historical records of population change and evolution to develop three main categories or stages of human development. These stages include: "The Age of Pestilence and Famine," "The Age of Receding Pandemics," and "The Age of Degenerative and Man-Made Diseases." Omran places these stages on a continuum assuming certain elements of progress that promote a society from one stage to the next. All societies can be placed into one of these categories as a way of understanding population dynamics, as well as the social, economic, and health attributes common to each type of society. Today, all three stages of epidemiologic transition exist on the planet, with western and industrialized countries theoretically in the "Age of Degenerative and Man-Made Diseases," while most developing nations exist somewhere between the other two stages.[1]

Towards the beginning of the twentieth century, the United States began to make a full transition out of the "The Age of Receding Pandemics" into "The Age of Degenerative and Man-Made Diseases." Prior to the adoption of wide scale sanitation and public health initiatives around the turn of the twentieth century, America was a nation that struggled with frequent pandemics of infectious diseases, such as tuberculosis, typhoid fever, measles, diphtheria, rubella, and infectious diarrhea. Approximately 44 percent of total deaths during this era were attributable to infectious diseases. As germ theory (the knowledge that viruses, bacteria, fungi etc. were the causes of infectious disease) was developed only toward the end of the nineteenth century, Americans had a limited ability to understand and control infectious diseases. However, once germ theory and nutrition were incorporated into public health policy, the rates of infectious diseases began to drop significantly.

In the early decades of the twentieth century, public health initiatives that remedied contaminated water, food supply, and unsanitary living conditions brought morbidity and mortality rates related to infectious diseases down significantly. About half of the decrease in total mortality was attributed to clean water technologies. Infant mortality rates dropped from over 200 per 1000 births in 1888 to approximately 120 per 1000 births in 1911.[2] According to Harvard economist, David Cutler, and Stanford Professor of Medicine, Grant Miller, approximately three-quarters of decreases in infant mortality, and two-thirds of decreases in child mortality in the early twentieth century can be attributed to clean water technologies.[3] Also, the illnesses with the highest correlations to mortality (tuberculosis, pneumonia and infectious diarrhea) were reduced significantly by improved hygiene and home-based treatment protocols (e.g. hydration and electrolyte replacement for diarrhea).[4]

It was at this point that Americans began to transition out of the "pandemic" phase and into the "degenerative" phase of human development, where "degenerative and man-made diseases displace[d] pandemics of infection as the primary causes of morbidity and mortality."[5] Advances in public health through widespread immunization programs and the availability of antibiotics (fully penetrating American society by the 1960s) also helped America to make a full transition into Omran's final category: "The Age of Degenerative and Man-Made Diseases." Importantly, Americans did not necessarily understand that transitioning out of the pandemic phase would mean degenerative and chronic illness would become society's next scourge. Instead, many Americans were under the impression that science and progress had delivered us into an age where sickness was a thing of the past, and health and wellness would reign supreme. Omran knew this to be a false impression, and many Americans are now beginning to understand that transitioning out of the pandemic phase was not without its costs.

There is no question that public health developments of the early twentieth century put America in a better place with regard to morbidity and mortality. More Americans are living longer lives. Parents no longer fear the arrival of one of the dreaded childhood illnesses, such as infectious diarrhea or diphtheria. With a few exceptions, most infectious diseases that were feared in the nineteenth century are now either rare or can be treated effectively with modern medical interventions. However, these great victories in the battle against germs have only created new, more complicated relationships with germs. Americans may no longer be helpless in the face of a deadly virus or bacterium, but they are just as much at the mercy of the microscopic world today as they were in the nineteenth century.

Interestingly, some of the same public health developments that led to the demise of deadly infectious diseases in the early part of the twentieth century may actually contribute to the epidemic of chronically ill children in America today. Public and private hygiene and sanitation initiatives aimed at controlling infectious diseases certainly reduced the impact of infectious pathogens, but some argue that we have become *too* sanitary. We have reduced our exposures to disease-causing germs, but we have also reduced our exposures to good, immune-building microorganisms. Also, antibiotics and vaccines have greatly reduced the infectious disease burden on the population, but they may also be contributing to widespread immune dysregulation, the biological precursor to chronic illness. These factors, in conjunction with other important cultural and sociological factors, may be responsible for the development of chronic illness in susceptible children. Additional factors include everything from the standard American diet, which is sometimes abbreviated SAD (an appropriate acronym), to exposure to environmental toxins. In the nineteenth century, we could blame illness on bugs. Today, our illnesses are of our own making.

One of the important observations that Omran makes in his population analysis is that societies in the degenerative phase have the technology and knowledge to prevent sickness (both infectious and chronic), yet sociological factors often preclude the effective prevention and management of degenerative illness. In other words, societies have it within their capability to control chronic illness, but social, cultural, and economic factors can impede a society's ability to effectively curb the development of such illnesses. Clearly, this is the case for chronic illness in America. It seems utterly confounding that a nation with resources as tremendous as the United States of America would have such high rates of chronic illness, especially among children. Yet, when you examine the root causes of chronic illness in children, it becomes overwhelmingly clear that these causes are factors that are deeply rooted in our culture, and therefore difficult to change.

As previously discussed, chronic illness in many American children may stem from underlying gut dysbiosis and immune dysregulation. Just as autism is believed to be the result of multiple genetic and environmental variables, many chronic childhood illnesses may result from a cocktail of environmental factors laid atop particular genetic susceptibilities. In many cases, genetics load the gun, and the environment pulls the trigger. What we are finding, however, is that certain environmental factors that contribute to chronic illnesses are so ubiquitous in American society, and their effects so overwhelming, that very few children have a genetic makeup that would allow them to escape unscathed. If the same environmental factors that make a child autistic are the same environmental factors that make another child develop ADHD or juvenile diabetes, then certainly "healthy" children who are exposed to the same environmental variables (but are not outwardly sick) could be affected on some level. A lack of disease symptoms does not mean that these children are not being affected by harmful environmental factors.

Environmentally derived gut dysbiosis and immune dysregulation can lead to illnesses such as autism or food allergies; however, many more American children suffer from gut dysbiosis and immune dysregulation that go undetected, simply because they are not yet symptomatic. This may be only a matter of time. Science supports the fact that environmental factors like toxin exposure or overuse of antibiotics cause biological and physiological damage in children with diagnoses such as ADHD and autism. There is enough new research to support the idea that even healthy children may experience similar biological damage, but with less severity or intensity. No genes can completely protect children from destructive environmental toxins; no genes work optimally with the standard American diet—a diet poor in nutrition and high in harmful substances; and no genes can fully withstand the immune modulating effects of excessive pharmaceutical usage and excessive vaccination. Genes are important for determining type, severity and onset of illness, but no genes can confer complete protection against ubiquitous, destructive environmental factors. America's epidemic of chronic childhood illness is *culturally derived*, and therefore, it is America's problem.

THE ENVIRONMENTAL FACTORS RESPONSIBLE FOR CHRONIC ILLNESS IN AMERICA'S CHILDREN

In recent years, a number of studies have correlated "western living" with the development of autoimmune or atopic disease.[6] The United States is not the only nation affected by the epidemic of chronic illness. For instance, "in the International Study of Asthma and Allergy in Children, the highest prevalences of asthma were in Australia, New Zealand and the UK, where in 2003 more than 20 percent of children aged 13–14 years reported asthma symptoms."[7] Much of the western lifestyle includes diet and health habits that have either been influenced by, or directly exported from, America. Several international studies have linked the American diet (as defined by increased consumption of processed and fast foods) with atopic disease.[8] International epidemics of immunological, inflammatory, and neurological disorders seem to be correlated with various components of western living. What exactly about western living is making so many people ill?

Hygiene is one of the most commonly implicated theoretical causes of western-associated chronic illness. Of all chronic illnesses, atopic (allergic) disease is probably the most studied by epidemiologists because it affects so many people, yet, no one knows what is behind the recent upward trends in the western world. As it became clear that allergies and asthma were on the rise, many researchers looked to the work of Dr. David Strachan and his "hygiene hypothesis" for answers. Initially, Strachan speculated that those children who were exposed to less infectious germs (e.g., through animals or other children) carried a greater risk for the development of atopic disease. Subsequent studies showed that rural children (exposed to microbes from animals and dirt) tended to carry a lower risk for atopy than urban children. The low-atopic profile of rural inhabitants is the basis for Graham Rooks' "old friends" hypothesis, which states that any microbial exposure (especially "friendly" or commensal bacteria) is important for the development of a healthy (nonallergic) immune system. Thus, many researchers speculate that the immune system needs to be primed by microbial exposure for proper function. Yet, a recent study looking at atopic disease in farmers, who are among the most rural of dwellers, found that they have a high risk for occupation-related atopic disease, which contradicts Rooks' "old friends" theory. As it turns out, these farmers may have developed atopic disease through pesticide exposure.[9] The point is that no one factor is likely to be responsible for chronic illness. In the case of these farmers, while they may have had good microbial exposures to protect them from atopic disease, their exposure to pesticides virtually negated this protection.

Researchers still cling desperately to the hygiene hypothesis and its corollaries because there is something truly intuitive about the theory. Developing nations have much lower rates of chronic noninfectious illness (e.g., allergic or autoimmune), while developed nations have high rates of chronic noninfectious illness. People in developing nations live in close contact with nature, whereas people in the developed world tend to live fairly removed from nature, in an artificial or hygienic setting. It seems to make intuitive sense that something about the artificial or hygienic setting causes these new forms of chronic illness.

Studies examining the link between the artificial setting (hygiene) and atopic disease continue to flood the scientific literature. These studies look at a variety of proxy measures for microbial exposure, such as number of siblings, day care, viral infection, washing and bathing, and household cleaning practices, in an effort to determine if lack of microbial exposure correlates with atopic disease. The studies that look for a hygiene explanation are many, the results are often conflicting, and few provide conclusive evidence of a link.

> Evidence of a link between atopy and domestic cleaning and hygiene is weak at best. Data published since the 1980s . . .show that our modern homes, whatever their visual appearance, still abound with a rich mixture of bacteria, viruses, fungi and moulds, as well as dust mites and other insects, and that our opportunities for exposure to these are quite likely to have increased rather than decreased, since a rising proportion of time is spent indoors.[10]

It is likely that the data conflict in these limited studies simply because hygiene and microbial exposure is only *one* variable in an epidemiological puzzle that contains many pieces. For example, a study that looks at microbial exposure in daycare settings and its relationship to the development of atopy is virtually meaningless if other variables such as antibiotic use during infancy or diet are not incorporated into the analysis.

Although the many hygiene studies prove inconclusive, this does not mean that microbes do not matter. On the contrary, microbial exposure is the single most important element of human immune function, and disrupted commensal microbial colonization in the gut plays a vital role in the development of atopic disease (and other chronic diseases). The problem is, most studies examine the impact of microbial exposure as an isolated variable, ignoring other important variables that impact the overall dynamics of the gut flora, and thus, the immune system. What is missing is a close examination of microbial exposures, or inputs, in the context of other environmental variables, such as pharmaceutical use, diet, and toxin/chemical exposures. Man, demonstrate a link between dysbiotic guts and chronic illness, and many more studies document the types of environmental factors that can contribute to gut dysbiosis, but few studies connect all of the dots.

The environmental factors that contribute to gut dysbiosis, immune dysregulation and downstream chronic illness are complex and vary by individual. Although American society is highly diverse, common cultural currents run through the lives of most every American. Elements of this common culture contribute to widespread gut dysbiosis and immune dysregulation. These factors can be grouped into five main categories:

1. **Medication/Drug Over-usage,** including prescription and over-the-counter medications.
2. **Exposure to Environmental Toxins/Pollution,** including heavy metals, electropollution, petroleum-based chemicals, and many other harmful synthetic substances.
3. **Diet and Nutrition** with an emphasis on the standard American diet and the many complex substances we consume every day.
4. **Habits and Lifestyle,** including everything from how we were born to what kinds of leisure activities we engage in.
5. **Excessive, or Improperly Administered Vaccines,** which pertains to the present standard childhood immunization protocol administered by most every state.

Not every American child is affected by each of these five categories. For instance, plenty of Americans do not consume the standard American diet, yet they may be exposed to pharmaceutical agents, receive a full recommended schedule of vaccinations, and live in neighborhoods that are toxically burdened. In some combination, most American children are touched by the above environmental factors.

Although these environmental factors can affect a child at any stage during their development, the most critical time is during the first few years of life, when a baby's immature immune system continues to develop. Researchers are discovering that the types and quantities of microbiota (microorganisms) that initially populate an infant's gut are of critical importance to the development of a properly functioning immune system. According to a 2007 article in the journal *Neonatology*, "Intestinal colonization . . . is essential for maturation of the gut-associated lymphoid tissue and the homeostasis of the intestinal epithelium and developmental regulation of the intestinal physiology. . . . Recent evidence demonstrates that deviations in gut microbiota may precede specific diseases later in life." Essentially, if an infant's gut is populated early on with pathogenic microbiota, or insufficiently populated with commensal bacteria, such as *Bifidobacteria*, then the immune system does not function properly. [11] Subsequent environmental assaults (toxins, infectious microbes, vaccine antigens, etc.) may be more than an infant's compromised immune system can handle. As the stability of a baby's immune system is exceedingly vulnerable during this time period, even the smallest environmental factors known to impact gut microbiota may impact the health of a child.

Many environmental factors can adversely impact an infant's gut microbiota. Perhaps the most important factor is the gut health of the baby's mother, and to a lesser degree, father. The microorganisms present in a mother's gut and vaginal canal at the time of birth are the same microorganisms that will colonize her baby's gut immediately during and after birth. The father's gut health is important in so far as he transfers his resident microorganisms to his partner through intimate contact. Mom's microorganisms can also be transferred to the baby via breastfeeding. Essentially, the health of gut and vaginal microorganisms of a pregnant mother plays a significant role in the overall health of her baby. A baby with balanced gut microbiota is better equipped to fight off the effects of environmental toxins, poor diet, vaccinations, and natural infections. Unfortunately, gut health is not something that is apparent or obvious to most pregnant woman. Subtle environmental factors influence the health of a mother's gut, and she may not be aware that simple actions that she takes can adversely impact the health of her gut microbiota. For instance, if she used certain pharmaceutical agents, such as oral contraceptives, NSAIDs (like ibuprofen, naproxen), acetaminophen, corticosteroids (asthma medications) or other steroids (e.g., prednisone), prior to or during pregnancy, then it is possible (although not certain) that her gut flora were negatively impacted.[12]

Theoretically, a breastfed baby has many advantages over a bottle-fed baby in that a breastfed baby tends to receive higher quantities of the "good bacteria" (such as *Bifidobacteria*) through breast milk, as well as critical immune factors. A breastfed baby can be protected against many infectious assaults, as the baby is offered passive protection (mother's antibodies) against certain pathogens via breast milk. However, a toxic mom, a mom who has a high level of toxins in her body, or a dysbiotic mom, may be passing along toxins and pathogens to her baby, which can impact her baby's health.[13] In this regard, there is some speculation that a bottle-fed baby might have some advantages. Although the recommendation is still that "breast is best," it is important to note that whatever microorganisms—good or bad—that are present in the mother can be transferred to the baby as well.

After a mother passes along her resident microbes to her baby, the baby's gut continues to be populated by other microbes in the environment. Studies in neonates confirm that the microbiota of infants vary significantly from one to the next, and a number of different factors are believed to cause this variation, including composition of mother's microbiome (microbes and metabolites in her body), mode of delivery (vaginal vs. Caesarean section), age of gestation at birth, and mode of feeding (breast vs. bottle).[14] Although the microbial composition of the gut tends to remain fairly stable after the first year of life, the microbiota will evolve and change according to environmental variables. For instance, if a baby is given certain pharmaceutical agents, such as ibuprofen, acetaminophen, or antibiotics, their levels of *Bifidobacteria* may be reduced while their levels of pathogenic bacteria may be elevated.[15] The following (figure 5) is a graphic illustration of how environmental variables can contribute to the

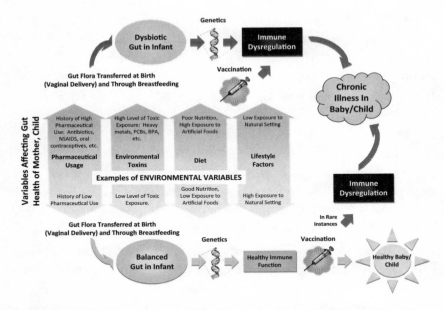

FIGURE 5: ENVIRONMENTAL VARIABLES THAT CONTRIBUTE TO GUT
DYSBIOSIS, IMMUNE DYSREGULATION AND CHRONIC ILLNESS IN
CHILDREN.

development of gut dysbiosis and subsequent immune dysregulation
and chronic illness in babies.

Interestingly, many of the environmental variables that negatively
impact the composition of gut microbiota are products of the modern
world, and more specifically, the twentieth century, especially the
American twentieth century. An explanation of how each of these environmental factors contributes to gut dysbiosis and immune dysregulation is critical for understanding the epidemic of chronic
childhood illness in America.

chapter 4

Factor 1— Medication Overusage

✦

PHARMACEUTICAL NATION

Perhaps the most significant factor that contributes to widespread gut dysbiosis is America's drug habit—that is to say, America's addiction to pharmaceutical agents. In 2008, U.S. drug sales totaled over $291 billion, and the number of "pill-poppers" continues to climb each year.[1] The number of prescriptions purchased from 1993 to 2003 grew 70 percent, while the U.S. population grew by only 13 percent.[2] Furthermore, Americans use more pharmaceuticals than any other nation in the world. In 2008, the U.S. spent more on pharmaceuticals than the U.K., Germany, France, Canada, all of Latin America, Japan, and the rest of the Asia combined! Between 40-50 percent of worldwide annual pharmaceutical sales are attributable to U.S. consumers. Japan, a nation with a population of approximately 130 million people (slightly fewer than half the US population) and the second biggest spender on pharmaceuticals, absorbed only a mere 9 percent of global pharmaceutical sales in 2008.[3] While many of these drugs are life-saving and an important part of many Americans' ability to function, it is an indisputable fact that there is a serious *overuse* of pharmaceutical agents in this country. Some pharmaceutical agents may be absolutely harmless to the gut bacteria, but certain drugs can wreak havoc when used incorrectly.

ANTIBIOTICS

Antibiotics are the most commonly prescribed therapeutic agent across all age groups in this country. Unfortunately, antibiotic use is also the most common cause of damaging alterations to gastrointestinal microbiota. That is not to say that all antibiotic use will result in gut dysbiosis. Plenty of people have taken antibiotics and seen their friendly gut bacteria levels return to normal shortly following cessation of therapy. The degree to which a particular antibiotic impacts gut microbiota depends upon the particular drug's spectrum of activity (broad versus narrow spectrum), pharmacokinetics, dosage and duration of treatment.[4] Furthermore, the degree to which a person can recover from antibiotic use (that is to say, recover their gut flora), may depend on other variables, such as genetics, diet, toxic exposures, etc. Nevertheless, antibiotics are changing the ecology of American guts, and few Americans know that it is even happening.

Statistics will tell you that Americans consume antibiotics like candy. Try to find someone in your circle of acquaintances that has not had at least one course of antibiotics in his or her life—it is a difficult person to find. Antibiotics are most commonly prescribed for everyday ailments such as ear, sinus, skin, and urinary tract infections. According to a review study sponsored by the Union of Concerned Scientists, outpatients (doctor's office visits) received 120 million courses of treatment of antimicrobials annually. This translates to an estimated 1.3 to 2.6 million *pounds* of antimicrobials (primarily antibiotics) used in outpatient settings every year. Inpatient (hospital) antimicrobial use estimates range from 550,000 to 1,100,000 pounds per year. Together, roughly 3 million pounds of antimicrobials are used in humans for therapeutic purposes every year.[5] Children are not excluded from this trend. "Data from 1992 indicated that by the age of 15 years, US children had received, on average, more than four courses of antibiotics to treat a single disorder, otitis media, a common ear infection."[6] We are a society that is heavily dependent upon antibiotics, yet we do not fully understand the broader medical and sociological consequences of these drug usage patterns. We have been in the age of antibiotics for more than sixty years, yet, we are only just beginning to connect antibiotic use to acute clinical problems, such as antibiotic-associated diarrhea. What is even more discouraging is that, as a society, we are only just beginning to grasp the link between the overuse of antibiotics and chronic illnesses.

It is important to note that antibiotics *are* lifesavers. Many infectious diseases would otherwise be deadly without antibiotics. But antibiotics do not come without costs. Medical practitioners have long understood that short-term consequences are associated with antibiotic use, but generally, these consequences are considered manageable, or acceptable, given the significant benefit of antibiotic therapy in combating infectious disease. The most commonly recognized acute clinical consequences of antibiotics include:

- Antibiotic-associated diarrhea, which often results from an overgrowth of *C. difficile*, noted pathogens;
- Decreased production of short-chain fatty acids—critical for many functions in the body, including neurotransmitter production and maintenance of intestinal integrity;

- Vulnerability to pathogenic microbes, especially immediately following the course of treatment;
- Impaired digestion, metabolism and detoxification capabilities.[7]

However, because they have not always been used judiciously in the American population, we are beginning to see the broader consequences of excessive use of antibiotics in America. Researchers are beginning to investigate the connection between the rise in chronic illnesses and the overuse of antibiotics. Dr. Natasha Campbell-McBride argues that many chronic illnesses are the result of alterations in gut microbiota from excessive antibiotic (and other pharmaceutical) usage. According to Dr. Campbell-McBride:

- Penicillins, the gold standard of antibiotics in America for decades, damage *Lactobacillus* and *Bifidobacteria* while promoting pathogens such as *Streptococci* and *Staphylococci*.
- Tetracyclines, the antibiotic given *chronically* to many teenagers in the 1980s and 1990s to combat acne, "have a particularly toxic effect on the gut wall by altering protein structure."
- Aminoglycosides and Macrolides—the mycins—negatively impact *E.coli* and *Enterococci*, both beneficial bacteria found in the gut[8]

There are dozens of different antibiotics and all of them have different profiles in terms of how they affect the gut flora. Some are narrower in activity and reduce certain strains of bacteria while leaving others untouched. Some antibiotics are effective at decreasing or eliminating the good bacteria (such as *Bifidobacteria* and *Lactobacillus* strains) while leaving certain pathogenic strains (such as *Klebsiella* or *Enterobacter* strains) untouched, while at the same time causing a proliferation of pathogenic yeast (like *Candida albicans*).[9] Use of amoxicillin has been associated with an increased rate of *Candida* growth.[10] Physicians have long known about the increased likelihood of *Can-*

dida overgrowth as a consequence of antibiotic therapy. In fact, in the 1960s, it was fairly common for physicians to prescribe an antifungal (e.g., anti-*Candida*) agent concurrent with an antibiotic to prevent the possibility of a secondary *Candida* infection. The most commonly used product contained both tetracycline (antibiotic) and nystatin (antifungal), commercially known as Mysteclin. These products have subsequently been removed from the market.[11]

Ear infections are the most common reason for antibiotic prescription in a pediatrician's office, but it is well established that antibiotics often do not help to clear the infection, and may have no efficacy in many human infections.[12] Although some initial steps have been taken by public health agencies to curb excessive antibiotic use, they continue to be used to treat children's ear infections, women's urinary tract infections, teenagers' acne, sinus infections and a whole host of other illnesses that may not necessarily need an antibiotic (because of the self-limiting nature or viral etiology of these infections). In addition, antibiotics are increasingly being used for their anti-inflammatory effects and may be used to treat nonbacterial diseases like asthma or rheumatoid arthritis.

Although antibiotic use in humans is excessive, it is only marginal compared to the amount of antibiotics used for agricultural purposes. In the 1950s, farmers discovered that feeding low doses of antibiotics to livestock would cause them to gain weight. Interestingly, antibiotics are used for "growth promotion and disease prevention" in livestock, yet, scientists do not know why subtherapeutic doses of antibiotics stimulate growth, nor do they know if antibiotic administration is even effective at preventing disease. In fact, it has been argued that this type of antibiotic use in livestock actually contributes to more infirm populations of animals. In the late 1990s, U.S. cattle received annually over 3.7 million pounds of antimicrobials, hogs received over 10.4 million pounds, and chickens received 10.5 million pounds for nontherapeutic purposes. These quantities represent a 53 percent rise in antimicrobial use in just 15 years, with poultry having the largest percentage increase (over 300 percent).[13]

These numbers are striking especially in light of the fact that humans consume about three million pounds of antimicrobials annually, a fraction of that consumed by livestock. Furthermore, the widespread use of antibiotics in livestock that are also commonly used in humans, such as penicillin and tetracycline, is a practice that is prohibited in Europe. In fact, in 2005, the EU prohibited the use of antibiotics in animal feed (although it is still given directly to animals through injections for therapeutic purposes). The EU is concerned about the long-term impact of subtherapeutic doses of antibiotics added to the human food supply. Yet, the U.S. does not seem to share any of these concerns. Or, perhaps powerful U.S. livestock interests who want to continue using subtherapeutic doses of antibiotics in livestock are marginalizing these concerns.

Antimicrobial use is not limited to humans and animals. According to a Union of Concerned Scientists report, antibiotics are also used (albeit in smaller quantities) on fruit crops to prevent blight. Over 43,000 pounds of antibiotics were applied to produce in 1999. New evidence also points to exposure to antibiotics in our drinking water. Multiple studies have examined the content of municipal drinking water to determine the level of detectable pharmaceutical agents being consumed by citizens through water supply. One study that examined tap water from nineteen U.S. water utilities serving over 28 million Americans found multiple pharmaceutical and endocrine-disrupting chemicals present in the water. Among the most frequently detected compounds were atenolol (beta-blocker used for cardiovascular conditions), carbamazepine (anticonvulsant/mood stabilizer used for bipolar disorder, epilepsy, schizophrenia, and ADHD), gemfibrozil (cholesterol/lipid lowering medication), meprobamate (tranquilizer), naproxen (NSAID, analgesic), phenytoin (antiepileptic, also used for psychiatric and heart conditions), sulfamethoxazole (antibiotic), and trimethoprim (antibiotic).[14]

The widespread use of antibiotics in animals and crops is problematic for human health for several reasons. The most commonly cited concern relates to the possibility of antibiotic-resistant bacteria resulting from common or low level use of antibiotics. Evidence points to the fact that antibiotic use in livestock can contribute to the development of antibiotic-resistant microbes, which can infect and sicken humans.[15] MRSA, an antibiotic-resistant strain of *staphylococcus* bacteria has received much attention in the press in recent years, as it has led to the deaths of many people. Also of concern is that people consuming antibiotics through their meat, fruit and water may be damaging their gut flora, or possibly growing antibiotic-resistant strains of bacteria themselves.

> One important realization must be that the reckless and largely uncontrolled use of antibiotics might not only change human society through the increased risks associated with multiple antibiotic resistance in pathogens, but also through irreversibly altering the symbiotic microbiome with which we have co-evolved. As we do not know the functions of many of these bacterial species in relation to human biology, we might already have started a large-scale genetic engineering experiment on our own symbiotics, with little or no knowledge of the future outcome in terms of human health.[16]

With the overuse of antibiotics, we are unwittingly participating in one of the greatest human medical experiments of all time, and our children are serving as the early predictors of a potentially grim outcome.

NSAIDS (NONSTEROIDAL ANTI-INFLAMMATORY DRUGS)

NSAIDs are anti-inflammatory pain medications that act as COX-inhibitors, which means they block the action of COX enzymes known to produce prostaglandins. Prostaglandins have many functions in the body, including promoting pain, fever, as well as protecting the lining of the stomach and intestine.[17] Over thirty types of nonsteroidal anti-inflammatory drugs are available on the market—perhaps the best known are ibuprofen (Advil, Motrin), naproxen (Aleve), and celecoxib (Celebrex). This class of drugs also includes aspirin (Bayer, Excedrin).

Over seventy million NSAID prescriptions a year are filled, while many more NSAID products (over thirty billion units) are sold over the counter.[18] NSAIDs are known to compromise mucosal cell integrity of the intestine, which leads to increased permeability (intestinal wall damage and leaky gut).

As previously discussed, increased intestinal permeability can lead to a cascade of allergic and inflammatory events. Studies have shown that NSAID-induced intestinal permeability and inflammation may occur in as many as 50-70 percent of patients.[19] A study examining the rate of gastrointestinal ulcerations among NSAID users found that 47 percent of the study population taking NSAIDs for rheumatoid arthritis had ulcerations in their intestines.[20] Studies have also shown that this intestinal permeability can be detected within twelve to twenty-four hours of ingestion, which implies that even occasional or intermittent use can be potentially damaging.[21] In a study of premature neonates given indomethacin (an NSAID), 30 percent of the infants experienced bowel perforation. Notably, indomethacin is the pain medication of choice in neonatal intensive care units. It is typically used as a life-saving measure for babies born with a congenital heart abnormality known as PDA (patent ductus arteriosus). [22] NSAIDs and aspirin are shown to degrade biofilm—the intracellular matrix formed by bacteria, fungi etc. (the "slime" on surfaces populated by microbes), thus they may work to degrade the protective biofilm of commensal bacteria in the gut, a critical part of the human inner ecosystem.

A study by Mohammed A. S. Alem and Julia Douglas at the University of Glasgow demonstrated that seven of nine drugs in the NSAID/aspirin category inhibited biofilm formation. These drugs included celecoxib, nimesulide, ibuprofen and meloxican and aspirin. Treatment with other COX inhibitors resulted in biofilms that consisted almost entirely of yeast cells.[23] In other words, these NSAIDs break down the important bacterial barrier (of commensal flora) that is so critical to a healthy digestive and immune system. If the biofilm (barrier) of good bacteria is broken down by NSAID use, then there is little protection from bad microbiota (yeast, pathogens, etc.) taking over. Without proper recolonization with good bacteria (through diet or supplements), gut dysbiosis is likely to ensue. Chronic NSAID use (or perhaps even acute use)—by both parents and children—is one likely contributor to the epidemic of gut dysbiosis and immune dysregulation in America. Because few acute complications are associated with NSAIDs in children, they are believed to be extremely safe and effective pain relievers. Pediatricians often recommend the administration of ibuprofen or something similar in children receiving vaccinations or suffering from high fevers or other pain. Unfortunately, the NSAIDs may be compromising the strength of the immune system when the body needs it most.

One other pain reliever is of importance with regard to gut dysbiosis, immune dysregulation, and the development of chronic illness: acetaminophen (Tylenol, Paracetomol). Tylenol has been shown to cause the depletion of glutathione in the liver, the body's detoxification headquarters.[24] Again, glutathione is an antioxidant found within every cell of our body and it is known to protect cells from oxidative damage (damage by free radicals/toxins). More specifically, glutathione helps move chemicals, drugs and other harmful substances out of the body. A body depleted of glutathione is considered to have impaired detoxification capabilities, and thus cannot effectively excrete heavy metals, endocrine disruptors (such as BPA) or other harmful substances that enter the body.

In recent years, the role of glutathione has moved to center stage among some autism researchers, as they are now finding that children with autism not only have impaired detoxifications capabilities, but they also have significantly lower levels of glutathione than neurotypical children.[25] Interestingly, Tylenol is among the most frequently recommended pre- and postvaccination pain and fever relievers. Thus, when our children's bodies need their levels of glutathione to be at their peak (to effectively excrete toxins associated with vaccination), we are giving them a medication that depletes their stores of glutathione. This is not to say that acetaminophen and vaccines *cause* autism, but it is likely to contribute to the total toxic burden experienced by children, both autistic and neurotypical.[26] One preliminary study out of the University of California at San Diego looked at the medical histories of eighty-three children with autism and eighty neurotypical children and found an association between post-MMR (measles-mumps-rubella vaccine) administration of acetaminophen and autism.[27] In other words, the researchers were able to draw an association between acetaminophen use after the MMR and autism, while they were not able to draw an association between autism and ibuprofen use after the MMR. Obviously, more research needs to be done in this area, but given what we know about acetaminophen's activity on glutathione, we ought to be careful about how it is used in the pediatric population.

OTHER PHARMACEUTICAL AGENTS

While antibiotics and analgesics, like NSAIDs and acetaminophen, are among the most commonly used pharmaceutical agents in this country, a whole host of other drugs can negatively impact microflora of the gut and our bodies' detoxification pathways. The commonly used drugs that have been implicated in gut flora damage include those in the steroid hormone category: oral contraceptives, some allergy and asthma medications, and steroids like prednisone or dexamethasone. Steroids have been shown to suppress immune responses, and promote intestinal yeast growth, both of which contribute to gut dysbiosis and immune dysregulation.[28] Many women in this country use oral contraceptives or allergy/asthma medications chronically before getting pregnant or giving birth, and it is possible that these medications altered their gut flora so as to affect the bacteria transferred to their children at birth.

According to Dr. Natasha Campbell-McBride, "many other groups of drugs, including sleeping pills, 'heartburn' pills, neuroleptics, cholinolytic drugs, cytotoxic drugs . . .cause different damage to the gut flora, digestive system and immune system."[29] The "heartburn" pills most commonly prescribed include a class of drugs known as proton-pump-inhibitors (PPIs), including products like Prevacid, Prilosec,

Nexium and others, which have been shown to negatively alter gut flora.[30] These drugs have also been associated with increased intestinal colonization of pathogenic microbiota such as *Klebsiella pneumoniae*, *Enterococcus spp.*, and *C. difficile*, among others.[31] Simplified, these drugs suppress the natural production of stomach acids (essential for digestion), which can result in a higher pH (making the pH more alkaline) in the stomach and portions of the gut. The problem with raising the pH in the stomach is that this allows certain pathogens to survive in what would otherwise be an inhospitable environment. Chronic use of PPIs alters stomach acidity and allows pathogenic challengers to compete with the good bacteria. Chronic use of PPIs creates an environment in the gut that is more hospitable to adaptive pathogens and less hospitable to the good bacteria.

This is most disturbing because this class of drugs has been used extensively in infants and children in recent years to treat the widespread symptoms of gut dysbiosis, such as reflux, abdominal pain, ulcers, eosinophilic esophagitis and other disorders. Proton pump inhibitors are the second most widely prescribed drug in America, and are the most commonly prescribed gastrointestinal medication in children. An estimated two million American children used gastrointestinal drugs in 2006, predominately PPIs. Furthermore, there has been a dramatic increase in the use of PPIs in infants in recent years, as more of the existing drugs have been approved for use in infants.[32] Many pregnant women take PPIs to help reduce gastrointestinal symptoms (such as heartburn, morning sickness) associated with pregnancy. Imagine the altered gut flora that would be transferred to a baby whose mother took "the pill," NSAIDs, and allergy medication all before getting pregnant, then continued to take a PPI for pregnancy-related heartburn, and a course or two of antibiotics to help with pregnancy-associated sinus infections. Once the baby is born, his reflux could be treated with a PPI and an NSAID. And thus the vicious cycle begins.

This is not an uncommon or unusual scenario. In fact, pharmaceutical use is so ingrained in America's cultural fabric that no one would question this sort of medication history, and many people could probably relate to it. The evidence supports the fact that pharmaceutical agents contribute to gut dysbiosis. The evidence also supports the fact that Americans are the most drug-"addicted" human beings on this planet. Thus, just by the nature of our citizenship, we are predisposed to poor gut health.

THE PHARMACEUTICAL INDUSTRY RISES

Why do Americans use so many drugs? The answer to this question is complex, but the story begins with the expansion of American pharmaceutical companies in the post-World-War-I era. In the wake of the Great War, and the devastation of European industries, American industries (including the pharmaceutical industry) experienced historic growth and expansion. It was during this era that a new system of commercial medicine emerged out of a singular medical discovery: antibiotics. When German scientists discovered the first marketable antibiotic, sulfanilamide, in 1935 (patented and marketed under the name Prontosil), it marked the beginning of the era of the wonder drug. American companies quickly developed sulfa drugs and their miracle cousin, penicillin. Sulfanilamides and penicillin could treat staph or strep infections without hospitalization or expensive medical bills, a sharp contrast to earlier treatments. Although infectious disease morbidity and mortality rates were already sharply declining by the time the sulfa drugs were introduced, the drugs further reduced morbidity and mortality, and they also provided a quality of life improvement for sick individuals. The ease and efficacy of these new drugs captured the loyalty and hopes of the American public. Authors Milton Silverman and Philip Lee elaborate:

> The germ killing sulfa-drugs and the antibiotics helped to slash the death rates from the once dreaded streptococcal diseases. . . . Similar victories were achieved against scarlet fever, erisypelas, streptococcal septicemia, meningococcal meningitis, staphylococcal infections and typhoid fever. . . . These new agents manifested a striking effect

in making recovery not only more certain but far smoother and quicker. Patients suffered less pain, tissue damage, and disability, and required less hospitalization—or none at all. As costly as some of these new drugs may have been, the total cost of medical care in the treatment of an illness was substantially lower, and patients were able to return to normal activity in a fraction of the expected time.[33]

Wonder drugs deeply affected the way that Americans perceived their health. Certain recovery from common infectious diseases enabled people to feel, probably for the first time in western history, that they had some degree of control over their own morbidity and mortality. It was out of God's hands, and into the physician's hands, as a physician could prescribe a wonder drug that could literally save one's life. Thus, Americans put their faith into the science and industry that provided them with this new feeling of confidence. Silverman and Lee describe the profound changes that Americans underwent in the wake of the antibiotic revolution:

> They found that many of the ills that had plagued them and their families for generations could be controlled and even cured by modern medical care, and they wanted that care for themselves and their children. The concept that good medical care is not a privilege but a right—an idea that was viewed as fantastic, and probably subversive, in the 1930s—had become broadly accepted as logical and obvious in the 1960s.[34]

Interestingly, this belief has only intensified since the middle of the twentieth century.

Faith in the power of pharmaceutical-based modern medicine is widely shared by Americans today, as evidenced by the fact that the vast majority of Americans go to medical doctors (MDs) for health issues (as opposed to naturopathic doctors, nutritionists, acupuncturists, or other alternative healers) and expect to walk away with a prescription. Health insurance companies typically reimburse patients only for services provided by medical doctors and will cover pharmaceutical agents, but not natural or homeopathic agents. Access to "good medical care" (provided by medical doctors) was one of the most passionately debated issues of the entire American Presidential election of 2008. Somehow, good medical care came to mean access to pharmaceuticals. Faith in the power of pharmaceuticals was forged with the introduction of antibiotics, as these drugs liberated Americans from many of their deepest fears and anxieties.

Real improvements in suffering achieved through minimal effort may have won the early loyalty of Americans, but the aggressive marketing power of America's pharmaceutical industry secured belief in drug therapy as *the* answer to all health ailments. Although there have been many wonder drugs developed since the first antibiotics, few have generated the kind of therapeutic miracle represented by antibiotics. The subsequent drugs developed to treat every sort of illness were marketed as if they were all wonder drugs or miracle cures. Pharmaceutical marketing (both direct-to-consumer and direct-to-physician) contributes to the belief, not only that there is a "pill for every ill," but that these pills can change your life for the better.

Americans continue to be bombarded by these sorts of messages every day. In 1991, direct-to-consumer (DTC) advertising of pharmaceuticals totaled $55 million. In 2006, U.S. pharmaceutical companies spent over $4 billion on DTC advertising and over $7 billion on advertising to physicians. Much of this spending increase is due to the lifting of restrictions on DTC advertising of pharmaceuticals that occurred in 1997. During the average day, Americans are bombarded by more than nine pharmaceutical advertisements on television.[35] Watch one hour of NBC's *The Today Show*, or ABC's *Good Morning America*, and see how many pharmaceutical advertisements you can count. Do these direct-to-consumer advertisements and marketing efforts work? Do they actually result in more prescriptions? You betcha. Several studies have shown that patients who ask for particular prescriptions from their physicians will receive it 50-80 percent of the time.[36] Since 1991, drug expenditures have increased at a rate of four times that of other medical expenditures (such as hospital or physician services), and drug industry profit margins have gone from 12 percent to 18 percent of revenues (while other Fortune 500 companies average 5 percent). [37] This is a truly American phenomenon. Direct-to-consumer advertising is allowed in only *one* other industrialized nation: New Zealand. It is banned in Europe! No wonder Americans are the greatest consumers of pharmaceuticals on the planet.

Pharmaceutical companies also aggressively court physicians in an effort to increase profitability. Each major pharmaceutical company has a sales force that is several thousand people deep, with GlaxoSmithKline exceeding all other rivals at nine thousand U.S. salespeople. According to Dr. John Abramson, author of *Overdosed America*, there is now one pharmaceutical sales person for every 4.5 office-based physicians. [38] Although some of the marketing to physicians, such as continuing medical education courses (CME) and office visits, is done with an air of legitimacy—educating the physicians on proper dosing and administration of particular drugs—a substantial amount of dubious marketing occurs among pharmaceutical sales reps. One former pharmaceutical sales representative, who spoke on the condition of anonymity, told of sales reps who frequently treated their physicians to strip club outings and $500 dinners. [39] Clearly, this sort of activity is the exception rather than the rule, but it does serve to remind us that pharmaceuticals are a business, like any other, and business is not always ethical.

Although not all physicians or American consumers are receptive to the messages of the pharmaceutical companies, the simple ubiquity of the message makes it a fundamental part of American culture today. While not every American adult or child will take pharmaceutical agents during their lifetime, there is no doubt that we, as a society, are swimming in drugs, literally and figuratively. Given what we know about the impact of certain pharmaceutical agents on the health of gut microbiota and our most fundamental detoxification pathways, it is high time we paid attention to our pharmaceutical culture and examine the ways in which it might be contributing to a nation of children suffering with gut dysbiosis and immune dysregulation.

chapter 5

Factor 2 — Environmental Toxins/Pollution

✿

CANARIES IN A SILENT SPRING — THE IMPACT OF ENVIRONMENTAL TOXINS

In 1962, Rachel Carson wrote *Silent Spring*, an examination of how pesticides were affecting the environment, with an emphasis on the devastation to wildlife. Carson used the metaphor of a spring without songbirds (or a "silent spring") as a metaphor for the insidiousness of environmental pollution. In other words, human destruction of the environment is often subtle and difficult to detect, until the damage becomes apparent through widespread human and wildlife disease and death. Carson, if she were still alive, would probably be sick to know that her prescient warning resulted in little change to our current habits of environmental destruction.

Like the absent songbirds that Carson believed to be the hallmark of wider degradation of the environment, American children are the canaries in the coal mine, or the early messengers alerting us that our way of life is toxic and seriously damaging to our health. We are all subjected to environmental toxins every day but children are especially vulnerable to their impact. Furthermore, children with gut dysbiosis and impaired detoxification capabilities are even more vulnerable to the damaging effects of toxins. Toxins are ubiquitous in American life. Many of us can weather exposure to environmental toxins like mercury, lead, arsenic, PCBs or perchlorate with little outward health effect because we have fully developed immune systems with all the necessary detoxification pathways (such as healthy commensal gastrointestinal and lung bacteria or normal glutathione levels) in place. Children with compromised or dysfunctional immune systems and inadequate levels of commensal bacteria cannot properly metabolize and detoxify these metals and chemicals. Consequently, they experience the toxicity to a much greater degree than healthy adults.

There are two main concerns with regard to children's exposure to environmental toxins. The first is the effect that environmental toxins have on the commensal bacteria and the immune system. Certain environmental toxins, like mercury, chlorine and fluoride, are believed to adversely affect commensal gut bacteria. Once the health of these bacteria is compromised, a child's body is left vulnerable to the direct impact of the toxins. Certain toxins have been associated with autoimmunity and the triggering of abnormal immune responses. Environmental toxins should be considered among the possible culprits in the epidemic of immune dysregulation in American children. The second concern with regard to toxin exposure is the direct impact that toxins, especially neurotoxins such as mercury, PCBs, perchlorate and many others, have on children's health. Even with properly functioning gut barrier and immune system detoxification capabilities, children can be adversely affected by exposure to these types of toxins.

Thousands, and perhaps even hundreds of thousands, of toxins present in our environment pose a real risk to the health of our children. For the hundreds of known and documented neurotoxins and the vast number of documented endocrine disruptors, there are an equal number (perhaps more) of toxins that we do not know much about. There are literally thousands of products that we consume every day in our food, cosmetics, and in the air and water, for which there is very little research regarding safety or level of toxicity. If there are safety studies, they are typically conducted by the manufacturing company of the particular compound, where a clear conflict of interest lies.

There is no question that many of these toxins are associated with chronic childhood illnesses. A vast body of literature supports the connection between various environmental toxins and chronic illness in children. Perhaps the most publicized connection exists between heavy metals and the development of neurobehavioral disorders such as autism and ADHD. Heavy metals (lead, mercury, cadmium, arsenic, chromium, manganese, aluminum) are everywhere in the American environment and most have been implicated in autism and ADHD (to a lesser extent). However, there are many more consequences of toxic exposure that scientists are only just beginning to understand.

Scientists are starting to coalesce around the notion that toxins can trigger autoimmune disease. As previously mentioned, most of the chronic childhood illnesses that are on the rise in this country are believed to have some autoimmune component. In her investigations for *The Autoimmune Epidemic*, Donna Jackson Nakazawa uncovered some of the more compelling connections between environmental toxins and autoimmunity. Among the many toxins implicated were household-name toxins such as BPA (bisphenol A, an endocrine disruptor found in some plastics, including baby bottles) and PCBs (highly toxic and ubiquitous industrial chemicals), but also lesser known toxins, like those found in everyday items such as hair dye or clothes that have been dry-cleaned.[1] According to Nakazawa: "Environmental toxins appear to mess with normal internal signaling pathways, making it difficult for our immune cells to recognize what is foreign and what is self—a bit like a covert enemy force sending up smokescreens and spreading disinformation."[2] One rat study published in the *American Journal of Pathology* in 2004 found that rats' immune systems "learned" to attack commensal bacteria (*Escherichia coli*) upon exposure to a particular chemical, dinitrophenol (mainly used in manufacturing).[3] To be sure, animal models do not always correlate directly to humans, but this information extrapolated to humans is of tremendous importance. This mechanism helps us not only to understand the role of environmental toxins in the etiology of autoimmunity, but it also illustrates how central the gastrointestinal system (and the microflora within it) is as the gatekeeper of human health and wellness.

The list of chemicals/toxins believed to trigger autoimmunity and chronic illness is long. The body of literature is vast. A number of these studies were described in chapter two. Here is another very small sampling of some of the recent research:

- A study published in *NeuroToxicology* in 2008 found that a flame retardant commonly found in humans (deca-BDE, a chemical used to fireproof household items) altered behaviors and brain development in mice. Mice that ate even very low doses of the chemical developed hyperactivity and adjustment difficulties that increased with age.[4] Separately, the Environmental Working Group detected this chemical in 65 percent of children and 45 percent of adults tested.[5]

- A study found that middle-income children exposed to pesticides during their first year of life had a four-to-tenfold increased risk of developing persistent asthma than nonexposed children.[6]

- A 2006 study in mice demonstrated that the contaminant TCE (trichloroethylene, a ubiquitous solvent made famous by the Woburn, MA, contamination that was immortalized in the book *A Civil Action*) was responsible for triggering autoimmune disease in exposed mice.[7]

Much of the world is polluted. Many people are exposed to the aforementioned toxins, yet Americans' relationship to chemicals is somehow different than that of other peoples. While many Americans are exposed to toxins like PCBs or mercury unknowingly, we are also a people who *willingly* consume toxins and contaminants daily through food and products assumed to be benign, or possibly even healthful. How did we get so chemical?

America's journey into rampant toxicity began with industrialization and exposure to byproducts of America's fledgling industries. The rate of production of toxins expanded exponentially after the First World War. The rise of chemical companies occurred concurrent with the rise of pharmaceutical companies, as many were one and the same. Prior to World War I, Germany dominated the chemical industry, but the war provided the opportunity for American companies to flourish. The 1920s were boom years for chemical companies as American chemists discovered new types of plastics, solvents, fertilizers and other chemicals with a multitude of commercial applications. The 1935 slogan of the Dow Chemical Company, "Better Things for Better Living. . . Through Chemistry" symbolizes the new chemical age that America created during this era.[8]

It was after the Second World War that America went through a chemistry revolution, where Americans began to put their faith in the concept of Better Living Through Chemistry. Randall Fitzgerald, author of *The Hundred Year Lie*, has marked this as the beginning of the "synthetics belief system," a time when Americans began to believe not only that all things were possible through science and chemistry, but also that products of science and chemistry were somehow *better* than natural products. Americans were so enamored with the new fangled products that came out of chemistry, such as cellophane, nylon, Teflon, and even Silly Putty, that the toxicity of all this chemistry was never seriously considered or evaluated.[9]

Ask any baby boomer about their memories of Melmac, and they will fondly recall the wondrous, unbreakable dinner plates that burst onto the commercial market in the 1950s. Americans rushed to the stores to buy themselves this new, exciting, and durable dinnerware, made of a plastic polymer known as melamine. Virtually every American household contained some pieces of Melmac. Fast-forward to the twenty-first century and melamine, our beloved Melmac, was found to be highly toxic when ingested. A 2006 scandal in China involving the adulteration of pet feed and milk with melamine led to the sickness of over a thousand babies (and two deaths) and the deaths of many animals.[10]

To be fair, the use of melamine dinner plates (still wildly popular in America, and still available for purchase at virtually every Target, Kmart or Walmart) is probably not harmful or toxic (as toxicity is related to ingestion); the story of melamine, however, illustrates our naïve trust in chemicals. New consumer products splash onto the market every day with flashy marketing and persuasive advertising, yet, few of us pause to consider, *what is this new product? Is it safe?* Some examples:

- **Sunscreen.** Early sunscreens (up until the 1990s) contained PABA, a chemical now believed to increase the risk of skin cancers when worn in the sun.[11] PABA has since been removed from the market for these (and other) reasons, but most Americans still wear chemical sunscreen every day. Do we know that the other chemicals in PABA-free sunscreen are indeed safe? Our dermatologists tell us that if we do not wear sunscreen every day, we will get skin cancer. Yet, an investigation of over one thousand brand-name sunscreen products by the Environmental Working Group found that four out of five products were ineffective or contained potential health hazards, and the top-selling brands (Coppertone, Neutrogena, and Banana Boat) were among the worst.[12] Furthermore, chronic sunscreen wearing can lead to vitamin D deficiency, an immune-suppressing condition.

- **Cell phones, PDAs and other wireless gadgets.** According to Mediamark Research, Inc., a consumer research organization, over 86 percent of American households now contain at least one cellular phone.[13] Many people also connect to the Internet wirelessly on their computers or via their PDAs (such as a Blackberry). Wireless technology has only been available to the public for a very short period of time. Must we wait for long-term epidemiological studies to emerge before we can determine if exposure to the electromagnetic fields created by wireless technology is safe? Some scientists are already ringing the alarm bells. According to Associate Professor of Environmental Health at Lincoln University, New Zealand, Dr. Neil Cherry, they are not safe: "Electromagnetic fields and radiation [associated with cell phone usage] damage DNA and enhance cell death rates and therefore they are a *Ubiquitous Universal Genotoxic Carcinogen* that enhances the rates of *Cancer, Cardiac, Reproductive and Neurological disease* and mortality in human populations [sic]. Therefore, there is no safe threshold level. The only safe exposure level is zero, a position confirmed by dose-response trends in epidemiological studies." [14] We all love our gadgets, but do we really know if exposing ourselves, or more important, our children to electromagnetic fields is not in some way detrimental to health?

Many products that we use every day may be harmful or may contain dozens of chemicals that we simply do not know enough about. Do you know for a fact that all of the ingredients in your toothpaste, shampoo, soap, mouthwash, makeup, deodorant, breakfast cereal, hand lotion, nasal spray, lip balm, diet soda, nondairy spread, shaving cream, bug spray, contact solution, and hair gel are safe? Yet, all of these chemicals enter your body, with unknown long-term consequences. These are items that you consume. This is not even taking into consideration all of the toxins that you are exposed to daily—everything from TCE in dry-cleaning to diesel exhaust—that we know to be toxic. We are barely two generations into the chemical and technological revolution—the long-term effects have not yet had enough time to emerge. American consumers continue to fall prey to sexy advertisements and persuasive marketing that convince us that we need these products in our lives. Better Living through Chemistry. Unfortunately, our culturally based habits of consumption are having devastating effects on our health, and particularly the health of our children.

Following are some disturbing facts regarding America's children and their toxic exposures:

- A recent study by the CDC found perchlorate (a toxic chemical in rocket fuel) in 97 percent of breast milk samples tested.[15] A Texas study discovered perchlorate levels in breast milk to be five times that of dairy milk. According to Philip and Alice Shabecoff, authors of *Poisoned Profits: The Toxic Assault on Our Children*, many more environmental contaminants have been found at unsafe levels in breast milk. "PCB concentration in breast milk is higher than the level that would trigger U.S. regulatory action if found in cow's milk."[16] Other substances found in unsafe levels in breast milk include: mercury, lead, flame retardant, dioxins and DDT (even though it was banned years ago).
- A 2009 Environmental Working Group study found 287 commercial chemicals in newborn babies' umbilical cord blood. Some of the chemicals included neurotoxins, carcinogens, and others associated with developmental delays.[17]
- Bisphenol-A, or BPA, a known endocrine disruptor, mimics the effects of estrogen, and is associated with cancers, early puberty, and brain damage among other adverse health problems. BPA can be found in many products used by infants and children. Several types of baby bottles are made with BPA. Liquid infant formula packages are lined with BPA. Cans of food are lined with BPA. "More than 6 billion pounds of BPA are used each year in resins lining metal cans, food packaging, hot beverage cups, and in blends with other types of plastic products." Laboratory studies have demonstrated that BPA in

packaging and bottles leaches into foods and beverages, especially when heated.[18]

- While most people know that mercury is a neurotoxin that can cause developmental delays, brain damage, and a variety of other devastating health problems, fewer people know of the many possible sources of mercury exposure. In 2009, the NIH published a review of children's environmental mercury exposures. Among the most common forms of exposure included: fish consumption (especially fatty, deep water fish like tuna or shark), coal-burning power plants, dental amalgams, thimerosal-containing vaccines, and medical waste incinerators.[19] In a report looking at children's daily exposure to mercury from dental amalgams, the estimated daily exposure to mercury ranged from 0.79 to 1.91mcg.[20] Also, some gymnasium floors contain a mercury catalyst used in a polyurethane finish that releases mercury vapor into the air. The latest discovery with regard to mercury exposure comes from Renee Dufault, a longtime environmental investigator of the FDA. Dufault conducted an investigation into the levels of mercury that can be found in high fructose corn syrup (HFCS). HFCS is the most popular sweetener in processed foods and drinks in America, including virtually all soft drinks. HFCS may contain mercury because mercury grade caustic soda is used in the manufacturing of some HFCS. In the study, it was determined that some of the samples (especially from a particular manufacturer) had levels of mercury as high as 0.57mcg/g. According to the EPA an average-sized woman should consume no more than 5.5 micrograms per day of mercury, meaning that the average American consumer (who, according to the US Department of Agriculture, consumes 49.8 g of HFCS daily) may be consuming *up to five times the upper safety limit of mercury every day through high-fructose corn syrup consumption* (assuming they consume HFCS that originated in particular manufacturers.)[21]

- Add up children's total mercury exposures from dental amalgams, HFCS, fish, and contaminated air and water, and it is
likely that many children's mercury levels far exceed government standards for safety. This level of exposure has real consequences for health, including developmental delay, decreased
IQ scores, and behavioral disorders, among others.

In hundreds of other ways, children are exposed to environmental
toxins on a daily basis. For more information see Philip and Alice
Shabecoff's *Poisoned Profits*.

A DIFFERENT KIND OF POLLUTION:
ELECTROPOLLUTION

Most people have heard about the alleged risk of getting brain cancer
from using cellular phones, yet few people take this risk seriously, at
least not enough to alter cell phone usage. Is the cell-phone-cancer
risk a real concern, or is it just another urban legend? And if cell
phones can be dangerous to our health, then what about other forms
of electromagnetic radiation? Should we be concerned about electromagnetic radiation as another form of pollution or toxic exposure that
can negatively impact the health of our children?

The truth is that the science surrounding the biological impact of
electromagnetic radiation is still emerging. Children's exposure to
electromagnetic radiation has grown exponentially in recent years
with the growth of wireless technologies, including everything from
WiFi to wireless baby monitors. Science is only just beginning to understand the potential consequences of children's exposure to electromagnetic radiation partly because these extremely high levels of
exposure have been around only for the last few decades.

What is electromagnetic radiation? Electromagnetic radiation
(EMR) or electromagnetic fields (EMF) are terms used to describe
exposure to certain waves or frequencies generated by electrical devices or electricity in general. Electromagnetic radiation can come in
the form of radio waves, microwaves, ultraviolet light, and x-rays,

among other forms. We are exposed to many types of electromagnetic fields/radiation in everyday life, including:

- Extremely low frequency (ELF) radiation, such as:
  - Electrical appliances
  - Electrical cords
  - Power lines

- Radio frequency (RF) radiation/microwave radiation, such as:
  - Cell phones and cell towers
  - Cordless phones
  - Broadcast transmission towers
  - Microwave ovens
  - Radar
  - Wireless networks (WiFi)
  - Wireless baby monitors
  - Wireless speakers, mice, printers and keyboards
  - Bluetooth devices

- Infrared — Remote controls

- Visible light

- Ionizing radiation
  - Ultraviolet radiation from the sun
  - X-rays
  - CT scans

It is well documented that high doses of ionizing radiation (e.g., CT scans and x-rays) can be quite damaging to human health. The medical literature is rife with evidence supporting the connection between ionizing radiation and human illnesses such as cancer.[22] Sickness and death attributable to radiation exposure from the atomic bomb and nuclear power plant accidents (like Chernobyl) are articles of historical fact. What is less well known is the impact of exposure to varied sources of radio frequency radiation or low frequency radiation, especially on children.

Most people are exposed to a tremendous amount of man-made electromagnetic radiation every day, especially that generated by radio frequency devices, but does all this exposure cause biological damage? We must remember that the human body runs on electricity. We are walking, talking, breathing electrochemical systems. Dr. Toby Watkinson of the Tobin Institute in San Diego, California, incorporates electro-chemical medicine, or energy medicine, into the treatment of his patients with chronic illnesses. Dr. Watkinson believes that energy and electrochemical factors are often overlooked by doctors when they treat illnesses. "We talk about the many different systems in the human body such as the gastrointestinal system, the cardiovascular system, and the immune system, but somehow we seem to forget that all of these systems run on electricity. The body is an electrochemical system. If something is damaging our electrical system, then the chemistry will not work." The communication that occurs within our body between cells, organs, and even microorganisms is mediated by electrochemical signals. Some scientists believe that exposure to seemingly harmless electromagnetic radiation, such as radio frequency radiation, can interfere with biological processes, and potentially lead to disease.

According to the 2007 Bioinitiative Report, written by the Bioinitiative Working Group, an international consortium of fourteen scientists, public health and public policy experts, a substantial amount of scientific evidence demonstrates that electromagnetic fields/radiation can be deleterious to human health. The authors of the Bioinitiative Report argue that there are several main areas where science has demonstrated a negative biological impact from electromagnetic radiation:

- Adult and childhood cancers
- Changes in the nervous system and brain function
- Effects on genes (DNA)
- Effects on the immune system
- Effects on stress proteins (heat shock proteins).

The Bioinitiative report is over six hundred pages long and examines the published body of scientific literature in detail. The report is free to the public and available at: http://www.bioinitiative.org.

Electromagnetic radiation may play a role in the etiology of chronic childhood illnesses in a number of ways. Perhaps the most powerful effect of EMR is upon the immune system. When the body senses exposure to electromagnetic radiation, it mounts an immune response much in the way that it would when it detects the presence of environmental toxins or pathogenic invaders. Studies have shown, for instance, that normal levels of exposure to radio frequency (e.g., that of WiFi) can cause mast cells (immune cells that release histamine) to be activated, triggering the onset of allergic type responses. According to the Bioinitiative Report, "Chronic provocation by exposure to ELF [extremely low frequency] and RF [radio frequency] can lead to immune dysfunction, chronic allergic responses, inflammatory diseases and ill health if they occur on a continuing basis over time." Many of our children's bodies are harboring chronic infections with bacteria, viruses or other microorganisms that their bodies are unable to kick out. Electromagnetic fields offer yet another chronic immune-stimulating exposure that can lead to chronic inflammation and oxidative stress (free radicals that can cause cellular damage). Chronic immune stimulation, inflammation and oxidative stress are central features of chronic illness in children.

Most American children are chronically exposed to electromagnetic radiation (EMR), some more than others. Think about the sources of EMR in a typical middle-class American home. In her home, a child could be exposed to cell phones, cordless phones, microwave ovens, televisions, radios, computers, electrical appliances, WiFi, and wireless electronics (baby monitors, speakers, printers). This is not even taking into consideration her exposures at school, at the mall, or in the outdoor environment, where cell towers and power lines provide ample exposure. According to the Cellular Telecommunications and Internet Association, there are approximately 270 million cell phone subscribers in America, and children are a growing proportion of those using cell phones and other wireless technologies. Given the ubiquity of wireless technology in our lives, it seems warranted that we further study the health implications of living wirelessly, especially with regard to children's health. In addition, children may be exposed to radiation through medical procedures. The radiation exposure of one CT-scan of a child's abdominal region is equivalent to two times the lifetime radiation exposure experienced by individuals living in the vicinity of the Chernobyl accident in the Ukraine.[23]

Fearing the health consequences of electromagnetic radiation almost seems like something that should be left to hypochondriacs and conspiracy theorists. Electronics and wireless technology have become such an integral part of our lives and our culture that it is difficult to imagine that they could be harmful. Like any other low-level toxic exposure, it is difficult to raise the alarm bells about EMFs if they are not creating acute health problems. This does not mean, however, that exposure is not harmful. For instance, exposure to the pesticides on a conventionally grown meal of vegetables may not cause any immediate health consequences, but this does not mean that the pesticides are not harmful to the body. We know that over the long term, exposure to pesticides can lead to chronic and even terminal health conditions. Similarly, exposure to EMFs may not cause acute clinical symptoms but may very well contribute to immune dysregulation over the long term. We may not break out in hives when we get near a WiFi transmitter, but this does not mean it is not stimulating the immune system into a chronically activated state. As a society, we need to sponsor more rigorous studies of the impact of EMFs on biological processes and make public policy changes accordingly.

Clearly, American children are heavily burned with toxins and environmental pollution. The greatest tragedy of all this toxic exposure is that we are simultaneously handicapping these children by weakening their natural detoxification defenses and immune systems with pharmaceuticals, excessive vaccinations, and anemic diets. The toxic burden of our children is tremendous, and when our children are forced to live in a toxic world with impaired natural defense mechanisms, there is an increased likelihood for epidemics of chronic disease.

chapter 6

Factor 3 — Diet and Nutrition

✦

YOU ARE WHAT YOU EAT: DIET MATTERS

Diet is an interesting part of the etiology of chronic illness because it can serve as both a help and a hindrance to good health, depending on content. A poor diet can surreptitiously contaminate the body with toxins and degrade the body's immune system, but a good diet can help protect the body against toxins and immunological damage. Much has been written about the health benefits of eating certain diets, including the Mediterranean diet or the Asian diet, as these diets tend to be higher in vegetables and good quality, lean protein. On the contrary, the American diet, long associated with high meat and starch content, has been associated with disease and poor health. While it is difficult to generalize about diet in a nation as diverse as the United States, the wide availability of commercial foods since industrialization has served to unify or homogenize the American diet to some degree.

Historically speaking, the American diet has never been particularly healthful. While Americans have long had the reputation of being well nourished, a more accurate description would be undernourished but overfed. Nourishment implies consuming food that serves as the basis of good health and strong constitution. Using eighteenth century standards, Americans of the Revolutionary era were considered well nourished because they were taller than their Europeans counterparts. However, taller does not necessarily mean well nourished. Eighteenth-century Europeans experienced acute spells of famine and political unrest that led to food scarcity and shorter statures. Food was simply more abundant in America, but this does not mean that Americans were receiving a balanced or even a healthful diet. [1]

The notion of a well-nourished American population is diminished further when put into the context of twenty-first century standards of nutrition. Prior to the industrial revolution, the diet of many Americans tended to be high in meats, like pork (or game in early America), and certain grains, like corn, and low in fresh fruits and vegetables. Food staples varied from region to region and across classes, but salted pork (and beef to a lesser degree) and either corn, potatoes, or coarse breads reigned supreme in the United States during the preindustrial era. Different regions and cultural groups had their own additional staples, such as dairy in New England or rice in the Southeast, but despite our agricultural heritage, the total human consumption of fruits and vegetables was relatively small. Industrialization did bring some level of variety to the American diet, but usually in the form of a variety of meats, and more processed grains. Historically, and culturally speaking, Americans were "carnivores of the first order."[2]

Eating five servings of fruits and vegetables a day (per the CDC's recommendations) may seem like a tall order for many Americans today, but it would have been downright laughable to Americans of the eighteenth and nineteenth centuries. "Early New Englanders thought of vegetables as sauces to accompany meats, much in the way applesauce accompanies pork today, and they commonly referred to them as 'garden sass.'"[3] This type of diet was not without consequences. The fact that meat and starches were the staples of the American diet, "made constipation the national curse for the first four or five decades of the nineteenth century."[4] Significant changes to the American diet over the next one hundred and fifty years would only make this problem worse, such that America would become known as "the most constipated nation on the face of the earth!"[5]

Changes to the American diet that came with industrialization and urbanization included the addition of more processed and refined foods, especially among the middle and upper classes. Breads were among the first foods to be "industrialized." In the 1840s, new flour milling techniques were applied to produce more refined, whiter breads. Prohibitive cost made the new whiter breads a mainly middle and upper class indulgence, but techniques developed in the 1870s opened up cheaper, whiter flours and breads even to the working classes. Some doctors of the late nineteenth century urged their patients to eat coarser, whole grain and unrefined breads to stave off constipation and other digestive ailments, but the desire for refined starches was too strong, and they soon became a staple in American diets.

Another interesting, and little noted, change to American lifestyles in the later part of the nineteenth century, especially among middle and upper class Americans, was the movement from home preservation of foods, through brining and pickling, to the procurement of processed preserved foods. For centuries, Americans (and most human societies, for that matter) relied on the process of culturing or pickling foods, vegetables and meats alike, to preserve foods so they could be eaten throughout the year. Many foods that were preserved at home were done using a process called culturing, or lacto-fermentation, which uses salt to preserve food in a brine dominated by lactic acid-producing bacteria. These lactic acid-producing bacteria are the same "good germs" that are a critical part of human gastrointestinal health. Common fermented or cultured foods in the American diet included home-brined or pickled meats, cabbage, cucumbers, corn relish, or watermelon rind.[6] Again, the American diet was not great in terms of overall intake of plant-based food (fiber), but the probiotic bacteria from brining and pickling may have at least provided people with some exposure to the beneficial bacteria necessary for good digestive health.

The consumption of cultured foods diminished in many American households, especially middle and upper class homes, with the introduction of the "icebox" (in the mid-nineteenth century) and the emergence of commercially available preserved foods. The icebox did diminish food preservation issues for Americans to some degree, but it was preserved food companies like Heinz, who burst onto the market in the later part of the nineteenth century, offering heat-processed alternatives to home-preserved foods, that truly impacted the culturing of foods among upper and middle class Americans. This is a significant development because heat-processing sterilizes food (eliminating all bacteria), where as culturing or fermenting actually grows the good bacteria. By the 1870s these good-germ-saturated foods were being edged out of the American diet by heat-processed foods that were steam-pressured (using heat rather than lactic acid to prevent spoilage) or preserved in vinegar. Thus, many upper and middle class Americans were becoming germ-free in their living conditions (moving into urban environments and away from good germ exposure in agricultural settings) while simultaneously removing vital germs from their diets. It is curious that the Americans that made the greatest number of changes to their diets during the industrial era were members of the upper and middle classes. Perhaps it is no coincidence that it was mostly upper class Americans that would be plagued by the modern malady of allergies (seasonal allergies or hay fever) during this same era. An increasingly processed and refined diet, low in fermented foods, may have contributed (in conjunction with other changing environmental factors like industrial pollution) to America's first cases of allergy.

Interestingly, many other cultures with far superior gastrointestinal health (and far fewer cases of chronic inflammatory illnesses) still incorporate some elements of cultured foods into their diets. "One striking observation [of ethnic cuisines] is that rarely are meals eaten without at least one fermented food, often a drink. . . . In Japan, it's not a meal without miso, soy sauce, pickles, all fermented products. In India, they drink soured milk every day, practically at every meal. In Indonesia, they eat *tempeh*, in Korea *kimchi* (a kind of sauerkraut) and in Africa porridge of fermented millet or cereal beers."[7] Many of these traditions, however beneficial for gastrointestinal health, are beginning to erode as American foods, habits, and tastes begin to infiltrate other cultures.

The American diet has long been low in fruits, vegetables and fiber necessary for good digestive health. As we know, digestive health is of critical importance to overall health, especially regarding the strength of the immune system. Poor gut health in America before the twentieth century meant susceptibility to infectious disease. Poor gut health in the twenty-first century means susceptibility to chronic disease. Our ancestors ate meat and potatoes and bread and butter just like we do, yet they were not afflicted with epidemics of cancer, heart disease and diabetes the way we are today. For children, there were not many chronic illnesses, other than the lasting effects of infectious diseases, like rheumatism from rheumatic fever. Americans could survive on these diets without developing cancer, diabetes, heart disease, autoimmune or other chronic diseases because they did not live in the toxic world that we live in today. Now, Americans eat a poor diet that reduces natural defenses against both infectious and chronic diseases *and* face a battery of daily toxic exposures (including pharmaceuticals) and other immunological assaults.

Clearly, American gastrointestinal health has never been optimal, but it appears to be worsening over time. The standard American diet prior to, and during, industrialization was not healthful, but it could be considered superior to the diet of contemporary Americans, simply because it did contain some cultured foods, and it also lacked the excessive processing and adulteration seen with more contemporary food. Contemporary American diets feature an overabundance of processed foods anemic in nutrition, and loaded with chemicals, stabilizers, additives, preservatives, and genetically modified organisms (GMOs). For most of these chemicals and new foods, we simply do not know if there are any long-term adverse effects of consuming them.

HOW AMERICANS EAT TODAY

Americans made some significant changes to their diets during the nineteenth century, but the twentieth century brought truly profound changes to the very meaning of food in America. If a nineteenth century American could travel through time to visit the kitchen of an average American family today, he would be shocked to find shelves stocked with items called food that are not really even food at all. Again, Americans are a diverse people and not everyone consumes the standard American diet; however, the types of food that are consumed by the vast majority of Americans are highly processed, nutrient poor, and eaten by people that prize convenience above all else. Following are some basic statistics concerning the standard American diet and American eating habits.

- In the 1990s, the average American consumed over 140 pounds annually of sugar with an additional 50 pounds of artificial (and potentially toxic) sweeteners on top of that. (Compare this to the 10 pounds consumed annually in 1821.)[8]
- According to Carol Simontacchi, author of *The Crazy Makers: How the Food Industry is Destroying Our Brains and Harming Our Children*, consumption of fresh produce is down, "with fresh apples down 75 percent, fresh cabbage down 65 percent, fresh potatoes down 74 percent, and fresh melons down 50 percent." While it is recommended by most nutritionists that one eat between 5 and 9.5 cup servings of

fresh fruits and vegetables per day, most Americans eat fewer than two servings.[9]

- Simontacchi also alerts us to the fact that Americans are consuming more unhealthful soft drinks and artificial foods than ever before. Simontacchi notes that "between 1960 and 1981, soft drink consumption increased 182 percent, food color consumption increased 1,006 percent, and corn syrup consumption increased 291 percent."[10] These rates of consumption have only increased in the last twenty years.

- Teenagers in particular consume vast quantities of soda or pop. Simontacchi writes that "the average teenage boy who drinks soda drinks three and one-half cans per day, and girls drink nearly that much."[11] Soft drinks are the single greatest source of dietary high-fructose corn syrup, the processed sweetener believed by some to be implicated in a variety of health conditions.

- The American diet is heavily dependent upon processed wheat-based products (pastas, breads, cakes, crackers, cookies, cereals) and dairy-based products (milk, ice cream, yogurt, cheese, butter) so that most Americans eat processed wheat and dairy items every day, sometimes at every meal. For many Americans, this repetitive exposure to milk and wheat products results in the development of intolerance to these foods (as in lactose intolerance and gluten intolerance, both undiagnosed epidemics in America).

In addition, according to other nutrition research:

- Over 72 percent of food energy consumed by Americans comes from dairy products (mostly processed), cereal grains (mostly processed), refined sugars, and refined vegetable oils (which notably cause oxidation), and alcohol. By all nutritional standards, this percentage should be inverted, where dairy, grains, oils and sugars should comprise a tiny portion of energy calories, and vegetables should comprise the bulk of energy calories. In addition, 100 percent of our energy should be coming from whole (unrefined/processed) foods, but the bulk of food that we consume is processed.[12]

- Americans consume high levels of refined oils, many of which contain omega-6 fats (e.g., corn, soy, canola oils) known to encourage inflammation. Omega-6 intake has increased from 1 kg a year a few decades ago to 12 kg per year. A body needs a balance of omega-6 and omega-3 oils (found in fish and some plants, such as flax), with a ratio of approximately 2 to 1 (omega-6 to omega-3). The average American ratio of omega-6 to omega-3 was 4:1 a few decades ago; today it is approximately 25:1.[13] There is even some speculation that the decreasing amounts of omega-3 fats in the American diet may adversely impact immune development during the fetal and neonatal periods, with inflammatory consequences (such as allergy).[14]

Furthermore, the food that we do consume, both processed and natural whole foods, has become so depleted of nutrients over the years that we have to work harder to nourish ourselves, even if we do eat good food. According to Randall Fitzgerald, analysis done by the US Department of Agriculture, found that "for every vegetable grown in the United States, every single nutrient that can be measured in each category of vegetable has undergone huge declines." This decrease in nutrients occurred because American soils have been overfarmed using modern chemically saturated and unsustainable agricultural techniques. Much of this depletion has happened in the last thirty years.[15]

More than 85 percent of the cereals (meaning grains like wheat, oats, rice) consumed in the US diet are highly processed refined grains. This is important because the processing of the grain removes the nutritious elements from the grains, leaving small particles of nutrient-poor flour that does little to nourish our bodies. When wheat is processed, 95 percent of fiber is lost, as well as 84 percent of iron, 95 percent of vitamin E, 82 percent of manganese, 80 percent of niacin, and 81 percent of vitamin B_2.[16] To add insult to injury, these processed grains are rapidly and easily converted into simple sugars in our bodies, upsetting blood sugar levels, but also providing perfect food for pathogenic microbes like *Candida albicans*.

The nutrient depletion that occurs in food processing is not restricted to grains, either. In the processing of tuna fish, for example, "the canning process removes 99 percent of vitamin A. . . 97 percent of vitamin B_1, 86 percent of vitamin B_2, and 45 percent of niacin, and it increases the level of oxidized cholesterol in the human body."[17] While the natural food becomes increasingly anemic, the food industry compensates for nutrient depletion by pumping in artificial nutrients, or "fortifying" foods with chemical vitamins, which are not readily used by the body the way natural vitamins would be.

In 2005, Dr. Loren Cordain, professor of health and nutrition at Colorado State University published a groundbreaking paper on the impact of the Western diet on health and disease. Dr. Cordain's paper looked at the massive gap between modern western diets (looking specifically at American-derived habits of eating) and our evolutionary requirements for nutrition and health. Evolutionarily and nutritionally speaking, our bodies are still stuck in the Paleolithic era, a time when humans were hunters and gatherers (eating minimally processed plant and animal foods). In other words, while human society has evolved to mass produce and process food at unprecedented rates, our bodies are still designed to eat as they did ten thousand years ago. Evolution is far too slow of a process to be able to keep up with the rapid changes in diet and food production that humans have created over the last 10,000 years, but the changes over the last century have left human bodies utterly confused. This biological confusion is what contributes to human disease because our bodies are unable to extract the necessary nutrients from the food that we consume. Thus, our bodies operate most efficiently on a Paleolithic-type diet, but we are all consuming a postindustrial diet, marked by processed, nutrient-poor food. It is only logical that our bodies are beginning to break down.[18] We are not receiving the nutrients we need for proper biological processes in the body and our bodies show the signs daily.

Besides the need for vitamins and nutrients, what does the type of food we eat have to do with the development of disease? Dr. Cordain maintains that our bodies need to maintain a certain pH balance (a balance between acidic and alkaline environments) in order to stave off disease. While the gastrointestinal system needs to be acidic to support the environment of the necessary lactic-acid-producing bacteria, the rest of the body needs to maintain a base or alkaline pH. "After digestion, absorption, and metabolism, nearly all foods release either acid or bicarbonate (base/alkaline) into the systemic circulation. . . . Fish, meat, poultry, eggs, shellfish, cheese, milk, and cereal grains are net acid producing, where as fresh fruit, vegetables, tubers, roots, and nuts are net base producing." The American diet is heavily skewed toward acid-producing food, which causes an imbalance in normal levels of pH.

> As a result, healthy adults consuming the standard US diet sustain a chronic, low-grade pathogenic metabolic acidosis that worsens with age as kidney function declines. Virtually all preagricultural diets were net base yielding because of the absence of cereals and energy-dense, nutrient-poor foods—foods that were introduced during the Neolithic and Industrial Eras and that displaced base-yielding fruit and vegetables.[19]

This chronic, low-grade pathogenic metabolic acidosis could also be looked at as a bodily environment that is ripe for disease.

American eating habits are extraordinarily important for gastrointestinal and overall health. The gut dysbiosis and immune dysregulation seen in so many children today with chronic illnesses are due in part to the types of foods that children eat. Because of the wide availability of junk food or nutrient-stripped, sugar laden, processed foods to American children, they are some of the biggest consumers of nutrient-poor food. Furthermore, the American marketing machine knows that children are vulnerable targets and market their products accordingly. What American child has not begged for sugar cereals based on the friendly cartoon characters on the box or the catchy jingle in the television ad? This problem becomes worse for low-income families because whole, nutritious food is expensive, and highly processed grains and sugars are cheap.

HOW DIET CONTRIBUTES TO GUT DYSBIOSIS AND IMMUNE DYSREGULATION

The microbiota in the gastrointestinal system consume the food we eat, too.

As alluded to earlier, some diets improve the balance of good bacteria in the gut, while others promote the growth of pathogenic bacteria. In a child that is already predisposed to gut dysbiosis through repeated pharmaceutical exposure, or other environmental toxin exposures, diet becomes exceedingly important to health outcome. Diet can alter the type of microbiota that dominate the gastrointestinal system in many ways. Diets high in sugar and refined grain, in particular, are known to promote the growth of pathogenic yeasts like *Candida albicans*. Some evidence indicates that diets high in sulfur compounds (found in dried fruit, white bread, alcoholic beverages, etc.) may promote the growth of potentially pathogenic microbes.[20] In addition, diets that are low in cultured foods (e.g., yogurt, kefir, naturally fermented vegetables) do not provide an opportunity to repopulate the gut with necessary probiotic ("good germs") bacteria.

Diets that contain high quantities of nutrient depleted foods (which describes the vast majority of food consumed by the average American child: Chicken nuggets, macaroni and cheese, white breads, white pastas, etc.) will deplete a child of essential vitamins and minerals necessary for proper immune function. The most basic biological functions in our bodies, from cell formation, to energy production, require nutrients from our diet. Nutrient-deprived diets deprive our bodies of the most basic building blocks required for immune cells production and function. Vitamins C, A, E, zinc, copper, magnesium, and many other nutrients deemed essential for immune health, are not easily assimilated into the body when they come in the form of synthetic vitamins packed into white bread or some other processed foodstuff. These vitamins are used more effectively when they come from whole foods. American children simply aren't eating enough fruits and vegetables or natural foods in general, so their bodies are chronically nutrient-deficient. As previously mentioned, even the vegetables grown on our soils are becoming depleted of nutrients. Immune systems cannot be expected to work without proper nutrition. A child who already struggles with gut dysbiosis is going to be at an even greater disadvantage if his diet is as anemic as most American diets because his gastrointestinal system cannot effectively extract these vitamins and minerals.

Excessive consumption of processed foods can contribute to gut dysbiosis, immune dysregulation, and chronic disease by introducing food toxins directly into the gastrointestinal system while simultaneously undernourishing the body. With a few exceptions, eating foods that are processed automatically means that there will be little to no exposure to protective probiotic bacteria because processed foods are pasteurized, sterilized, irradiated, sanitized and packaged so that all microbes stay out, good and bad. Without the protective probiotic bacteria to help protect the gut lining and process the ingested toxins, we are left utterly helpless against food-toxin damage.

TOXINS IN OUR FOOD

Our children have a tremendous toxic burden with regard to chemicals in their environment. They are exposed to all sorts of toxic petroleum-based substances, heavy metals, volatile-organic compounds, all with detrimental health effects. What is most shocking is that American children receive a good portion of their toxic burden through the food they eat. American agriculture is heavily dependent upon the use of nitrogen fertilizers, herbicides and pesticides for the production of fruit, vegetables and grains. A substantial portion of these toxins make their way into our children's bodies with significant consequences. For instance, organophosphate insecticides widely used on crops can cause damage to the brain and nervous system, particularly in those whose central nervous system is developing, namely, fetuses, infants, and children. "For infants six to twelve months of age, commercial baby food is the dominant source of unsafe levels of OP [organophosphate] insecticides. OPs in baby food apple juice, pears, applesauce, and peaches expose about 77,000 infants each day, to unsafe levels of OP insecticides."[21]

The dangers of pesticides and insecticides is well known, but what is less well known is that the many processed foods we eat every day (that we believe to be "safe" or even "healthy") contain ingredients that are actually quite harmful, especially if consumed in large quantities. Of the thousands of food additives and new processed foods that Americans consume every day that may be adversely affecting their health, there is only very limited research on what these additives actually do once in the body. Industry and government standards for demonstration of safety are minimal and poorly enforced. However, a few studies are beginning to emerge, and the news is not good. For example, studies demonstrate a link between certain food additives and intestinal permeability, the physiological condition that leads to allergies and other health problems.

Widely used emulsifiers, such as carrageenan and certain sugar esters, are believed to contribute to intestinal permeability and other gastrointestinal problems. Emulsifiers are additives that make products stay "mixed together." They make foods creamier, frothier, smoother, and prevent separation of different ingredients in processed foods. Most of us are not even aware that these products are in our food, but they are ubiquitous in the American food supply. They are in breads, ice cream, yogurt, mayonnaise, salad dressings, cookies, cakes, whipped cream, infant formula and many, many other foods. Some common food emulsifiers that you might read on food labels include: mono- and diglycerides, polysorbates, succinylated monoglycerides, esters of monoglycerides, carrageenan, soy lecithin, and many others. Many food additives have not been studied extensively in humans, in fact, most have received only perfunctory safety approval. New research is demonstrating that many of these additives are not safe at all.

A study published in 2001 in Environmental Health Perspectives, a National Institutes of Health publication, demonstrated that carrageenan, a seaweed and an additive in many processed foods (including dry soup and dip mixes, baby cereal bars, milk substitutes, ice cream, lunch meats, etc.), is associated with intestinal permeability, intestinal neoplasms (cancerous-like growth), ulcerations, and other adverse gastrointestinal effects.[22] Sugar esters, a large category of surfactants (emulsifiers) used widely in foods, cosmetics, soaps, shampoos and many other consumer products, have also been associated with increased intestinal permeability. A study done at the University of Guelph in Canada found that a particular type of sugar ester, sucrose monoester fatty acids, can contribute to greater intestinal permeability and increased impact of food allergens.[23] Sodium caprate/caprylate, another food and drug additive used as a binder, emulsifier and anticaking agent has also been shown to increase intestinal permeability. It has been studied for its ability to enhance absorption of small molecules (pharmaceutical agents) precisely because of its ability to cause intestinal hyperpermeability. These additives are a mere sampling of the thousands of substances added to our foods, drugs, and beverages, but many more simply have not been studied.

Some other examples of food additives that are believed to add to our children's overall toxic burden include:

- MSG, or monosodium glutamate, a flavor enhancer known to be an excitotoxin (acting on the nervous system, can cause neuron damage). A recent study demonstrated that MSG combined with aspartame (artificial sweetener, such as NutraSweet) and two different food colorings caused nerve cells to stop growing.[24]
- Trans fats or hydrogenated fats/oils, present in many processed goods, are shown to increase inflammation, and "interrupt normal brain function in everyone from children with ADHD to adults with depression or dementia."[25]
- Certain additives in children's drinks can be damaging in particular combinations. Beware of the combination of sodium benzoate/potassium benzoate and ascorbic acid (vitamin C) found in many children's juices and soft drinks, as the combination is believed to produce the highly potent carcinogen benzene.[26]

- Other potential toxic additives include: BHA and BHT (preservatives, possible carcinogen); nitrates/nitrates (preservatives, potential carcinogen); artificial colorings, such as "red dye #" or "blue dye #" (potential carcinogens); and many other additives.

SOYBEANS AND OTHER GENETICALLY MODIFIED ORGANISMS

One of the lesser-known potentially dangerous foods for American children is soy. The soybean is seen by many as a terrific health food, as it is high in protein, low in fat and is promoted for its "heart healthy" qualities. Although soybeans and soy byproducts have been grown and processed in the United States since the 1930s, soy has only recently become a significant part of the American diet. Most of the soy consumption in the United States today comes in the form of processed soy products, including meat and dairy substitutes, soy lecithin, soy flour, soybean oil and other soy byproducts that are ubiquitous in processed foods. It can be found in everything from granola bars to fast food hamburgers and cupcake frosting. The use of soy in the U.S. exploded in the 1990s at the same time that Monsanto, an agricultural biotech company, developed genetically modified soybeans that would be resistant to their particular brand of herbicide, *Roundup*. Currently, it is estimated that approximately 90 percent of soybeans grown in the United States are genetically modified.

Americans are consuming an inordinate amount of genetically modified soy products on a daily basis in their diet. An estimated 18-25 percent of American infants are fed soy formula during their first year of life, usually because of an intolerance or allergy to cow's milk.[27] Research indicates that this may not be such a good idea. Soy consumption has been associated with impaired iodine absorption (a mineral essential for the prevention of hypothyroidism and developmental delays), as well as other mineral deficiencies (such as calcium, magnesium, iron and zinc). Again, vitamin and mineral deficiencies can compromise a child's development, particularly with regard to the nervous system and immune system.[28]

ιe, may precipitate certain health issues, but many Ameri-
ncerned about possible health risks associated with consuming genetically modified soy. Of all plant products, soy has the greatest
percentage of genetically modified crops in the country. However,
many other crops have undergone genetic engineering, especially
canola (55 percent), cotton (79 percent), and corn (52 percent). Genetically modified organisms (GMOs) are those that have had genes
from other species "injected" into their DNA in order to modify their
final product. This is typically done to make a plant resistant to insects,
herbicides, or to prevent spoilage by extending life. This is the ultimate
industrialization and commodification of agricultural products.

While no one really knows the true consequence of human consumption of genetically modified organisms, preliminary animal
model research and epidemiological studies are beginning to sound
some alarm bells to potential hazards. The plain truth is, no one—
not the FDA, not the CDC—is tracking the potential health impacts
of consuming GMOs. Yet they can be found in 75 percent of
processed foods in America.[29] What are the particular health concerns
associated with the consumption of GMOs? The following is a list of
concerns raised by Andrew Kimball, executive director of The Center
for Food Safety in Washington, D.C.

- Antibiotic Resistance: Antibiotic resistant genes injected into
  the GMOs during testing and development are contained
  within genetically modified produce. There is speculation that
  this could lead to a transferring of such genes to microorganisms in the human gut, leading to the presence of antibiotic
  resistant germs in our guts.
- Allergies: There is also speculation that genetically modified
  foods may cause allergic reactions. Cross-reactivity has been
  demonstrated in laboratory animals. Some researchers believe
  that the widespread peanut allergies seen in America in recent
  years may be the result of cross-reactivity to genetically modified soybeans.

- Weakening Immune Response: According to a rat study published in *Lancet*, rats fed on a genetically modified diet (as compared to controls on a non-GMO diet) had "underdeveloped organs, lower metabolism, and a less robust immune system."
- Loss of Nutrition: The FDA determined that genetic engineering can result in "undesirable alteration in the level of nutrients" in food.[30]

The potential dangers associated with GMOs has led the vast majority of Europe to declare itself GMO-free, where GMO crops are banned throughout. When considering that these new epidemics of chronic health conditions in American children are strongly correlated with immune dysregulation, the role that GMOs might play in etiology should be vigorously examined by medical science.

chapter 7

Factor 4 — Habits and Lifestyles

AMERICAN HABITS AND LIFESTYLES

The one environmental factor that most mainstream pediatricians will agree contributes to chronic disease in children is the American way of living. This explanation incorporates the "hygiene hypothesis" and sedentary indoor lifestyles, both of which are widely accepted among physicians as potential contributors to disease.

Although the science examining the link between lack of microbe exposure and the development of chronic disease is still emerging, many scientists and historians agree that improved hygiene, facilitated by improved public and private sanitation, coupled with urbanization, may provide some source of explanation for the increase in chronic inflammatory disease. Studies have shown that rural populations that migrate toward cities (including rural European immigrants migrating to American cities in the nineteenth century) develop allergies and asthma at a rate much greater than those who continued to live rurally.[1] These trends give credence to the microbe/hygiene hypothesis, but we know that the hygiene hypothesis does not provide the whole picture.

With the work of Louis Pasteur and other scientists on the germ theory in the late nineteenth century, upper and middle class Americans became increasingly aware of the dangers of germs, and slowly began to make lifestyle choices that would avoid them. Hygiene habits such as frequent bathing and laundering were incorporated into American lifestyles toward the end of the nineteenth century, especially among upper and middle class families.[2] Interestingly, as previously discussed, upper and middle class Americans were disproportionately affected by allergies in the nineteenth century. It would seem that avoidance of dirt and exposure to natural microorganisms is somehow implicated in the development of atopic disease. Clearly, the science does not support this hypothesis as a *sole* causative agent, but perhaps low exposure to outdoor (e.g., soil, animal) microorganisms is contributing to gut dysbiosis and immune dysregulation on some level.

Human beings living in the western world have experienced a rapid change in lifestyle over the last century and a half, but biologically, we are the same beings that we have been for thousands of years. Our bodies have not yet adapted to modern lifestyles, yet we expect them to operate properly despite this fact. "Because of the slowness of adaptive evolutionary machinery, of particular interest according to this perspective are lifestyle factors that either witnessed a rapid change in recent times or represent an obvious departure from the conditions that prevailed for most part of our evolution, i.e. factors likely to exemplify the discordance between our 'Stone Age' genes and 'Space Age' living conditions."[3]

Changes to American lifestyles over the last century and a half have significantly reduced contact with our natural outdoor habitat. This means we have lower exposure to soil organisms, like particular strains of beneficial *Lactobacillus* bacteria found in soil. The change in the *quality* of exposure is likely to impact the types of bacteria that colonize our guts, and epidemiological studies examining the protective benefits of rural living (free from chemical/pesticide exposure)[4] tend to support this notion. Thus, while we do not have lower *total* microbe exposure, we do have *different* microbe exposure. Research demonstrates that the types and diversity of microbes that colonize our guts is of critical importance. Thus, if we do not have the "right" kind of bacteria colonizing our guts (e.g., multiple soil organisms) then the "wrong" kind of bacteria colonize our guts (e.g., *clostridia* class of bacteria), leading to gut dysbiosis, immune dysregulation and eventually chronic illness.

Modern activities anchor us indoors rather than outdoors. Most Americans work, eat, and sleep indoors. Our leisure activities, including television, video games, computers, and even sports, tend to be indoors. Activities that were commonly done outdoors less than a century ago, such as travel and shopping, have moved indoors. We live distantly from our natural outdoor habitat and this can impact the qualitative characteristics of the microbiome (microorganisms living within us), but other "outdoor" exposures may be equally important.

Recent research has highlighted the importance of vitamin D, a vital immune-supporting hormone acquired through sun exposure (and to a lesser extent, diet), to health and wellness. Dr. Michael Hollick, Professor of Medicine, Physiology and Biophysics at Boston University School of Medicine, has written extensively on the subject of vitamin D deficiency in America and has found that the majority of Americans (especially those living above 35 degrees latitude, or north of Georgia) are vitamin D deficient. In two separate studies, 52 percent of Hispanic and black adolescents in Boston, and 48 percent of white preadolescent girls in Maine were found to be vitamin D deficient.[5] This is significant because vitamin D deficiency has been linked not only with rickets, but with many chronic illnesses ranging from autoimmune diseases like multiple sclerosis to bone diseases like osteoporosis. Vitamin D is of critical importance to the proper functioning of the immune system. The immune system of a child with gut dysbiosis will be further impaired by a lack of vitamin D. Thus, vitamin D (through sunlight or diet) may not be solely responsible for the development of chronic illnesses in children, but a deficiency will exacerbate an already dysregulated immune system.

American children tend to spend the bulk of their days indoors often engaged in passive activities associated with the computer or television. According to a study conducted by the Institute for Social Research at the University of Michigan, American children ages six through seventeen spend over fourteen and a half hours watching television, nearly three hours on the computer, and less than one hour engaged in outdoor activities each week.[6] Indoor-bound children reflect larger trends in America. According to the Environmental Working Group, "People spend 65 percent of their time in their houses, and 25 percent in some other indoor environment. Transit takes from 5 to 7 percent of the time, and usually less than 5 percent is spent outdoors, studies show."[7]

All this time indoors reduces children's exposure to natural sunlight critical for vitamin D, but it also reduces their exposure to important natural microorganisms, and instead exposes them to indoor toxins. Indoor pollution is known to be more toxic than any outdoor pollution. The Environmental Working Group has cautioned that indoor air pollution levels are "many times higher than those from the outdoors, even when compared to city air where trucks and factories belch pollution." Furthermore, indoor time is usually spent engaging in sedentary activities, at the expense of exercise, which provides important defense against oxidative stress and inflammation.[8]

On average, American children today spend fewer hours outdoors than ever before in human history. When they do go outdoors, they are typically lathered in vitamin D-blocking sunscreen. According to a study conducted by Dr. Hollick in 1987, SPF 30 sunscreen reduced serum levels of vitamin D by 99 percent.[9] This means that even if you do go outside to "get some vitamin D," if you are wearing sunscreen, you will not actually get vitamin D. What's more, sunscreen may contain toxic chemicals that need to be processed and excreted. If a body's detoxification capabilities are handicapped (gut dysbiosis, compromised immune system), then the toxins can accumulate in the body and cause further harm. Recent studies have also found that the nanomolecules of zinc oxide and titanium dioxide in sunscreen can kill off beneficial microorganisms. These are the same beneficial microorganisms (in our bodies and our environment) that are so critical to the detoxification process. So, we send our children outdoors (for one hour a week) lathered in sunscreen full of chemicals and assume that this is healthy for them. Our relationship with the sun and the outdoors needs to be reevaluated.

BIRTH AND INFANT FEEDING

In addition to lack of time spent outdoors, subtle components of modern American life may predispose a child to gut dysbiosis, immune dysregulation and subsequent chronic illness. Some researchers have proposed the idea that how babies are born may influence their health as growing children. There is tremendous controversy over the importance of mode of delivery (how babies are born) with regard to long-term health outcomes. In 1965, about 5 percent of births were done through a Caesarean section, by 1975 approximately 10 percent were C-section, and by 2006 the rate had reached over 31 percent. In fact, the C-section is the most common hospital procedure in operating rooms in the United States.[10] With the number of C-sections performed in America today, this debate is of incredible importance.

Researchers believe that as a baby descends through the birth canal, she is "inoculated" with bacteria (such as *Lactobacillus*) that are critical for the early development of the immune system. Babies delivered via Caesarean section are not inoculated with their mother's bacteria in the same way, and may instead first become inoculated with bacteria present in the hospital surroundings. Consequently, babies born via C-section tend to have different mixes of bacteria in their gut as compared to babies born vaginally. "It has been shown that bacterial colonisation of the gut in infants born by Caesarean delivery differs from that in infants born by vaginal delivery; for example, a lack of Bacteroides spp, bifidobacteria, and lactobacilli has been shown in their faecal specimens."[11] Antibiotics are given routinely to mothers perinatally to prevent operation-associated infections, and it is possible that this course of medication also adversely affects the gut health of the infant.

Other studies have demonstrated differences in immune cell activity between babies born vaginally or by C-section. As gut dysbiosis and immune dysregulation are so central to the development of chronic illness in children, it is possible that the differences in gastrointestinal bacteria and immune cell activity based on mode of delivery play some role in the development of (or lack of) chronic illness. At least one study demonstrated a statistically significant increase in risk of atopic asthma in children delivered by C-section.[12] A subsequent, and much larger study, found a statistically significant increase in risk for asthma and hay fever among children born by C-section, but this correlation was not found for atopic dermatitis.[13] Another study in Germany concluded that Caesarean delivery might be a risk factor for infant diarrhea and sensitization to food (e.g. food allergy) in those families who have a history of allergy.[14]

Unfortunately, because of the many variables leading to the development of atopic disease, these studies, although interesting, are not entirely convincing because they incorporate only a few variables. More meaningful studies have looked at the overall impact of mode of delivery on actual immune cell activity and immune responses, rather than disease development. A study conducted in Finland in 2007 found that children born via C-section not only had different fecal bacterial makeup, but they also developed different immunological pathways than their vaginally delivered peers. The babies delivered by C-section had lower fecal bacterial cell counts, demonstrated stronger humoral immune response (as opposed to cellular immune response), and demonstrated higher levels of immune cells such as IgA-, IgG-, and IgM-secreting cells. Science has not provided definitive evidence that Caesarean section results in increased risk for disease (although correlations seem to exist); however, the preliminary findings that babies born via C-section may develop altered immune responses certainly merits more research. Even with the preliminary data on C-sections and gut bacteria, doctors in many other nations routinely recommend the administration of probiotic supplements to babies born via C-section.

Furthermore, preterm delivery (often associated with incubator/ NICU exposure, antibiotics or other pharmaceuticals, and delayed breastfeeding) has been correlated with delayed colonization of the infant gut with probiotic bacteria, such as *Bifidobacteria*, and a much a higher risk for the development of some chronic illnesses, such as asthma and ADHD.[15] Delayed or altered colonization of the infant's gut with appropriate bacteria could lead to immune dysregulation and the development of disease. However, many additional variables affect the health of a preterm infant (e.g., many are born without fully developed lungs) that make it difficult to draw correlations between gut bacteria, immune dysregulation and the development of chronic disease in preterm infants. Again, the differences in gut bacteria and the subsequent development of chronic illness in babies born prematurely warrants additional research. What all of this research does tell us is that the gut bacteria are important to the immune system and alterations in the gut bacteria may have lasting immunological implications.

Another interesting component of American birth culture that may have implications for infant health and wellness is the widespread use of pitocin (synthetic oxytocin, the natural labor hormone) for labor augmentation in U.S. hospitals. A study published in *Obstetrics and Gynecology International* in 2009 found that the administration of pitocin to laboring mothers actually results in decreased glutathione levels in their newborn babies. Glutathione is the critical cellular antioxidant that helps us detoxify and effectively deal with oxidative stress (from toxins, immunological assaults, etc.). According to this study, babies born to women administered pitocin during labor may have reduced detoxification capabilities shortly after birth.[16] Unfortunately, this is the same time that the Vitamin K shot and hepatitis B vaccine are administered, both of which contain ingredients (such as aluminum hydroxide and formaldehyde in hepatitis B or benzyl alcohol in Vitamin K) that may increase oxidative stress in the newborn. More studies need to be done to confirm the potential danger of administering these therapies to babies with decreased glutathione levels.

Just as we have altered the way we routinely deliver babies in the United States, we have also altered the way that we feed infants. In the nineteenth century, most women breastfed their babies, and those who did not, fed their babies cow's milk or early forms of artificial infant formula. In fewer cases, wet-nurses may have been used. For hundreds of years, American women breastfed their babies well into the second year of life, as it often worked as an effective form of birth control. Today, it is estimated that approximately 70 percent of American women at least attempt to breastfeed their newborns, but the numbers drop substantially after the first few months of life. The CDC reports that by three months, roughly 30 percent of mothers still nurse their babies. Historically, breastfeeding an infant for the first year of life was a near ubiquitous phenomenon, but today, fewer than 20 percent of American mothers nurse a full year. This is a tremendous increase in breastfeeding compared to recent decades. In the 1970s, breastfeeding rates plummeted so that only 25 percent of mothers *ever* breastfed their babies at all. Some socioeconomic variables also correlate with breastfeeding rates. Lower rates of breastfeeding occur in certain populations, including unmarried women, black and Latina women, rural populations, and those who are less educated or earn a low income.[17] Certainly occupation and employment factor greatly into these statistics, as does education and awareness of the benefits of breastfeeding. It is therefore safe to assume that the vast majority of American babies over three months old are receiving some form of artificial milk substitute in lieu of breast milk, possibly at the expense of immune health and function.

Breastfeeding rates are significant because the decision to breast-feed an infant may have important implications for immunological development in the first year of life. It is believed that breast milk contains important immune factors that are responsible for modulating antigen exposure (e.g., helping to develop oral tolerance) and stimulating immune system maturation. Numerous studies have compared breastfed babies to formula-fed babies in an effort to find clinical differences based on early diet. As medical science has concluded that breastfed babies have clear health advantages over formula-fed babies (i.e., resistance to infectious disease, and lower risk of chronic diseases, etc.), most medical doctors now recommend breastfeeding infants for as long as reasonably possible. However, research has not yet fully elucidated the impact of formula feeding versus breastfeeding on the subsequent development of chronic illnesses in children. Yet, like the mode-of-delivery studies, researchers have been able to show differences in gut bacteria and immune cell activity between breastfed and formula-fed babies, which has implications for the development of chronic illness.

Breastfeeding is believed to benefit an infant's developing immune system in many ways. First, passive immunity (protection from certain pathogens) in the infant is established by breastfeeding, as a mother passes her antigen specific antibodies (specific to certain infectious agents) from her breast milk to her baby. This affords a nursing baby a certain level of protection from infection. Second, viable bacteria (such as the beneficial *Bifidobacteria*) and DNA from many other bacteria present in the mother's gut are transferred from the mother's intestines (via an endogenous cellular route) to breast milk. This process may serve to imprint the baby's immune system with information regarding which microbes are friendly and which ones are foes. Essentially, the baby's immune system learns how to interface with its environment from "information" transmitted through breast milk.[18] Assuming there are no abnormal immune dysregulating influences in the baby's life (e.g., exposure to environmental toxins, or possibly over-vaccination), then breastfeeding can be viewed as an important part of the immune system maturation process. Lack of breastfeeding may not be harmful to an infant, per se, but the infant will not receive the continuous immunological "education" that comes from breastfeeding.

This transfer between mother and baby is an area of emerging science, but animal models have provided some interesting insights. For example, nursing mice given probiotic fermented milk (e.g., milk kefir that contains good bacteria) showed improved immune function, and this benefit was transferred to their pups via nursing. Apparently, the offspring of mothers fed fermented milk showed increased secretory IgA (an important immune factor produced in mucosal linings) in their intestinal fluid, a sign that breastfeeding had transferred the immune boosting benefits of the fermented milk ingested by their mothers.[19] This study is significant because it demonstrates how breastfeeding and maternal diet can positively impact a child's developing immune system. On the other hand, a poor maternal diet (e.g., one high in *Candida*-feeding sugars) could result in the transfer of pathogenic microbes and microbial DNA that would not be of benefit to a child's developing immune system. More detailed research in this area would help to elucidate to what degree maternal diet and gut dysbiosis shape and alter a child's developing immune system. It is plausible that poor maternal diet and the microbial conditions for gut dysbiosis could be transferred to an infant via breastfeeding with implications for the development of chronic illness.

The natural rhythms of birth and infant feeding that are a critical part of the development of an infant's immune system and health have been significantly altered by the modern world. A mother whose body is imbalanced (gut dysbiosis and immune dysregulation) may pass these imbalances on to her baby, who is then faced with additional environmental challenges, such as pharmaceutical agents, harmful chemicals, excessive vaccinations and infectious disease. This baby will have a compromised immune system and an inability to effectively handle these environmental assaults. In another scenario, a mother who has a perfectly balanced inner ecosystem but has a Caesarean section, and cannot or chooses not to breastfeed her baby, will not transfer the immune building benefits of her gut flora and breast milk onto her baby. Thus, her baby will not have the advantages he could. The picture regarding breastfeeding and mode of delivery is complicated. While breastfeeding and vaginal delivery seem to be of importance to the healthy maturation of an infant's immune system, this may be true only so long as the mother herself is "ecologically" balanced.

THE ROLE OF STRESS

Perhaps it is capitalism and the enterprising spirit, or perhaps it is personal or social expectations to achieve the American Dream, but cultural elements make Americans a busy and stressed out people. While some cultures are admired for their ability to sit, relax and enjoy life, Americans are known for their ability to let life pass them by while they are busy working. The best time to witness this frenetic pace of life is at mealtime. To witness an American eating is to witness a culture on the go. Many American meals are eaten on the road, at work, and often standing up. Incidentally, this is not a new phenomenon. According to one European visitor to America in the nineteenth century, the American national motto was "Gobble, gulp, and go." In fact, "foreigners often remarked on the eerie silence that reigned at American dinner tables, as diners seemed to concentrate on getting the tiresome burden of stuffing themselves out of the way in as short a time as possible."[20] This may speak to the culinary inadequacies of American cooking, or more likely, it speaks to American values and priorities, which tend to be more focused on working, and less focused on living.

America is an incredibly stressed nation. The following are some statistics compiled by the American Psychological Association that provide a barometer of the current level of stress in America:

- A recent survey found that Americans are deeply affected by stress, with 53 percent of Americans reporting feeling stress-associated fatigue, 60 percent reporting feelings of irritability

or anger from stress, and as many as 52 percent reporting that
they lie awake at night because of stress.

- About half of Americans report overeating or eating unhealthy
foods as a way to manage stress, and 39 percent of Americans
find themselves skipping meals as a result of stress. About one-
fifth of Americans drink alcohol to manage stress, and 16 percent smoke as a way to deal with stress.[21]

To be sure, stress begets unhealthy behaviors (such as unhealthy
eating or alcohol use), but stress alone is enough to cause damage to
the body. What does all of this stress do to our bodies? When a person
experiences stress their adrenal glands put out a stress hormone called
cortisol. Increased production of cortisol can depress the immune system and stimulate the release of the body's sugar stores into the bloodstream. These surges of sugar can encourage the growth of *Candida*
just as much as direct sugar consumption. Stress may encourage the
growth of pathogens, but it can also wreak havoc on the good bacteria
in our guts. Animal models have demonstrated that animals subjected
to stressful stimuli (in one case, the separation of a young rhesus monkey from its mother) resulted in shedding of *Lactobacilli* — essential
commensal bacteria. Furthermore, human studies have demonstrated
that stressful situations are correlated with a decrease in *Bifidobacteria*
and *Lactobacillus*, and a rise in pathogenic bacteria, such as *Bacteroides fragilis*. Theories have proposed that the release of cortisol or
norepinephrine might impact the growth of potentially pathogenic
bacteria in the gut.[22] Furthermore, stress has been shown to increase
intestinal permeability and exacerbate underlying gastrointestinal vulnerabilities (such as a predisposition to inflammatory bowel disease).[23]

Thus, stress can be a significant factor contributing to gut dysbiosis
in Americans. A pregnant woman who experiences significant stress
in her life may affect the balance of her inner ecosystem, which can,
in turn, affect the inner ecosystem of her baby when he is born. This
child may then be predisposed to a dysbiotic gut and compromised
immune function when he comes into the world. Like diet and toxic
environmental exposures, stress is just one more compounding factor

in our culture and our environment that may predispose our children to chronic illness. In the last century and a half, we have drastically changed our environment, and "as human ecology changes, so does our microbiota."[24]

There is no doubt that microbiota in the human gut are of tremendous importance to the development and maturation of proper immune function. Every day, scientists continue to learn new information regarding the specifics of host-microbe interaction in the gut. The clinical implications of these discoveries are profound. If we can understand and catalog the role of microorganisms in relationship to genetic, biochemical and physiological processes in the human body, we will achieve a new height in our understanding health and illness in the human body.

Over the last few decades, scientists have slowly begun to unravel the mysteries of microorganisms in the human body, but much work remains to be done. In 2006, the NIH began work on what has become known as the Human Microbiome Project, a government-funded project that is the germ equivalent of the Human Genome Project. The project aims to study the final frontier in human biology—the microbial cells present in and around the human body. The project is extensive and involves initiatives such as sequencing the genomes of bacteria, and mapping bacteria communities present in various sites in the human body. The next great scientific and medical breakthroughs may come from discoveries made regarding the role of microorganisms in the human body. They are a critical, but often forgotten, part of human biology whose time has come.

Clearly, we need to understand the role of microorganisms in our body and our environment if we are ever going to understand the etiology of chronic illnesses like asthma, ADHD, autism and many others. We know that microorganisms are a critical piece of the puzzle regarding the rampant immune dysregulation in children today. However, they are not the only piece. It is important to remember that gut dysbiosis and immune dysregulation often occur as a result of a perfect storm of different environmental factors. Following are two diagrams that visually depict how different environmental variables alter the

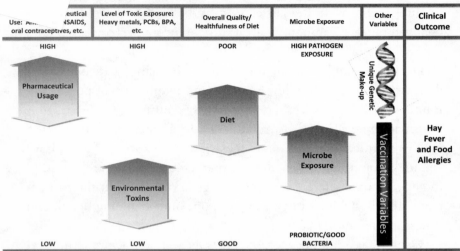

...ental Variables for Child A* That Result in Allergies as a Clinical Outcome

* For illustrative purposes; not all variables represented

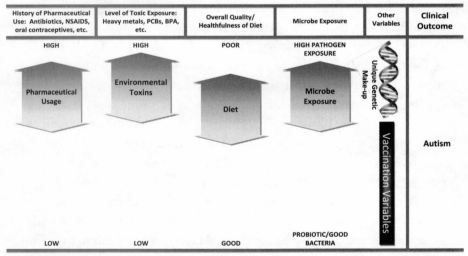

Environmental Variables for Child B* That Result in Autism as a Clinical Outcome

* For illustrative purposes; not all variables represented

FIGURES 6 AND 7: ALTERATIONS IN ENVIRONMENTAL VARIABLES IMPACT CLINICAL OUTCOMES.

course of health and wellness for any given child. In these illustrations, the environmental exposures of Child A result in the development of hay fever and allergies, while a different set of environmental exposures for Child B might result in the development of autism. (See figures 6 and 7.) The final environmental variable that has not been addressed is that of childhood immunization.

chapter 8

Factor 5 — Immunizations and the Immuno- compromised

✿

Vaccination is such an important, yet controversial and emotional topic that it must be discussed with great care and caution. Few topics in contemporary America can raise tempers and drive antagonism as quickly as that of childhood immunizations. The very conversation is rarely cordial or civil, and often brings out the worst in people. The national debate over vaccination has rapidly devolved into a national argument where lines have been drawn and sides have been assigned.

You are either provaccine or antivaccine, and there seems to be little space for people who want to discuss the subject with honesty and candor, devoid of emotion. There are vaccine advocates who call people who don't vaccinate their children "parasites" and "leaches," and there are vaccine safety advocates who send hate mail and stalk certain vaccine advocates. This antagonistic exchange loses sight of the very reason for the vaccination program: the health and safety of our children.

This needs to change, as the health and welfare of our children, and the future of our country, may depend on our ability to calmly and rationally discuss America's current childhood immunization policies and programs. Unfortunately, this country lacks an effective forum for discussing such a complex and emotional topic. The mainstream media might even enjoy the fight between opposing sides because it makes for good, scintillating news. The sound-bite-oriented nature of our culture and society makes discussing complex issues like childhood immunization programs difficult. Scientific publications tend to avoid publishing pieces that even remotely challenge or question the established vaccine protocol out of the (rational) fear that such discussions might impact the current high childhood immunization rates, with unknown consequences.

Peer-reviewed journals tend to avoid scientific articles if they are in any way critical or speculative about vaccines. One well-respected physiologist who published an article on the subject of gastrointestinal disease and autism was repeatedly warned by the scientific journals to which he submitted his article of the "dangers of talking about vaccines." He was even told to change his article and remove portions that raised some interesting questions about vaccination protocols. His article was eventually published in a respected peer-reviewed journal, after he had edited out some relevant commentary on vaccines.[1] Debate is healthy, but a hyped-up media and an overly cautious scientific community have left us devoid of a meaningful and comprehensive debate about vaccination in America. Instead, we have an angry shouting match, leaving confused parents unsure of where to turn.

The great vaccine debate is not new in America, but it has become reinvigorated in recent years, especially as American parents watch the prevalence of so many chronic illnesses climb year after year. In particular, parents of children with autism are putting a spotlight on our current vaccine program, as many claim that their children regressed into autism following certain childhood immunizations. Again, no one claims to know for sure what causes autism, but these parents are asking themselves, "Can vaccines be a piece of this puzzle?" Governmental and healthcare authorities repeatedly and quite adamantly rebut, "No," citing multiple scientific studies. Yet, this has not stopped parents from questioning and urging their leaders and the scientific community for more information regarding the safety, efficacy and long-term impact of America's vaccination program. Although the vast majority of American parents still fully vaccinate their children, the rising numbers of children with autism whose parents point to vaccination as a possible etiological suspect is giving pause to an increasing number of concerned parents. Why do we continue to debate the safety and efficacy of childhood immunizations in America, and how can we move this debate forward?

A BRIEF OVERVIEW OF THE GREAT VACCINE DEBATE

Dr. Paul Offit, Professor of Pediatrics at UPENN, Chief of Infectious Disease at Children's Hospital of Philadelphia, and patent holder on the universally recommended RotaTeq (rotavirus) vaccine, argues that the great divide in America over vaccination began with some unfortunate mishaps in America's early vaccine programs. According to Dr. Offit, these early failures of vaccines prevented a perfect trust from being established between vaccine science and parents.[2] Dr. Offit is himself a central figure in the great debate, as he has written and lectured extensively about the lack of connection between childhood illnesses and vaccination. Parents of children with autism (and other vaccine safety advocates) have become quite incensed by Dr. Offit's dismissive attitude toward their many claims that their children's autism is in some way connected to vaccines. The antagonism is so great between Dr. Offit and these groups that he recently published a book to defuse their attacks both on him, and the vaccination program. His book, *Autism's False Prophets* (2008), discusses the great lengths to which parents of children with autism go to heal their children. Many parents blame vaccines for their children's development of autism, and Offit sympathetically chalks this up to the desperation that these parents feel as they search for answers to explain why their child is autistic. Offit's attempts to defuse the debate seem to have backfired, as many parents of children with autism view his book as condescending and perhaps even insulting.

Part of this vaccine debate deadlock comes from the fact that more and more children are being diagnosed with chronic illnesses of unknown etiology, and vaccines make for a plausible culprit. We may be at record-high immunization rates today, but American parents have long been skeptical of the safety of vaccines. Dr. Offit has argued that this fundamental distrust in vaccines began in the mid-twentieth century with what is known as the Cutter Incident. In the early stages of polio vaccine development, a company known as Cutter (who was not the only manufacturer implicated) inadvertently allowed live and active virus into the polio vaccine they produced, when the vaccine was supposed to contain killed virus. As a result, tens of thousands of children were inoculated with live virus, leaving thousands sick, 164 severely paralyzed, and 10 dead.[3] Offit believes that this incident set the stage for distrust between the vaccine manufacturers and the public. He argues that people have never truly trusted the process of vaccination. This phenomenon dates back to the nineteenth century, when public health officials went door to door inoculating citizens of both the U.S. and the U.K. with smallpox "vaccine" (which at the time involved scratching one's arm and exposing it to pus from a person infected with cowpox). This crude method of vaccination caused some people to become sick, but it also generated a lot of fear and skepticism among the public.

The Cutter Incident may be an important event in the history of vaccines that impacted public perceptions about vaccine safety, but it is not the only incident that occurred in America. Additional bumps along the vaccine road have, to a degree, weakened American trust in vaccines. In the 1960s, some children who were inoculated with an early killed measles virus vaccine experienced a severe sickness now known as atypical measles upon exposure to the wild type virus. As many as 160,000 children developed the more severe atypical measles as a result of this particular type of vaccine mishap.[4] However, both the Cutter Incident and the atypical measles outbreak involved infecting vaccine recipients with infectious diseases. More recently, vaccines have been implicated in acute neurological and immunological injuries and the development of chronic illnesses.

In 1982, a documentary entitled *DPT: Vaccine Roulette* aired on network television, examining claims of vaccine injuries sustained from the DTP shot (DTP, for diphtheria, tetanus, and pertussis). Adverse affects associated with the DTP shot included high fevers, encephalitis and other neurological events. Arthur Allen, author of *Vaccine*, argues that the airing of this documentary marks the birth of the Vaccine Safety Movement, the organization of parents, and some clinicians, to reevaluate the safety of our childhood immunizations based on a growing number of adverse events experienced by vaccinees. The safety of the DTP vaccine had been questioned for decades, as it had caused severe neurological damage in a small subsegment of vaccine recipients. Dozens of lawsuits had been filed against DTP manufacturers by the time the FDA looked into reformulating the DTP vaccine. In 1996, the DTP vaccine was replaced with the DTaP vaccine (which contained acellular rather than whole cell pertussis), a vaccine with an improved safety profile, including fewer incidences of neurological damage.

As parents became more aware that vaccines can, in rare instances, cause acute injury, they began to pressure lawmakers to offer some sort of governmental or corporate compensation should such an injury occur. In addition, pharmaceutical manufacturers sought protection from mounting lawsuits. In 1986, Congress enacted the National Vaccine Injury Act, designed to ensure a stable supply of vaccines while simultaneously reducing the financial liability of vaccine manufacturers regarding vaccine injury lawsuits. In 1988, The National Vaccine Injury Program was launched, which provided an alternative for the vaccine injured to seek compensation without having to directly sue the manufacturers. The program is funded by a $.75 tax on each dose of vaccine purchased in the U.S. Between 1988 and 2008, over $875 million was awarded to individuals found to be vaccine injured by the vaccine court. For claims of injuries suffered before 1988, over $900 million was awarded. Nearly $2B worth of vaccine injury compensation might just be enough to cause some parents to approach their child's vaccination with caution.[5]

The vaccine court system is a testament to the fact that vaccine injury can and does happen. Many parents understand this risk as they agree to vaccinate their child, as it is commonly believed, and routinely explained by pediatricians, that vaccine injury is extremely rare, and the benefits of vaccination outweigh the risks of not vaccinating. However, more recently, the risk profile of vaccines seems to have expanded to include not only "extremely rare" acute injuries (such as encephalitis/brain damage or anaphylaxis), but to include autism, multiple sclerosis, Guillain-Barré syndrome and other autoimmune disorders. Vaccine-induced autism seems to be the leading claim against vaccines currently, with over 5,500 claims filed with the vaccine court, awaiting adjudication. This is the number of claimants who have taken the time to bring suit to the vaccine court; many more parents claim that their children's autism is in someway linked to vaccination.[6] It is important, however, to put this number into context, as millions of children have been vaccinated in this country whose families have not filed claims with the vaccine court, or who simply have no problems with vaccines.

About two decades after the establishment of the vaccine court, *New York Times* reporter David Kirby wrote a bestselling book on the subject of mercury and vaccines. Kirby's book, *Evidence of Harm*, published in 2004, served to stir the vaccine pot further by lending credence to those who claimed that the ethylmercury preservative (more commonly known as thimerosal) in vaccines was responsible for injuring children. Kirby presents the story of parents who believe their children were vaccine injured in a sympathetic light, lifting them out from underneath the label of antivaccine zealot. Mercury was removed from most (although not all) childhood vaccines in 2000, but Kirby's book nonetheless reinvigorated the mercury-autism-vaccine debate. As of 2009, this debate had not been put to rest, despite the fact that mercury is present only in a few vaccines (including the influenza vaccine and a few select others).

Clearly, a significant number of American families feel that vaccines in some way caused or contributed to their children's chronic illnesses. It is no wonder that many other American parents continue to be spooked by the immunization program, fearing routine childhood vaccination could contribute to the development of autism or other debilitating disorders. While some parents may be aware of the Cutter Incident, or have some distant understanding of the remote possibility that an acute vaccine injury is possible, this is less likely to be the cause of vaccine fears. The more likely reason for the recent distrust in vaccines is the loud and incessant voices of parents of vaccine injured children and alleged vaccine injured children, many of whom are autistic, who believe that vaccines were the trigger that sent their child off the cliff toward regressive autism. The debate surrounding vaccines has been alive and well in America for quite some time, but it is reaching a new crescendo, and this is due largely to the voices of parents of children with autism and children with vaccine injuries.

Perhaps the highest profile parents of vaccine injured children include Barbara Loe Fisher, author and head of the vaccine safety advocacy group, National Vaccine Information Center; and Jenny McCarthy, celebrity author and board member of Generation Rescue, a nonprofit autism organization. These mothers, among an entire legion of equally dedicated parents, continue to, quite literally, *beg* public health authorities and the scientific community to more closely examine the safety and efficacy of America's childhood vaccines. Both mothers believe that their children were injured by vaccination and experienced severe and lasting disabilities as a result (encephalitis and subsequent ADHD/learning disabilities for Fisher's son Chris, and autism for McCarthy's son Evan). Parents like Fisher and McCarthy often like to say that they are not antivaccine, but are for more sensible and individualized approaches to immunization.

Yet, for all the efforts of McCarthy, Fisher, and the many other vaccine safety advocates, there seems to be little movement in Washington or among vaccine manufacturers to investigate their claims that vaccines contribute to severe disabilities and chronic illnesses. The resistance on the vaccine advocacy side of the debate appears to very strong, and a serious reevaluation of America's childhood immunization program seems unlikely. The opinion leaders on this side of the debate, such as Dr. Paul Offit, tend to be quite dismissive of parents like Fisher and McCarthy, believing that they are somehow mistaken about the etiology of their children's illnesses, or that they are endangering children's lives by challenging the vaccine status quo. They believe that questioning vaccines may have dire consequences in terms of reduced vaccination rates and recurrences of deadly childhood diseases. This is certainly a real possibility that should be carefully considered. Outbreaks of infectious diseases like measles typically follow declining vaccination rates. Vaccine advocates fear the return of dangerous infectious childhood illnesses, but vaccine safety advocates fear that the current vaccination schedule may be causing immunological and neurological impairment in a large percentage of American children.

It seems strange that these two sides cannot talk considering the common fears and objectives of each side. One side fears deadly and dangerous infectious childhood illnesses (like pertussis, polio and meningitis) and the other side fears an epidemic of severe and debilitating chronic illnesses (like autism, inflammatory bowel disease, diabetes and SIDS—sudden infant death syndrome). Both sides want healthy and safe children. No parents want their children to suffer with whooping cough (pertussis). No parents want their children to suffer with autism. Vaccine advocates will continue to fight to protect America's children from infectious diseases, and vaccine safety advocates will continue to fight until they see the right kind of scientific studies (unbiased, comprehensive and designed with their concerns in mind) that demonstrate that vaccines do not contribute to chronic illness in children. These two sides need to get together—*today*—so that no child need suffer from dangerous infectious disease *or* debilitating chronic illness.

Many vaccine advocates argue that science has proven vaccines to be safe and that there is no established link between vaccines and chronic illnesses like autism. Unfortunately, the science that exists that "proves" the safety of vaccines (e.g., disproving a link between the MMR vaccine and autism) is not satisfactory to many parents of children with chronic illnesses. Quite a few studies have examined the link between neurodevelopment and certain vaccines (e.g., the MMR), and none of these studies has demonstrated a link. Yet many parents of children with autism believe that these studies are poorly designed, and they are crying out for more comprehensive studies. For example, a study published in *Pediatrics* (the journal of the American Academy of Pediatrics) in February 2009 that looked at the impact of thimerosal (mercury preservative in vaccines) on neuropsychological performance in children ten years after exposure concluded that:

> The lack of consistency among the results of our study and other available studies suggests that an association between thimerosal exposure through vaccination in infancy and neuropsychological deficits is unlikely or clinically negligible.[7]

This study is often cited as *proof* that thimerosal does not cause neuropsychological problems. This study found no statistically significant difference in neuropsychological performance between the two groups of children that were examined. The fundamental flaw with this study, according to vaccine safety advocates, is that *both* groups of children in this study received thimerosal, just in different doses. The first group received 62.5 micrograms of ethylmercury from their infant vaccines, while the second group received 137.5 micrograms of ethylmercury from their infant vaccines. One could argue that there was no statistically significant difference in neuropsychological performance in the two groups because they both received thimerosal—and no evidence indicates that clinical outcomes in human children exposed to thimerosal are altered depending on the dose of thimerosal, especially within such a narrow range.

Vaccine safety advocates cry foul and argue that this study should have involved a control group, or a group that did not receive any thimerosal in their vaccines at all, and even better, another control group that did not receive any vaccines at all. Vaccine advocates argue that this study helps to put to bed the concern that thimerosal causes neurological problems. No one seems to be able to agree on whether or not vaccine-related thimerosal causes neurological or other cellular damage in children. There is no question that this issue needs to be sorted out, but other issues concerning vaccines need to be addressed, and arguing over thimerosal tends to distract from these other concerns. While it is certainly possible that thimerosal damages a subset of children (in some cases triggering autism), it is a false assumption to believe that vaccines that do not contain thimerosal are necessarily safer. Thimerosal has been a central focus of the vaccine debate for over a decade. Yet its removal from most vaccines (except the flu vaccine and a few others) in 2000 leaves many wondering: If thimerosal causes autism, developmental delays and other health issues, then why are the prevalences of these illnesses and disorders continuing to rise?

Could it be the thimerosal that is still contained within the flu vaccines (recommended to be given annually to every child six months or older and to pregnant women) that causes these problems? It is possible, but it is important to remember that likely many factors contribute to chronic illnesses and disabilities in children. Vaccines may be one of those factors, with or without thimerosal. We will never know to what degree vaccines (or thimerosal) play a role in the epidemic of chronic childhood illnesses until we study populations of vaccinated versus unvaccinated children to look for relationships between vaccines and health issues.

One of the more recent concerns about vaccines is that certain vaccines (or perhaps too many vaccines or an inappropriate combination of vaccines) may negatively affect children who have preexisting health conditions like a mitochondrial disorder or certain metabolic imbalances. The Hannah Poling case brought this issue into the national spotlight in 2008. Hannah Poling is a ten-year-old girl who allegedly developed autism after she received five vaccines (for nine diseases) in one day at the age of nineteen months. After Hannah's family brought suit against the vaccine manufacturers, the vaccine court ruled that Hannah's "autism-like symptoms" were "significantly aggravated" by vaccinations but primarily because she had what they termed an "underlying mitochondrial disorder." The vaccine court ruled in favor of the Poling family and will be awarding compensation for her vaccine injury.[8]

It is still unknown as to whether Hannah had a preexisting mitochondrial disorder or whether the vaccines themselves caused her mitochondrial disorder. Regardless, the Hannah Poling case raises a number of important questions. Could vaccines cause mitochondrial disorders? If vaccines can be harmful to children with underlying mitochondrial disorders (as the Poling decision implies) then should we be screening all children for these sorts of underlying conditions prior to vaccination so that no children develop autism unnecessarily? If so, how do we screen children in a cost-effective and noninvasive manner? Furthermore, should we start by conducting studies to determine the prevalence of underlying mitochondrial disorders in the pediatric population? Have we learned anything from the Hannah Poling case? Can her experience help us to redesign public health policies so that we can protect the most number of children from harm? Despite the obvious opportunities for learning presented by this case, it seems to have caused only more division and contention over the entire vaccine question.

As a nation, we are absolutely paralyzed and unable to determine one way or another if vaccines contribute to chronic illness because vaccine advocates and vaccine safety advocates cannot agree on what studies must be done to establish safety. The vaccine advocates say that all necessary studies have been done. According to a number of studies, MMR does not cause autism, they say. Case closed. Vaccine safety advocates argue that the studies done to date are flawed, paltry, biased, and do not address some of their fundamental concerns and questions regarding the safety of vaccines.[9] For instance, they would like to see more expansive studies that look at the immune system's response to many vaccines at once.

No studies examine the immunological impact of administering five or six or more different vaccines to an infant at the same time. Plenty of studies look at immune response (presence of antibodies) to one, two, or even three vaccines administered simultaneously, but none simulate the real life immunological response of a six-month-old baby who is taken to the pediatrician's office to receive the hep B, flu, IPV, DTaP, and HiB vaccines, all in the same visit. Furthermore, studies tend to assess immunological response by looking for the presence of antibodies. Few studies look at the long-term impact on other immune cells or immune function (such as Th1, Th2 or Th3 responses). These would be exceedingly difficult studies to run, especially because of the wide number of variables involved in vaccination and immune response. This does not mean, however, that we should stop trying to gather more information.

Vaccine safety advocates also say that they would like to see specific studies that look at the combined physiological impact of certain vaccine adjuvants and additives, such as aluminum, mercury, bovine serum, formaldehyde, and many other substances contained within vaccines. They would also like to see how environmental factors (such as antibiotics, acetaminophen or toxin exposure) might impact a child's response to vaccines. In addition, some would like to examine glutathione levels in early infancy to see if young babies are physically equipped to detoxify upon vaccination. And finally, they would like to see studies that compare vaccinated to unvaccinated children. This is perhaps one of the most commonly cited criticisms of vaccine safety studies: no long-term (or epidemiological) vaccine safety studies that compare fully vaccinated to completely unvaccinated children in America exist. Many parents believe either that certain vaccines (such as DTaP or MMR) or perhaps even the entire vaccine schedule cause some form of immune dysregulation in their children, leading to chronic illness. Yet there is *not one* comprehensive study published in a peer-reviewed journal that examines this claim by parents.

Given the availability of modern medical health records, a comparison of the health of unvaccinated children to the health of vaccinated children is entirely feasible. Why doesn't this study exist? It is not just antivaccine zealots or vaccine safety advocates who are calling for this type of study. One of the most respected women in American public health, Dr. Bernadine Healy, former head of the NIH (National Institutes of Health) and the American Red Cross, has similarly called for such a study. In a recent article, Dr. Healy stated:

> Less than a year ago, the National Institutes of Health put out a call for expanded research on vaccine safety that contains many of the very things that parents are asking for: examination of the way the immune system handles different vaccines, the impact of nonvaccine components (like mercury and aluminum), and better understanding of susceptibility to vaccine side effects. The government laid out the need for markers that might predict vulnerable groups and proposed research on the comparative effect of different vaccine schedules and combinations of vaccines. This work is long overdue; shockingly, so is a study comparing groups of vaccinated and unvaccinated children.[10]

Dr. Healy may be interested in initiating détente in the war over vaccines, but most other health officials continue to drag their feet. The American Academy of Pediatrics (after years of pursuit by vaccine safety advocacy groups) has finally agreed to look into the issue of vaccine safety, while simultaneously continuing to recommend that more and more vaccines be added to the existing childhood immunization schedule. Public health officials and pediatricians just want to do their job: protect America's children from harmful infectious diseases, and they are sick and tired of the vaccine safety advocates getting in their way. But vaccine safety advocates are a dedicated and passionate group of individuals, and they are not going away.

What are we to do? At a minimum, we need to reevaluate the value and necessity of vaccinating America's children with all of the current recommended vaccines. To date, there has not been a rigorous assessment of the safety and efficacy of our existing immunization program. To be sure, individual vaccines have been extensively studied for safety and efficacy (some more than others), but there have been *no* studies conducted in this country that examine the safety and efficacy of the entire vaccine program as it exists today. A child born in America today will receive multiple doses of fifteen vaccines by the time they are six years old (and the majority of these are given before two years of age). Just thirty years ago, when the prevalence of chronic illness in children was low, children received only seven vaccines. (See table 4.) Yet, we have never evaluated the long-term impact of such a vaccine schedule, and no country in the world vaccinates as much as the United States. (See table 5.) It is not unreasonable for American parents to expect governmental leaders to reevaluate our vaccine program.

There may be *just* fifteen diseases that a child is vaccinated against by the time they are six years old, but there are at least thirty-four different vaccines for these diseases—each manufactured differently, containing different components—made by different manufacturers. Any given child might have a completely different mix of vaccines than another child treated in a different pediatrician's office. The protocol is one size fits all, but actually, different vaccines are used throughout the country. For instance, a child being vaccinated for Haemophilis Influenza Type B could either receive ActHiB (Sanofi Pasteur), Comvax (Merck), HibTITER (Wyeth), OmniHiB (Glaxo-SmithKline), or PedVaxHiB (Merck). Each of these vaccines contains different ingredients in different combinations. The variables in any given child's vaccination schedule are tremendous. Not only does each child have a different genetic makeup, a different immunological profile (including different and diverse populations of gut bacteria),

TABLE 4. IMMUNIZATION SCHEDULE 1979 VS. 2009—MANDATORY IN MANY STATES FOR SCHOOL ENTRY[11]

	1979	2009 (number in parentheses indicates the number of doses)
Vaccines mandated by most states for school entry	MMR DTP Polio	Hepatitis B (3) Rotavirus (3) DTaP (3-4) Hib (3-4) Pneumococcal (3-4) Polio (3-4) Flu (every year) MMR (2) Varicella (2) Hepatitis A (2) Meningococcal (1) (for certain high risk groups)

TABLE 5. U.S. MANDATED VACCINES COMPARED TO OTHER DEVELOPED NATIONS[12]

Vaccine	Percent of 30 Developed Nations that Mandate this Vaccine:
DTP	100 percent
Polio	100 percent
MMR	100 percent
Hib	93 percent
Hepatitis B	60 percent
Pneumococcal	37 percent
Varicella	13 percent
Rotavirus	10 percent
Influenza	7 percent (USA and Canada Only)
Hepatitis A	0 percent (USA only)

and a different environmental toxic burden, but they are each getting different cocktails of vaccines. It is an incredibly complex picture to be able to tease out what any one vaccine might be doing in a particular child's body.[13] Thus, the only way to truly evaluate whether or not America's vaccination program contributes to chronic illness in children is to compare vaccinated to unvaccinated children. This study should have been done decades ago.

In the meantime, parents are anxious because they do not feel that public health officials or many doctors take their concerns seriously. When asked by a parent, "What do all of these vaccines do to my child's body?" most pediatricians explain that a child's immune system can process thousands upon thousands of antigens (substances foreign to the body) at any given moment with no problem. Why should multiple vaccines, which contain only a few antigens, cause any problems? This is the patent response given by most pediatricians and soldiers of science. It may be true that the human immune system routinely processes thousands of antigens at any given moment, and it can handle multidimensional immunological assaults with little problem, yet vaccination is not a normal type of antigen presentation to the immune system. The truth is most pediatricians do not know what the full schedule of vaccines does to children other than theoretically protect them from infectious disease. Before we can begin to answer this question, more comprehensive research is needed to understand exactly how a fully vaccinated child's immune system differs from an unvaccinated child's immune system.

There is much justification for this research, beyond the speculation that vaccines contribute to chronic illness in children. Vaccines present a much more complicated interaction between the immune system and antigens than any naturally occurring body/antigen interaction. First, today's vaccines bypass parts of our normal "innate" (or nonspecific) immune system, which includes the mucosal surfaces of our nose, eyes, mouth, gastrointestinal system, etc. Instead, vaccines are presented directly into the bloodstream or subcutaneously (under the skin), which skips over key parts of a body's immune response located in these mucosal surfaces.[14] Second, vaccines contain many unnatural components, including elements that are genetically engineered, that the body would never encounter in the natural world, that are injected either directly under the skin or into the bloodstream. Third, it is still unknown as to whether the many antigens within a given vaccine beside the pathogenic antigens (e.g., bacterial toxin or virus) are truly inert. In other words, most vaccines contain other ingredients besides the virus or bacterial toxin that have not been studied long term to establish safety. Some of the substances (potential immunogens) within vaccines include: residual proteins or molecules from animals used to culture (grow) the vaccine viruses and bacteria — these include chicken embryo, mice brains, and monkey kidneys; genetically engineered DNA from viruses; various synthetic components, such as potassium glutamate (related to MSG), aluminum hydroxide, and polysorbate 80; human albumin (human blood plasma); soy peptone broth (a culture medium); and many, many other components. Where are the long-term studies that indicate that *injecting* these components into a body does not stimulate an autoimmune response, for instance?

In response to the claim that a child's immune system can handle any number of vaccines simultaneously, it is not so much that the infant's body is overwhelmed by exposure to multiple antigens at one time (as occurs with multiple vaccinations in one visit), rather it is what types of antigens are presented, in what combination, and how they interact with the immune system that matters. In other words, it is not the quantity of antigens, but the quality of antigens, and how they interface with our defense system. For example, when a child eats lunch at school, she may be simultaneously exposed to thousands of naturally occurring antigens, such as wheat, peanut, sugar, apple, streptococcus bacteria, rhino viruses, mold, parasites, plastic particles, food particles from her neighbor's lunch, sand and dust from the playground, etc. The immune system is designed to effectively process these exposures and respond appropriately depending on perceived danger of the antigens.

When a child is injected with multiple antigens from vaccines, the quantity of antigens will notably be smaller (a drop in the bucket compared to an average school lunch), but the quality of the antigens is significantly different, and the very mechanism of injection skips the part of the immune system that is typically the first responder to antigen presentation. Even the most basic immunology textbook highlights that the route of contact between antigen and immune system matters: "Route of contact . . . can influence the qualitative nature of a response; for example, an immunogen [substance capable of producing immune response] that contacts the intestinal mucosa typically evokes the production of a different type of antibody than would be produced if it entered through the bloodstream, and this can affect subsequent events in the immune response."[15] There is much discussion in the scientific community about how vaccines may cause a Th2 skew in the immune system, which may be related to the types of immune responses generated by vaccines as compared to natural infections. In other words, certain vaccines have been shown to elicit a Th2 response, which is a type of white blood cell (helper T-cell 2) that needs to be in balance with another type of white blood cell known as a Th1 cell (helper T-cell 1) in order for the immune system to operate properly. Repeated stimulation of Th2 types of responses (by vaccines), it is theorized, may disrupt the balance between Th1 and Th2 responses, causing immune dysregulation (which is clinically associated with illness).

Studies have demonstrated that some vaccines call up the Th2 side of the immune system's response, while others call up the Th1 side of the immune response.[16] Many children with chronic illnesses, such as asthma or allergies, tend to have a Th2 skew to their immune system. Other children with autoimmune disorders, such as juvenile diabetes or rheumatoid arthritis, have been found to have a Th1 skew. This dysregulation of T-helper cells (or *lack* of regulation) could happen for a number of reasons, but vaccines are certainly a suspect. A Th2 skew could result from low levels of gut *Lactobacillus* (good bacteria), which are known to help regulate the T-cell responses, or from repeated immunization with vaccines that call up Th2 responses, or *both* of these factors could be involved.[17] Currently, the American childhood immunization schedule is loaded with vaccines that stimulate a Th2-type response (e.g., hepatitis B, polio, measles), although Th1 stimulating vaccines (such as the whole-cell pertussis vaccine) do exist in the schedule.[18] Dr. Kenneth Bock has noted in his book *Healing the New Childhood Epidemics*, "We are a Th2 skewed society." Dr. Bock elaborates:

> This skewing [in favor of Th2 cells] can be caused by a variety of factors—including, for example, stress, and yeast overgrowth—but the primary factor that now appears to cause this skewing toward Th2 dominance is the presence of toxins. Mercury in the body promotes excessive activity of Th-2 cells. So does lead. So does aluminum. These heavy metals aggravate and overexcite the immune system, resulting in allergy, impaired immunity, and in autoimmunity, in which the immune system inadvertently attacks healthy tissues and organs.[19]

Toxins (e.g. aluminum) in vaccines have long been suspected of dysregulating (e.g., causing a Th2 skew in) the immune system. The fact is, we just do not know to what degree the toxins in vaccines, or other additives, such as animal tissue, may be responsible for our children's immune systems going haywire. Immune dysregulation may be largely due to children's heavy exposure to environmental toxins, making toxins in vaccines negligible. Because of the epidemic of immune dysregulation in this country, it is absolutely imperative that we study *all* factors that might play a causative role. If vaccines do cause the immune system to become dysregulated, then we need to figure out how to prevent this from happening through modifications to vaccines, or by fortifying the body's immune system so that it does not respond to vaccines in this manner. If further research vindicates vaccines, then we need to educate the public about this reality. We cannot abandon vaccines, as they are so critical to the prevention of infectious disease, yet we cannot continue to administer vaccines if they are in some way causing epidemics of chronic illnesses in children.

MORE THAN JUST MERCURY: EVIDENCE INDICATING THAT VACCINATIONS MAY PLAY A ROLE IN CHRONIC CHILDHOOD ILLNESSES

Many parents claim that their child's routine vaccines were in some way responsible for their child's chronic illness or disability. Their observations and experiences watching their children respond adversely to vaccines should be taken into consideration. These experiences could be quite helpful in guiding scientists to a better understanding of the precise mechanisms of multiple vaccinations in individual children (with particular genetic polymorphisms/variations, for example).

Parents argue that there is a great need for more research on the long-term immunological consequences of vaccines in children. But, is there any *scientific* reason to believe that vaccination might be adversely affecting children's immune systems? A review of vaccine history and current scientific literature reveals a tremendous amount of evidence linking vaccination to immunological dysregulation in vaccinees. A mountain of evidence demonstrates that some vaccines cause autoimmunity, allergic disease, encephalitis (swelling of the brain), mental retardation, behavioral disorders, inflammatory conditions and many other adverse events. In fact, most early (experimental) versions of vaccines had to conquer these sorts of adverse events before they could be licensed for use in the public. It is not such a far stretch of the imagination, therefore, to believe that today's vaccines might cause immune dysregulation or contribute in some way to the autoimmunity or immunological dysfunction that is arguably at the epicenter of today's chronic illnesses in children.

The following is a brief historical catalogue of ways in which vaccines have been linked directly to degenerative human health conditions, autoimmune diseases or other serious adverse events.

Animal Tissues and Autoimmunity. Researchers by the names of Maurice Brodie and John Kolmer created two separate polio vaccines in the 1930s that were tested on twenty thousand children throughout the country. Kolmer's vaccine killed nine children (and paralyzed more) and Brodie's vaccine caused allergic encephalitis, which is an acute inflammation of the brain that occurs when T-cells are sensitized to attack myelin components (an autoimmune reaction against brain tissue causing brain damage). Part of the reason this happened is because the researchers used monkey brains to grow the viruses that would then be injected into human subjects. Researchers subsequently discovered that viruses grown in animal brains can cause the human immune system to attack its own brain tissues (autoimmunity to brain).[20] This was found to be the case in rabies vaccines grown in rabbit brains, [21] and other vaccines grown in mice brains (including a West Nile virus vaccine).[22]

Despite these findings, mouse brains are still used in the production of commercially available vaccines, such as the Japanese encephalitis vaccine.[23] Just recently, Japan suspended routine immunization with the Japanese encephalitis (JE) vaccine because of a number of serious vaccine-induced adverse events, including a case of acute disseminated encephalomyelitis (brain inflammation leading to brain damage). Researchers speculate that the mouse brain protein in the vaccine may cause the human immune system to attack its own brain tissues. Seven cases of this same illness (vaccine-induced brain damage) were documented in the 1990s.[24]

The polio virus in the IPV polio vaccine used today is grown in monkey kidneys and calf blood serum. Other animal tissues and cells are also involved in the manufacturing of vaccines. Some vaccines contain glycerol, derived from cow fat, and gelatin and amino acids derived from cow bones. In addition, "the growth medium for viruses and other microorganisms may require cow skeletal muscle, enzymes and blood."[25] Residual animal tissues and cells in vaccines have been found to cause autoimmunity to human brain tissue in vaccinees. This is fairly well-established science. New science tells us that autoantibodies to brain (and other) tissues have been found in children with autism. The question remains, could any of our childhood vaccines be, in some way, contributing to this type of autoimmunity?

Guillain-Barré Syndrome and the (first) Swine Flu Affair. In 1976, reports that a virulent form of a swine flu was emerging in the United States (believed to be similar to the influenza virus that killed millions of people in 1918) resulted in the rapid vaccination of forty million Americans against this virus. Shortly after the vaccination program began, reports of deaths and other adverse events associated with the vaccine began to pile up at the CDC. According to the CDC, there were 181 deaths reported following swine flu vaccination (142 of which occurred within forty-eight hours of immunization). A direct link between the vaccine and the deaths has not been established, yet it is possible that the vaccine in some way precipitated a fatal event in some of the vaccinees.[26] Over five hundred people developed Guillain-Barré syndrome (GBS) as a direct result of the vaccine, and twenty-five people subsequently died from GBS. Guillain-Barré syndrome is a debilitating, and sometimes deadly, autoimmune disease that affects the peripheral nervous system.

There were four thousand injury claims, $1.3 billion in compensation was requested, and the federal government eventually paid out approximately $100 million to flu shot recipients.[27] The CDC was so concerned about the relationship between the swine flu vaccine and GBS that they completely halted the vaccination program in December—before flu season was even in full swing. Ironically, the swine flu never materialized, which is why this is often referred to as the Swine Flu Affair or the Swine Flu Fiasco. "Epidemiologists wondered if the cause of so many people developing GBS after getting the swine flu vaccine might have been a residual protein taken from the myelin of embryonic chicks [egg protein] that existed in the vaccine through all its manufacturing stages"[28] The association between GBS and the swine flu vaccine may seem like a fluke or one of those typical bumps in the history of vaccination; however, in later years (1992, 1993 and 1994), a number of Americans would develop GBS after receiving their annual influenza vaccine. There may be something about how the influenza vaccine is manufactured that increases the risk of an individual developing an autoimmune disease like GBS. Two scientists, John Harley and Judith James, have shown that "molecular mimicry between a protein in a virus and a protein in the body could lead to autoimmune disease."[29] In other words, it is scientifically plausible that the certain proteins (virus or animal) found in vaccines can cause autoimmunity in vaccine recipients. Most recently, the HPV (human papilloma virus) vaccine known as Gardasil has been implicated in the development of GBS in a number of vaccinees. At least thirty-one girls since 2006 reported the development of Guillain-Barré Syndrome after receiving the Gardasil vaccine.[30]

Strep Vaccine and Autoimmunity. In the 1960s, efforts to develop a vaccine for group A streptococcus (which causes strep throat) were disastrous, as the developed vaccine caused innoculees to generate antibodies against their own tissues, including their brains and heart, another case of vaccine-induced autoimmunity. Five people died during the trials of this vaccine, and further plans for development were scrapped.[31]

Current Scientific Research Linking Immune Dysregulation and Vaccination. A diverse body of research investigates how vaccines may contribute to immune dysregulation. In examining this literature, it is important to remember that vaccines are unlikely to be the sole causative agent of immune dysregulation in children. They may be one part of a larger group of predisposing factors (including genetics, environmental toxins and gut dysbiosis) that contribute to the epidemic of immune dysregulation. Following is a brief overview of some of the more intriguing findings regarding vaccination and immune dysregulation:

- Over the last two decades, the medical literature has become littered with studies documenting cases of autoimmune diseases triggered by vaccination. In 2000, Drs. Yehuda Schoenfeld and Anabel Aharon-Maor of Tel Aviv University performed a review of the medical literature documenting vaccine-induced autoimmunity. They found over 138 cases of vaccine-induced autoimmune disorders that were documented in peer-reviewed literature (as opposed to simply reported to VAERS or similar).[32] An example of a typical case of vaccine-induced autoimmune disease includes a case documented by researchers in 2008, at the Sao Paulo University School of Medicine in Brazil, where they described a twelve-year-old girl who developed a deadly neurological autoimmune response following her third dose of hepatitis B vaccine. The young girl (who was taking no drugs and who had no relevant previous medical history) developed a seizure attack and unconsciousness after vaccination. An autopsy "revealed cerebral edema with congestion and herniation and diffuse interstitial type pneumonitis." [33]

- Multiple studies have demonstrated that ethylmercury (thimerosal found in some vaccines, such as flu shot) and methylmercury (mercury found in fish) are immunosuppressive and cause a Th2 skewing of the immune system.[34] Flu shots are mandated by many states to be given annually to anyone six months or older. The immune skewing effect of mercury is a perfect example of how multiple environmental factors may contribute to immune dysregulation in children. In this case, children exposed to mercury through diet, vaccines and other environmental sources could experience a Th2 skewing—or immune dysregulation associated with allergies, asthma, autism, and other inflammatory illnesses.

- A study published in the journal *Neurology* in early 2009 found an increased risk of central nervous system inflammatory demyelination (destruction of nerve tissue) with the Energix B vaccine (GlaxoSmithKline's hepatitis B vaccine) but not for other hepatitis B vaccines. The study looked at 349 children with acute CNS inflammatory demyelination and compared them to 2,941 matched controls to see if the affected children had higher rates of vaccination with hepatitis B vaccine. The investigators found no strong correlation between acute CNS inflammatory demyelination and hepatitis B vaccination, but they did find that those affected were more likely to have received the Energix B vaccine. The investigators concluded that the Energix B vaccine did indeed increase the risk of developing acute CNS inflammatory demyelination. Further study of this connection is necessary to confirm this association; however, it does remind us of the many variables in a given vaccination program. Multiple vaccines are given for any one disease. Some preparations may present higher risks of adverse events.[35]

- Researchers in France recently uncovered the connection between aluminum adjuvants used in vaccines and a condition known as macrophagic myofasciitis (MMF). MMF, first reported in France in 1998 (where over 200 cases were identified), "is defined by the presence of a stereotyped and immunologically active lesion at deltoid muscle biopsy," the location on the body where intramuscular vaccine injections are given. "It was recently demonstrated that this lesion is an indicator of long-term persistence of the immunologic adjuvant aluminum hydroxide within the cytoplasm of macrophages at the site of previous intramuscular (IM) injection [with hepatitis B, hepatitis A and tetanus vaccines]." In other words, aluminum hydroxide (an immune response stimulator in vaccines) has been found concentrated at the site of vaccine injection (the deltoid muscle). When a vaccination containing aluminum hydroxide is given, the aluminum hydroxide is supposed to dissipate in the body over time. In the case of patients with MMF, the aluminum stays right at the injection site, never dissipating, causing their immune systems to switch into a chronic state of activation. MMF is associated with a host of systemic problems. Many patients with MMF report symptoms similar to chronic fatigue syndrome (CFS), a disorder believed to be caused by immune dysregulation (chronic immune stimulation). In the study, nineteen of nineteen patients with MMF had received aluminum-containing intramuscular vaccinations (in the deltoid muscle) in the preceding months (ranging from one month to seventy-two months). One-third of patients with MMF develop autoimmune diseases, such as multiple sclerosis. These patients show signs of an immune system that is unable to shut itself off, and a Th2-skew to their immune function. Interestingly, the World Health Organization has called for the performance of epidemiological studies to understand the prevalence and pervasiveness of MMF. If a significant prevalence of MMF and associated autoimmune diseases and immune dysregulation is found in the general population, public health officials may be required to reevaluate the use of aluminum adjuvants in vaccines. [36]

- A recent study in Canada found that children who delayed their first DPT (diphtheria, pertussis, and tetanus) shot by more than two months halved their risk of developing asthma by age seven. Children who delayed all of their first three doses had an even lower risk. The researchers examined the health records of 11,531 children who received at least four doses of DPT. The researchers speculate that early childhood immunization promotes stimulation of Th2 cells and delaying vaccination may mitigate this effect to a degree.[37]

Animal models also demonstrate how vaccination can induce autoimmunity or immune dysregulation:

- A 2004 study published in *Biomedicine and Pharmacotherapy* found that non-autoimmune mice injected with adjuvant oils (used in a limited number of vaccines, mostly experimental), such as squalene (MF59) and Bayol F, developed lupus-related autoantibodies. (Lupus is a debilitating autoimmune disease.) The authors urge caution about the use of adjuvant oils in human vaccines given their potential to induce autoimmunity.[38] Numerous other studies support the induction of autoimmunity in animals receiving injections of squalene.[39] Adjuvant oils have long been used in veterinary vaccines and experimentally in human vaccines to increase the immune response in recipients. Although squalene is not licensed for use in the U.S., it is currently being used in vaccines that are in clinical development for HIV, herpes simplex, Cytomegalovirus (CMV) and hepatitis B.[40] It has also been tested as a possible adjuvant for use in influenza vaccines. Some researchers and many veterans believe that the use of squalene in some batches of anthrax vaccine administered to soldiers in the first Gulf War in the early 1990s contributed to a chronic illness now known as Gulf War Syndrome.[41]

- A study published in the *Journal of Autoimmunity* in December 2008 found that rabbits and mice immunized with peptides from the Epstein-Barr virus developed autoimmunity. The animals developed high levels of lupus-like autoimmunity (83 percent of rabbits and 43 percent of mice) and were found to have low levels of white blood cells (also immune dysregulation).[42] This study builds on previous work linking the Epstein Barr Virus to autoimmune disease through the mechanism of molecular mimicry.[43]

DOES THE AMERICAN CHILDHOOD IMMUNIZATION PROGRAM CAUSE CHRONIC ILLNESS?

Vaccines are associated with adverse events such as autoimmune diseases, acute and chronic inflammatory illnesses, and even death. These facts are indisputable. Over eighty years of vaccine history and medical research supports these facts. This is why there is the Vaccine Adverse Event Reporting System (VAERS), a government-sponsored ı devised to track all reported adverse events from vaccines, and the Vaccine Compensation Program. Approximately $2 billion has been paid out to thousands of victims of vaccine damage. We know that vaccines can cause severe damage in a very small proportion of the vaccinated population. What we do not know, however, is the degree to which vaccines also cause more subtle, difficult to track changes to the immune system in the wider population. Does the American vaccine schedule in some way contribute to the epidemic of immune dysregulation in our most highly vaccinated segment of the population, our children? Medical research has established that vaccine-induced immune dysregulation (in the form of autoimmunity, Th2 skewing, inflammation, etc.) occurs in some people, and it is plausible that a more subtle or subclinical form occurs in many more. Yes, it is plausible, but we need to study fully vaccinated versus completely unvaccinated children and look closely at how the immune systems in each group function before we can answer this question with certainty.

When put into a larger environmental context, an overloaded vaccination schedule, in conjunction with other environmental factors that tax our immune system (such as diet, toxin exposure, lifestyle, etc.), may be contributing to an epidemic of immune dysregulation in America. Our understanding of vaccine safety is extremely binary. We believe that vaccines are either 100 percent safe or they cause severe damage, but we do not consider the possibility that there may be a *spectrum* of damage between "safe" and "severe" that is both chronic and insidious.

Let us look at some preliminary studies that examine the relationship between vaccination and chronic illness or developmental disabilities. In recent years, the hepatitis B vaccine has come under quite a bit of scrutiny in this regard. The October 2008 issue of *Toxicological &Environmental Chemistry* contained a study that demonstrated a *nine times* higher risk of developmental disability in boys who were vaccinated with a full series of hepatitis B vaccine as compared to boys who had not been vaccinated with the hepatitis B vaccine at all. "This study found statistically significant evidence to suggest that boys in the United States who were vaccinated with the triple series hepatitis B vaccine, during the time period in which vaccines were manufactured with thimerosal, were more susceptible to developmental disability than were unvaccinated boys."[44] Another study published in *NeuroToxicology* in October 2009 found that infant primates vaccinated with a hepatitis B vaccine within twenty-four hours of birth demonstrated abnormal early neurodevelopmental responses as compared to unvaccinated controls.[45] In September of the same year, researchers at the University of New York at Stony Brook published a research abstract in the *Annals of Epidemiology* that noted that newborn boys vaccinated with the hepatitis B vaccine had three times the risk of developing an autism spectrum disorder.[46]

After years of pleading with public health authorities (to no avail) to conduct a vaccinated versus unvaccinated epidemiological study, Generation Rescue, one of the country's most visible autism and vaccine safety advocacy groups, decided to sponsor their own study. The study, completed in late 2008, compares health outcomes (such as presence of ADHD, autism, etc.) of vaccinated versus unvaccinated children in two states, California and Oregon. The vaccine and health outcome information was gathered by telephone survey. Their findings, quite disturbing, merit further examination with more rigorous epidemiological studies. A total of 11,817 families were surveyed providing a study population of 17,674 children, ages 4-17. In the entire study group, 991 children were recorded as completely unvaccinated. Although telephone surveys are subject to recall errors or other biases, they are the methodology used by the CDC to determine prevalence of neurodevelopmental disorders such as ADHD. The study found:

- Vaccinated boys were 155 percent more likely to have a neurological disorder than unvaccinated boys.
- Vaccinated boys were 224 percent more likely to have ADHD.
- Vaccinated boys were 61 percent more likely to have autism.
- Among older vaccinated boys, ages 11-17 (about half the boys surveyed):

- Vaccinated boys were 158 percent more likely to have a neurological disorder.
- Vaccinated boys were 317 percent more likely to have ADHD.
- Vaccinated boys were 112 percent more likely to have autism.
- Vaccinated boys and girls were 120 percent more likely to have asthma.
- No differences in neurodevelopmental disorders were noted in girls.

Generation Rescue makes the following comment regarding the outcome of this study on their website:

> Generation Rescue is not representing that our study proves that the U.S. vaccine schedule has caused an epidemic in neurological disorders amongst our children. We are a small non-profit organization. For less than $200,000, we were able to complete a study that the CDC, with an $8 billion a year budget, has been unable or unwilling to do. We think the results of our survey lend credibility to the urgent need to do a larger scale study to compare vaccinated and unvaccinated children for neurodevelopmental outcomes.[47]

There are other anecdotal reports of unvaccinated children faring better than vaccinated children with regard to chronic illness and developmental disorders. An article published by United Press International in 2005 reported on the large medical practice Homefirst Health Services, located in Chicago, IL, which claims to have no cases of autism among the many unvaccinated children in their practice. Most Homefirst patients do not receive any vaccinations. "We have a fairly large practice. We have about 30,000 or 35,000 children that we've taken care of over the years, and I don't think we have a single case of autism in children delivered by us who never received vaccines," said Dr. Mayer Eisenstein, the director of the centers and a vocal vaccine safety advocate. In a practice of this size, considering national prevalence estimates of autism at 1 in 100, they should have seen many children with autism go through their practice. If you count only the 15,000 children delivered (at home) by Homefirst who have been followed from birth on with no vaccinations, there should be at least 150 children with autism, but there are none.[48] According to Dr. Eisenstein, asthma is also virtually nonexistent in his practice.[49]

Similar findings have been reported among the Amish in Pennsylvania, a cultural group that typically refuses many medical interventions, including vaccination. The "no autism in the Amish" story, however, has been dismissed by many, including the former CDC director Julie Gerberding, because the Amish tend to have a homogenous gene pool. No such gene pool exists for the patients of Homefirst Health Services. Yet, this is only anecdotal information, and its credibility is questionable until subjected to rigorous statistical and epidemiological analysis. It is also important to remember, vaccines are only one piece of the immune dysregulation puzzle. Many other environmental factors may work in conjunction with excessive vaccination to cause immune dysregulation and resulting chronic illness.

THE CONNECTION BETWEEN VACCINATION, GUT DYSBIOSIS, AND IMMUNE DYSREGULATION

One of the concerns about the current vaccination schedule is that many children receiving vaccines could technically be considered immunocompromised because of an ongoing state of gut dysbiosis, nutritional deficiency, toxic overload and other environmental variables that affect our immune system. Unfortunately, vaccines are intended for the immunocompetent. In fact, many manufacturers list on their vaccine labels that vaccines are contraindicated for those who are immunocompromised. This is particularly true for live virus vaccines. For example, the prescribing information given to physicians for Merck's MMR II (shot for measles, mumps and rubella) states that the MMR II is contraindicated for "patients receiving immunosuppressive therapy"; or those with "primary and acquired immunodeficiency states," such as AIDS; cellular immune deficiencies (e.g., low natural killer cells); and hypogammaglobulinemic and dysgammaglobulinemic states (altered or reduced levels of immunoglobulins/antibodies). Furthermore, it states that active measles virus infection and measles inclusion-body encephalitis (measles infection causing brain swelling, often deadly) has been reported in immunocompromised individuals who received the vaccine.[50] Thus, patients whose immune systems are damaged or poorly functioning should *not* receive this or other live virus vaccines because of documented adverse events associated with vaccinated immunocompromised individuals.

The CDC recommends that children with congenital immunodeficiency (an inherited condition where the body's ability to produce antibodies is impaired) or other types of severe immunodeficiency should not receive certain vaccines, especially live attenuated virus vaccines. This caution is offered because there is a higher probability of an adverse event occurring from vaccination (for example: severe, chronic, and even fatal gastroenteritis associated with the rotavirus vaccine).[51] It is extremely rare for a child today to have congenital immunodeficiency, and few would be considered clinically immunocompromised (like an AIDS patient), but many American children do have some degree of immunodeficiency because of an impaired ability to produce antibodies (caused by gut dysbiosis and toxin exposure). Thus, it merits further study as to whether children should be screened for immunocompetence prior to vaccination.

Gut dysbiosis and toxin exposure can affect the body's ability to produce antibodies (immunoglobulins such as IgG or IgA) necessary for healthy and normal immune responses. Many studies have looked at the immune function of children with autism to determine if it differs significantly from normally developing children.[52] In one University of California study involving over five hundred children ages two to five years, children with autism were found to have significantly lower levels of IgG and IgM antibodies as compared to controls (normally developing peers). Furthermore, low levels of these antibodies seemed to correlate with autistic behaviors. For instance, children with low levels of IgM or IgG antibodies tended to have a higher incidence or intensity of autistic behaviors, such as stereotypy or lethargy.[53] These abnormalities in immunoglobulin levels may occur as a result of gut dysbiosis or exposure to environmental toxins. Dr. Natasha Campbell McBride explains how immunoglobulin deficiencies and subsequent immunodeficiency can be caused by gut dysbiosis:

> In the cell wall of *Bifodobacteria* (the good bacteria largely populating the human colon) there is a substance called Muramil Dipeptide which activates synthesis of one of the most important groups of immune system cells — lymphocytes. As a result, a healthy gut wall is literally infiltrated, jam-packed with lymphocytes, ready to protect the body from any invader. Scientific research shows that in people with damaged gut flora there are far fewer lymphocytes in the gut wall, which leaves it poorly protected. . . . Lymphocytes in the gut wall produce immunoglobulins. The most important one in the gut is Secretory Immunoglobulin A (IgA). Secretory IgA is a substance which is produced by lymphocytes in all mucous membranes in the body and excreted in body fluids. It is found in breathing passages, nose, throat, bladder, urethra, vagina, saliva, tears, sweat, colostrum, breast milk and of course the mucous membranes of the digestive system and its secretions. Its job is to protect mucous membranes by destroying and inactivating invading bacteria, viruses, fungi, and parasites. . . . When the healthy gut flora is compromised the number of cells producing IgA falls and our ability to produce IgA is reduced. . . . As a result their gut wall has poor ability to defend itself from fungi, viruses from vaccinations or the environment, bacteria and parasites.[54]

As previously discussed, environmental toxins can directly impact the health of gut flora, reducing beneficial bacteria. If healthy commensal bacteria are in low numbers in the gut (because of gut dysbiosis or toxin exposure), then the human body cannot mount an effective immune response against natural infections *or* vaccines. In some cases, the consequence is chronic infection, such as recurrent ear, sinus or respiratory infections. In other cases, the immune system becomes so dysregulated that a cascade of atypical inflammatory or autoimmune activities in the body begins. Interestingly, children with autism almost universally suffer from chronic infections or other atypical immune activity, such as overactive immune response.

According to the Autism Research Institute and the Lyme-Induced-Autism Foundation, many children with autism are in a state of chronic inflammation, where their immune systems are unable to shut off or kick out pathogenic invaders, such as:

- *Borrelia* bacteria or other bacteria associated with Lyme disease and coinfections
- *Streptococcus* bacteria, associated with a condition known as PANDAS: Pediatric Autoimmune Neuropsychiatric Disorders Associated with Streptococci
- Measles virus (as was found by Dr. Wakefield in the biopsied intestines of children with autism)
- Herpes viruses
- Epstein-Barr virus, among others.

Chronic inflammation and autoimmunity are increasingly recognized as central to the pathophysiology of autism in many afflicted children. Laboratory tests currently offered by companies such as Metametrix, Great Plains Laboratory, Doctor's Data, Genova, and others have been used widely to detect which sorts of pathogens have set up camp in individuals with autism. Parents who have recovered their children from autism often claim that recovery came only as soon as they were able to identify the resident pathogens, and then regulate their child's immune system enough to be able to effectively battle the pathogens. These children spend every day fighting an immunological battle. Parents have used all sorts of antimicrobial products and treatment protocols, including antibiotics, antifungals, natural herbal antimicrobial remedies, homeopathic remedies, and many others, to help their children battle the germs camped out in their guts and other tissues. Those who recover their children from autism have regulated their immune systems and beat the "bugs." And thousands of children have recovered.

There are children with autism who have never been vaccinated. Clearly, for these children, vaccination played no role in their condition. Again, autism and other chronic inflammatory illnesses most frequently occur as a result of a perfect storm of environmental and genetic factors. For some children, environmental factors such as antibiotic use, maternal health, and environmental toxins played a larger role in their disease etiology. For others, vaccines played a leading role. There are many parents of children with autism who argue that vaccines caused their child's autism, or that they regressed into autism shortly after being vaccinated—most often with a live attenuated virus. This story is told time and again within the autism community. It is unknown to what degree vaccination could be a sole causative agent in the development of autism, but it has certainly played a significant role for many who struggle with chronic immune dysregulation. If vaccines cause autoimmunity, Th2 skewing and other dysregulations of the immune system, then they could certainly play a role in the etiology of autism as well as other chronic inflammatory childhood conditions.

A Tragic Case Study Illustrates the Disastrous Potential of Underrecognized Immune Dysregulation

In a tragic case study documented in 1999, a seemingly healthy twenty-one-month-old boy developed measles inclusion-body encephalitis (MIBE), a severe neurological event, resulting in brain damage, eight and a half months after receiving the MMR vaccine. Lab work determined that the measles virus that had caused the inflammation in his brain and body was the vaccine strain. He had no other evidence of infection (no rash, fever, etc.) after the MMR shot or prior to the onset of MIBE. There was no prior evidence of immunodeficiency in this boy, but upon hospitalization for MIBE, they found that he had dys-gammaglobulinemia, which refers to abnormal levels of certain im-munoglobulins/antibodies. Also of interest, this boy also had evidence of oral thrush (*Candida* of the mouth) and a *Candida*-related diaper rash. While hospitalized, he had repeated seizures and was found to have *Campylobacter upsaliensis* in his blood, and he died after fifty-one days in the hospital.[55]

According to his medical history, this boy was considered normal prior to MIBE, but his imbalanced levels of antibodies, *Candida* in-fections and *Campylobacter* in the blood are clear clinical indications that he was immunocompromised. This boy had no other patholo-gies, such as HIV or leukemia, that could be responsible for compro-mising his immune system. The investigators who examined this boy's case agreed that they could not find evidence of any sort of classic immunodeficiency syndrome, and attributed his case to some un-known or unspecified "primary immunodeficiency" (like a congenital immunodeficiency) without ever investigating possible environmental factors that could have precipitated his condition. It is uncertain whether this boy was immunocompromised prior to his MMR shot, which would have precipitated a chronic battle with the measles virus, or whether the MMR *caused* this boy to become immunocompro-mised, since measles virus is known to suppress the immune system, but something in his experience caused immunological impairment that ultimately resulted in his death. This boy was unable to effectively fight the measles virus he received from a vaccination, and it led to a tragic neurological consequence. The point of this story is that chil-dren with immune dysregulation may not have commonly recognized signs or symptoms of immunodeficiency, and exposure to infectious agents, either naturally or through vaccines, can have disastrous con-sequences for them.

Very few doctors would consider a thrush infection or a *Candida* diaper rash outward signs of immunodeficiency that should be inves-tigated prior to vaccination. In fact, few worry about vaccinating im-munocompromised or sick children. The CDC recommends that clinical signs of infection (including low grade fever, diarrhea, ear infection, etc.) should *not* preclude vaccination. This is because enough studies have been done in vaccinated immunocompromised patients with few cases of severe adverse events occurring immediately following vaccination. However, few studies actually follow these patients long term to see if problems develop later, or evaluate how effectively the patient's immune system is able to fight the infection.

Typically, researchers use antibody response or antibody levels as an indication that the vaccine worked. If the antibody levels are there, the vaccine is considered effective. If no serious adverse event occurs within twenty-four, forty-eight or seventy-two hours (and sometimes as long as several weeks) later, then the vaccine is considered safe. As the prior case study illustrates, a lack of immediate adverse event does not mean that the child's immune system is effectively managing the vaccination. This boy experienced an adverse event *eight months* after immunization. Interestingly, many parents of children with autism report that their children either immediately or slowly developed autism after a live virus vaccine, a possible indication that their bodies were struggling to fight off the infection because they were immunocompromised at the time of the vaccination.

Although this case study represents an *extremely* rare sort of event, the clinical story is significant because it is not unlike the bizarre immunological dysfunction that is seen in children with autism. This boy's chronic battle for over eight months against the measles virus is similar to the chronic infections suffered by children with autism. What Dr. Andrew Wakefield found in the intestines of children with autism was a chronic infection with live measles virus of the vaccine strain.[56] Other studies have found chronic infections with varicella zoster virus (chickenpox). A similar case reported in the literature in 2005 describes a previously healthy four-year-old boy who developed a chronic infection with varicella virus for over a year and a half, a finding considered "extraordinary" by the investigators.

Typically, varicella is no longer detectable in the blood within weeks of acute infection. The investigators were unable to explain the reason for the boy's chronic infection; primary immunodeficiencies, such as HIV and congenital issues, were ruled out. They did note, however, that the boy had a history of chronic ear infections and some asthma symptoms, which are signs of immune dysregulation, prior to the chickenpox.[57] These are two very rare studies published in the literature, but they reflect a larger trend of underrecognized immune dysregulation in American children that can lead to severe consequences, such as adverse reactions to vaccines, severe acute and subclinical chronic viral infections, and even regressive autism. It is unknown how many American children with immune dysregulation are battling subclinical chronic infections, but it is a phenomenon that merits further investigation, given the disastrous consequences demonstrated by these case studies.

What these case studies provided for investigators was the opportunity to do an immunological work up on seemingly healthy patients that had an adverse response to a virus or a live virus vaccine. No one fully understands why some people respond adversely to vaccines while others are fine. Many immunocompromised patients have received the measles and chickenpox vaccines without serious adverse events. Yet, cases like these should force us to closely examine why these boys, and many children with autism, were unable to kick out the viruses. The measles case study, and other rare occurrences like it, does not prove that immunocompromised children will develop MIBE or measles infection after receiving the MMR, nor does it indicate that all seemingly healthy children are in some way immunocompromised, but it does make us reflect on our existing one-size-fits-all immunization protocol. Given the epidemic of immune dysregulation in this country, we can no longer assume that all children who appear to be healthy are necessarily immunocompetent, or that every vaccine is appropriate for every seemingly healthy child on the same standardized schedule. Perhaps it is time for us to take a more individualized approach to childhood immunization so that we can protect the greatest number of children from harm.

What's Mercury Got to Do with It? Tying Mercury, Autism, Vaccination, Gut Dysbiosis and Immune Dysregulation All Together

In recent years, the debate over vaccines has become increasingly focused around the role of mercury. Many parents of autistic or vaccine-injured children hold the mercury preservative in vaccines — thimerosal — responsible for damaging their children. Some vaccine safety advocates seem as if they are obsessed with mercury. David Kirby's book *Evidence of Harm* only heightened the anxiety over mercury in vaccines. An interesting twist in the mercury-autism story occurred in 2000, when the vast majority of mercury was removed from childhood vaccines. A notable amount of mercury still exists in vaccines, if you consider the cumulative effect of yearly flu shots from the age of six months on, but this amount pales in comparison to the quantities of mercury injected into children prior to 2000. Yet, despite the removal of the vast majority of mercury from the infant immunization schedule, rates of autism continue to rise at breathtaking rates.

That autism rates continue to climb, despite the removal of much of the thimerosal, only highlights that autism has a profoundly complex etiology. As previously discussed, mercury may affect some children, and not others, depending on the health and vitality of the individual's detoxification pathways. A child with gut dysbiosis, immune dysregulation, and low levels of glutathione cannot effectively clear toxins (chemical, metal or biological) from their body — which makes a vaccine a toxic assault on their body, especially if it contains mercury. Vaccines containing thimerosal may be of little consequence to a child with a healthy gut and a healthy immune system. Again, the friendly bacteria in the gut help to detoxify mercury in the body; if we do not have these friendly bacteria, we are unable to excrete the mercury and it is stored, in various forms and locations, throughout the body, resulting in physiological problems.

If a child cannot properly process toxins like mercury, then *no* amount of mercury, even the small amount in flu shots, is safe for that child. Furthermore, some researchers speculate that pathogenic microbes that inhabit the gut in lieu of the friendly bacteria actually use minerals and heavy metals to create a matrix known as a biofilm to bind colonies of their brethren together. Biofilms exist throughout the body, and can thus serve as an additional way for a body to store heavy metals. Formation of biofilms with mercury or other metals may present another toxic burden on the body, as it is difficult for the immune system to overcome pathogenic biofilms. It is plausible that mercury from vaccines can be retained in the bodies of children with certain physiological imbalances (gut dysbiosis). Exposure to mercury, even in small doses, could then be considered harmful.

Does this then mean that thimerosal-free vaccines do not play a role in the etiology of autism? Not necessarily. Again, a child with gut dysbiosis and immune dysregulation may have difficulty processing *other* toxins found in the vaccines, such as aluminum. Vaccines can also provide a vehicle for infectious agents to enter the body (such as measles virus) and precipitate chronic infection, as illustrated in the case studies of the two boys who could not kick out their infections. They can also stimulate immune dysregulation by repeatedly presenting an unusual immunological challenge to the body while the immune system is still developing and maturing. As previously discussed, vaccines have been associated with autoimmunity, Th2 skewing and generalized dysregulation of the immune system. These events occur with or without thimerosal. Further research is necessary to determine exactly *how* vaccines work to dysregulate the immune systems of particular children, but it is clear that the more dysbiotic the gut, the greater the immune dysregulation that will be seen.

We do not give vaccines in a vacuum. Every vaccination occurs within a particular environmental context that can be either helpful or harmful to the body's management of that vaccine. If the human body did not have to deal with other environmental burdens, such as poor nutrition, chemical toxins, stress, etc., then vaccines might be readily tolerated by all children. Unfortunately, this is not the world that we live in. Environmental burdens can actually make vaccines ineffective or toxic to us. For example, exposure to environmental toxins has been shown to reduce a body's immune response to vaccines and impede its ability to produce antibodies. In one study, rhesus monkeys were exposed to polychlorinated biphenyls (PCBs) and then injected with sheep erythrocytes (red blood cells) to see if toxins modified the monkey's ability to build antibodies to the sheep cells. What the researchers found was that the PCBs did, in fact, reduce the antibody response to the sheep cells in the monkey (along with other immunological changes), leading to the conclusion that environmental toxins can contribute to the dysregulation of our immune systems. Perhaps vaccines are inherently less effective and more harmful when administered in a toxic world.[58]

When Vaccinating Babies, Genes and the Environment Matter

Toxic exposures have been shown to negatively impact immune responses during vaccination, but evidence also indicates that other types of environmental factors might be able to mitigate this influence. For example, breastfeeding influences the development of an infant's immune system, and it can even modulate vaccine responses in infants. Studies have shown that some breastfed babies develop different, more robust responses to vaccines than formula fed babies. One study found that breast-fed babies "induced higher serum antibody responses to *oral* polio vaccination but not to other systemic vaccines." But the breastfeeding question is complicated because while some studies demonstrate an immunological benefit with regard to vaccination and reduced atopic disease, other studies have shown the opposite results. This may have to do with the health of the baby's mother, and her gastrointestinal health in particular. The DNA of microbiota in a mother's gut can be transferred to a baby's gut via breast milk (via "an endogenous cellular route").[59] These transfers could impact the development of a baby's immune system in a positive or negative way, depending on maternal gut health. Thus, breastfeeding could be an important way to mitigate some of the immune dysregulating influences of our modern world, including vaccination, but only if the lactating mother has good gut health.

Each child responds differently to each vaccination. There are scientific explanations for this that are not currently incorporated into public health immunization protocols. The current vaccine protocol is standardized for all children, but children have a multiplicity of genetic and environmental variables that predetermine whether or not the vaccines will work for them, and whether or not they will respond adversely to the vaccines. Children with gut dysbiosis often lack the healthy bacteria that produce key immune cells (e.g., lacking antibody producing lymphocytes, or T-cell regulatory capabilities), and thus may not be able to stimulate appropriate immune responses to vaccination. The consequences of this early immune dysregulation can include reduced efficacy of vaccines, and the development of chronic illnesses later in life.

Dr. Patrick G. Holt and Dr. Julie Rowe of Telethon Institute for Child Health Research in Australia argue that it is important to understand factors that precipitate early immune dysregulation as it determines outcomes with regard to vaccine efficacy and the long-term health of children:

> There is some evidence to suggest that delayed Th1 maturation may reduce the capacity of children at high risk of atopy to respond to vaccination efficiently in infancy. In response to BCG [Bacillus Calmette-Guerin] vaccination [tuberculosis vaccine not mandated in US] in infancy, for example, failure to develop long-lasting delayed-type hypersensitivity responses to tuberculin was associated with increased risk of atopy at 12 years. In addition, children who develop atopic dermatitis had a reduced ability to respond to pneumococcal vaccinations. With regard to the DTP vaccine, it has been observed that infants at high risk of atopy had specific responses to tetanus toxoid that were consistently more Th2 skewed, displaying higher Th2/Th1 ratios. . . . Furthermore, in another study we have shown that in vitro proliferative responses to tetanus toxoid during infancy were inversely related to the atopic phenotype.[60]

These studies are important because clearly children with an increased risk of atopy (as determined by genetics, microbiota in the gut, or other factors) may have a reduced response to vaccines and a higher likelihood of developing chronic illnesses, such as allergies or asthma, later in life. Perhaps we should be screening children for these variables and making modified vaccine schedules that mitigate the risk of developing chronic illness for these children.

The American vaccine program does not need to be scrapped. Instead, it needs to be reevaluated, and as Dr. Bernadine Healy argues, more research needs to be done to assure the public that the vaccination schedule is as safe as it can possibly be for our children. If, however, vaccines are definitively proven by medical science to cause immune dysregulation, then we need to determine how we can mitigate or prevent the immune dysregulation in vulnerable children. Many alternative practitioners argue that vaccine damage can be prevented by a) adding high doses of vitamin A and vitamin C supplements prior to and following vaccination b) assuring that no child who is ill or on antibiotics is ever vaccinated and c) not giving Tylenol or other glutathione depleters anywhere near the vaccination. It is possible that a safe vaccine protocol can be established so that all children are protected against horrible diseases like Haemophilus influenza type B and pertussis, but additional steps or new elements may need to be added to the existing protocol. This may include removing some of the nonessential vaccines from the schedule.

DÉTENTE: MOVING AWAY FROM CONSPIRACIES AND TOWARD SOLUTIONS

Some people argue that vaccine manufacturers, in collusion with corrupt government officials, are trying to force people to vaccinate *just* so they can make money. While this is certainly a possible scenario, there are a lot easier ways to make money than through vaccines. No pharmaceutical company *really* wants to be in vaccine manufacturing. It's not a terribly profitable business, and the associated liability is enormous. In fact, most manufacturers have tried to get out of vaccine production at one time or another simply because it is an ugly business with not much upside. While there may be collusion between the vaccine manufacturers and the federal government to try to cover up some of the potential damaging effects of vaccines in an effort to limit liability and to protect the immunization program, no pharmaceutical company wants to bring this liability upon themselves.

Safe and effective vaccines are extremely difficult to make, expensive, and not terribly profitable. According to the Jordan Report, a vaccine report put out by the National Institution of Allergy and Infectious Diseases, "The costs of vaccine development have been estimated to range generally from $300 million to $800 million. [In 2006,] Costs for development of live attenuated influenza vaccine may have exceeded $1B. Few private firms are willing or able to make those kinds of financial commitments."[61] When they do make these kinds of commitments, return on their investment is not guaranteed. For example in 2004, after much pressure to rapidly produce influenza vaccine for the upcoming flu season, the vaccine manufacturer Chiron was forced to shut down their influenza production facilities because the British government and the FDA found that their plant was contaminated with *Serratia marcescens*, a mildly pathogenic strain of bacteria. The risk of contaminated vaccines must be prevented, even if it means that the manufacturer loses out. Flu vaccines are notoriously difficult to develop and produce, and they must be done on an extraordinarily tight timeframe. In this particular scenario, Chiron lost on all accounts. In 2000, Wyeth, another vaccine manufacturer, stopped producing DTP vaccines (when they were asked to remove thimerosal), as retooling their factories to remove thimerosal from the production process would have made production of the DTP shot cost prohibitive.[62]

In 1967, twenty-six companies made vaccines in the United States. In 2006, there were four manufacturers (Merck, Sanofi, Glaxo-SmithKline, Wyeth) producing the bulk of our vaccines (two others, Chiron and Medimmune, manufacture flu vaccine). The companies that do make vaccines have to be large enough to shoulder the tremendous liability should something go wrong. Some of the original vaccine makers consolidated through mergers and acquisitions, but others, such as Eli Lilly, Pitman-Moore, Pfizer, Cutter, and Parke Davis, dropped out. Pfizer does still make vaccines, but only for pets and livestock, a market infinitely less vulnerable to litigation.

To illustrate the point further, preventative medicine is never as profitable as the treatment of chronic illness and the vaccine business could not survive without external financial, governmental and legal support. In 2005, vaccines "made up 10 percent or less of the sales of the four big companies." Without the support of government (e.g., the NIH subsidized a new $150 million flu vaccine plant for Sanofi-Pasteur) and private donors, such as the Bill and Melinda Gates Foundation, and protection by the federal government from liability (e.g., the 1986 Vaccine Compensation Act), more vaccine manufacturers would likely drop out.[63] The development and marketing of vaccines *is* a money-making enterprise, but it is also high risk and carries a high probability of product failure. The federal government and other sources of external support enable this industry to even exist. We would not be able to have a national health program to protect us from infectious diseases were it not for this liaison.

However, this liaison should not protect the vaccine industry if they are producing vaccines that are not safe, nor should it allow the federal government to mandate excessive vaccines because of their close relationship with the vaccine industry. We can waste our time looking for the political economy conspiracies within government and the vaccine industry, or we can instead put pressure on the appropriate authorities to do the research necessary to ensure that our childhood immunization program is as safe as it can possibly be. Of course the federal government and the vaccine industry are in collusion. They have to be to make the whole concept of massive public immunization work. But it is our responsibility, as citizens, to ensure that this collusion does no harm. As there is mounting evidence of harm associated with our existing childhood immunization program, it is now time for us to pressure our leaders to rigorously examine the safety and merit of this program as it exists today.

Again, vaccines are only one piece of the complex puzzle of chronic childhood illness. Conditions like autism are the result of a number of environmental variables all working together to create vulnerabilities in our immune systems that lead to larger physiological dysfunctions. A study published in the journal *Pediatrics* in 2000 reminds us of this important fact. The study looked at the presence of atopy (or allergic disease) in families with an anthroposophic lifestyle as compared to other, more typical, American families. An anthroposophic lifestyle is one that encourages the use of natural methods for the promotion of health and wellness. These families typically do not use many vaccines, pharmaceuticals or other modern healthcare interventions. As the authors describe it, "Anthroposophic lifestyle includes the restricted use of antibiotics and vaccinations, and the increased consumption of fermented vegetables that promote the growth of lactobacillus plantarum." In this study, most of the children with an anthroposophic lifestyle had been vaccinated, but only with the tetanus and polio, and much later than typical children.

After comparing differing environmental factors, the researchers found that children with an anthroposophic lifestyle have lower rates of atopy than their age-matched conventional-medicine-using peers. (See table 6.)[64]

A similar study conducted in 2005 and published in *Pediatric Allergy and Immunology* compared the gut microbiota of children with an anthroposophic lifestyle with that of their conventional peers. The researchers found that the children with an anthroposophic lifestyle had a greater diversity of *Lactobacilli* (probiotic bacteria) in their fecal samples as well as higher levels of other probiotic bacteria, such as *Enterococci*.[65] These bacteria levels were negatively correlated with the presence of atopic disease. The anthroposophic children with better profiles of fecal bacteria also had lower rates of atopic disease. It all comes back to the gut. Many lifestyle factors affect the gut flora with meaningful clinical consequences.

Now What?

In order to diffuse the great vaccine debate and create a national childhood infectious disease management program that is universally trusted, a few key steps need to be taken:

TABLE 6. CHILDREN OF ANTHROPOSOPHIC LIFESTYLE VS.
CONVENTIONAL PEERS

Environmental Factors	Anthroposophic Children	Conventional Peers
percent of children had received antibiotics	52 percent	90 percent
percent of children vaccinated for MMR	18 percent	93 percent
percent consuming fermented vegetables	63 percent	<5 percent
Consumption of organic or biodynamic food	Higher	Lower
Clinical symptoms of atopic disease	13 percent	25 percent
Bronchial Asthma	5.8 percent	17 percent
Positive Skin Prick Test (IgE test indicating allergy)	7.2 percent	13 percent

1) We need to monitor the long-term effects of our current childhood immunization program by conducting a large unbiased epidemiological study comparing vaccinated to unvaccinated children. We also need to fund and support extensive laboratory research to elucidate the full immunological impact of the existing vaccine program in children.

Recent developments in Congress indicate that these are not such outlandish ideas. In May of 2009, U.S. Representative Carolyn Maloney (NY) and U.S. Representative Christopher Smith (NJ) introduced into the House, H.R. 2618: *Vaccine Safety and Public Confidence Assurance Act of 2009.* This bill proposes the establishment of an independent vaccine research and surveillance agency that will be charged with improving vaccine safety and public confidence in vaccines. The authors of this bill indicate that the current surveillance of vaccine safety (limited to acute adverse events) is inadequate and that public confidence in vaccines will continue to erode until vaccines are studied for their role in chronic illness. Although the specifics of proposed studies are not detailed in the bill, there is mention of the need for additional long-term epidemiological as well as in vitro laboratory studies pertaining to vaccine safety.

Should this bill make its way through Congress and into the implementation phase, the new vaccine research and surveillance agency needs to first focus on epidemiological studies looking at chronic illness.

These studies should include large numbers of children with well-documented health and mental health records. Researchers should document other lifestyle factors that might impact gut and immune health, such as history of antibiotic or other pharmaceutical use, diet and nutrition, family history, and potential toxin exposures. This study has to be designed in collaboration with parents of children with chronic illnesses such as autism.

2) We need to better understand the immune function of fully vaccinated children as compared to unvaccinated children.

The scientific literature indicates that vaccines do alter a body's immunological pathways. The degree to which this is clinically or epidemiologically meaningful has not been determined with certainty. Studies evaluating the immune function of the two groups should be comprehensive and reflective of real-life immunization experiences. Researchers need to use clinical parameters (symptoms, clinical history) as well as laboratory parameters (antibody response, T-cell function, etc.) in the analysis. If the above epidemiological study requires us to make modifications to the existing immunization program, the information necessary to guide these decisions will come out of this type of research.

3) We need to invest more research dollars into immunology.

We know so much about the human body and the immune system, yet we understand so little. We currently operate in a vaccine-based paradigm, where we believe that most serious infectious diseases can best be prevented through vaccination. Is this true? A paradigm shift is in order. Insight into how we might be able to avoid (or treat) infectious diseases without vaccination by controlling, regulating or fortifying immune responses might just be the wave of the future. But we will never realize this future until we make an investment in it. The NIH's Human Genome Project, or the Human Microbiome project are great models for the type of commitment we need to make to understanding immunology in the twenty-first century. Let us initiate the "Human Immunology Project." The bottom line is, more research needs to be done. The great divide between those who trust vaccines and those who do not needs to be narrowed, and this will never occur until more research elucidates the impact of vaccination on children's developing immune systems.

We live in a toxic world. Everything we do, everything we eat, touch, taste, smell, and see is potentially toxic to our bodies, which struggle to adapt to these new and hostile surroundings. The good news is that it is within our power to turn this epidemic around. If we can isolate the environmental variables causing our children to be sick, then we can eliminate or modify these factors so that our children can grow up in a safe and healthy world.

chapter 9

Healing the
Children

People with chronic illnesses are notorious for trying anything and
everything in an effort to recover. Sometimes their efforts pay off,
sometimes they do not. But following the trail of those who have recovered from chronic illness can provide important insights into the
etiology of particular illnesses. It may seem like an unscientific or cir-
cuitous way to get at the root cause of a particular illness, but it is the
approach taken by millions diagnosed with chronic illnesses—illnesses that are called chronic precisely because there are no well
known or established cures.

Millions of children are affected by the epidemic of chronic illness in this country. Luckily, thousands of trailblazing children have

recovered from their illnesses—the very same illnesses that their doctors told them they would have for life. In the case of chronic childhood illnesses like autism, allergies, or asthma, it has long been
assumed that the best that any one patient could hope for would be
to effectively manage the symptoms of the illness. This is no longer
the case. The cures exist, and recovery happens, it just tends to happen
outside the conventional western medical paradigm.

In this chapter you will read the stories of families who have recovered their children from chronic illnesses: two children with food allergies, one child with allergies and asthma, and two families with
children with autism. These children did not rely on conventional
western medicine to heal them and they had to venture out onto the
fringe of socially acceptable or understood treatment protocols. This
can be difficult to do, especially if your pediatrician or friends and
family do not support your efforts. But they did it, and their children
are reaping the benefits every beautiful, illness-free day of their lives.

THE RECOVERED

Anaphylactic Allergy: Jack

Peanut anaphylaxis, the severe and life-threatening allergy to peanuts,
is something that every parent dreads for their child. A child who experiences an anaphylactic reaction to a particular food may experience swelling, difficulty breathing, hives, sweating, heart rate changes,
diarrhea, or other severe symptoms. In some cases, exposure to even
the smallest airborne particle of peanut can cause a child's throat to
swell and their blood pressure to drop, and they can lose consciousness. If appropriate rescue measures are not taken shortly after exposure to the allergen, an anaphylactic reaction can be deadly.

Jack is one of those unfortunate kids who developed a severe allergy
to peanuts. When Jack was nineteen months old, he had his first taste
of peanut butter and quickly ended up in the hospital. Upon ingesting
a small amount of peanut butter on a cracker, Jack's face swelled, he
broke out in large hives, and his eyes swelled shut. Jack was rushed to

the hospital where he was given Benadryl and steroids, and monitored closely. He recovered from this severe allergic reaction, but his parents soon learned that many elaborate precautions would have to be taken to ensure that this sort of thing did not happen again.

Jack's parents, Suzi and John, went to extraordinary lengths to educate teachers, schools, caregivers and family members about the danger that peanuts posed to Jack. Suzi even considered homeschooling because she was concerned about the risk of exposure in a school setting. According to Jack's physicians, even exposure to an airborne particle of peanut could have deadly consequences for Jack. There were other exposures throughout Jack's childhood. The mere act of opening a jar of peanut butter would make Jack itch, swell and turn red. Jack learned to always carry an epi-pen, an emergency shot of epinephrine that could save his life in the event of accidental exposure.

While Suzi and John did everything they could to protect Jack from accidental peanut exposure, they simultaneously began to look for answers as to why Jack developed this allergy in the first place. Jack's family has no history of food allergies, no autoimmune disease, or other indications that his allergy might somehow be a function of genetics. They took Jack to see many allergists throughout Ohio and Michigan, looking for answers. It was here that they learned that Jack's IgE (immunoglobulin E) levels for peanuts were off the charts. The allergists could validate that Jack did, indeed, have a severe peanut allergy, but they were not able to provide much comfort beyond this knowledge. The only answer they got from allergists was to "stay away from peanuts, and carry an epi-pen."

Unsatisfied with the answers offered by conventional medicine, Suzi took Jack to see a homeopath. Unsure as to whether or not the homeopathy was helpful in addressing Jack's peanut allergy, Suzi also took him to see a naturopath, Dr. AnnAlisa Behling, who practices an allergy elimination technique called NAET, or Nambudripad's Allergy Elimination Technique. NAET is a treatment developed by a physician and acupuncturist, Dr. Devi Nambudripad, that helps relieve people of allergies and many other health issues. The technique is derived from principles of energy medicine and traditional Chinese medicine, where certain acupressure points are manipulated in order to help the body release allergic and immune-based reactions. Ultimately, NAET helps to balance and regulate the body's immune responses.

Jack worked with Dr. Behling for about a year to address the underlying immune dysregulation that manifested itself in a severe peanut allergy. By the end of the year, Jack could put a spoonful of peanut butter in his mouth with no problems whatsoever. In the eyes of Suzi and John, this was nothing short of a miracle, given the severity of their son's previous reactions to peanuts. In the course of Jack's yearlong NAET treatments, they also learned that Jack had other sensitivities (such as salt, yeast, and egg) that may have been affecting his health in more subtle ways. Jack was treated for all of these sensitivities and is now a healthy and allergy-free nine-year-old. Jack and his family no longer worry about the life-threatening possibility of peanut exposure. Now, Jack is able to be a normal carefree kid—the way kids should be.

Food Intolerances: Cole

Food sensitivities or intolerances are often overlooked by many doctors because they are not considered to be true allergies (IgE-mediated). This does not mean they are not clinically meaningful. Many people with food sensitivities do not even know that they have them, but they can suffer from serious health problems if these sensitivities are not addressed. Cole, a ten-year-old boy into cooking and Tai Kwon Do, was one of these individuals. Although he was never diagnosed with food allergies in the traditional sense, his health and early childhood were quite severely impacted by his body's inability to tolerate wheat and dairy.

Cole's mother Katrina was not immediately aware that her son had food intolerances. As a newborn, he had eczema on his body and she recalls that he was a pretty "gassy" baby, subtle signs that his body was not responding well to certain food antigens in breast milk or formula. Cole had other signs of immune dysregulation, including chronic ear infections in his first year of life and an allergy to certain antibiotics. He was also chronically constipated as a baby.

Katrina took Cole to see the pediatrician many times over the next several years for stomach pains, gas, constipation, and diarrhea. Unfortunately, the pediatrician was not able to do much for Cole, aside from recommending that he drink a nondairy formula known as Alimentum. In the meantime, his bowel symptoms continued unabated. By the time Cole was four years old, Katrina made the connection between Cole's dairy consumption and his bowel symptoms. Because dairy is usually consumed daily in a child's diet, it can be hard to isolate this as a contributor to particular health symptoms. By using the diet elimination and challenge technique, Katrina determined that dairy products would cause Cole to have explosive diarrhea. Katrina took Cole to see an allergist, who gave him the gold-standard allergy test—the IgE skin prick test. This test concluded that Cole was not allergic to dairy. This did not seem to add up. Katrina could reproduce the diarrhea symptoms in her son by giving him dairy, and make the symptoms go away by removing dairy, yet the allergist assured her that her son was not allergic to dairy.

Feeling discouraged at the lack of answers from his pediatrician and his allergist, Katrina took Cole to see a pediatric gastroenterologist when he was five years old. It was here that Cole received the less conventional food allergy test, the IgG test, which can help to determine if someone has sensitivities or intolerances to food. Sure enough, Cole's IgG test indicated that he was very sensitive to both dairy and wheat. With IgG test in hand, Katrina immediately removed wheat and dairy from Cole's diet. Within forty-eight hours of these diet modifications, Cole's abdominal pains, diarrhea and constipation cleared up. Clearly, dairy and wheat were a problem for Cole, even though several prior medical doctors assured Katrina that they were not his issue.

Because of this discovery, Cole went dairy-free and wheat-free for four years. At birthday parties he would skip the pizza and take his own wheat-free, dairy-free desserts. Katrina would pack him special foods wherever he went, so that he would not be exposed to the troublesome food. As far as Katrina and Cole were concerned, this was no way for a kid to live.

Katrina had read about a local chiropractor, Dr. Mark Joachim in Norwalk, Connecticut, who practiced an allergy elimination technique known as BioSET. BioSET, developed by Dr. Ellen Cutler, is similar to NAET but uses different instruments and protocols. BioSET utilizes acupressure, enzyme therapy and laws of quantum physics to help redirect and reprogram a body's immune responses to ordinarily benign substances like food. Essentially, BioSET practitioners manipulate the flow of energy in the body in order to modulate immune responses. Cole went through the full BioSET allergy-elimination protocol over the course of several months, and by the time he had finished the protocol he could eat wheat and dairy with no observable symptoms—no diarrhea, no constipation, no abdominal pain. Katrina also used BioSET to clear her own allergies, allergies that she developed as an adult. For her family, Katrina believes that BioSET was "a lifesaver." Cole can now go to school, birthday parties, pizza parties and do all of the normal kid activities without worrying about the consequences of his allergic reactions.

Katrina often wonders how she and her son developed allergies to food.

As a child, Katrina did not have any known food allergies, nor did her husband (although they both now wonder if they had undiagnosed allergies like Cole). Certainly, neither of them experienced symptoms as severe as Cole's when they were children. Yet, Katrina has an unusual past that might provide clues into how members of her family developed dysregulated immune systems.

Katrina grew up near Valley Forge, Pennsylvania, less than seventy miles downwind of Three Mile Island, the site of the worst nuclear reactor accident in U.S. history. The Three Mile Island nuclear reactor meltdown occurred in the spring of 1979. Radioactive gas leaked from the plant, although no one knows exactly how much gas escaped. Several decades later it was determined that there was an increased incidence of certain types of cancer (including lung cancer and leukemia) as well as other health conditions among people living directly downwind of the nuclear plant. A little over a year after the accident, Katrina's mother, who was thirty-five at the time, was diagnosed with multiple sclerosis (MS). There was no other family history of autoimmune disease or MS. Katrina and her family moved away from Pennsylvania when Katrina was sixteen, but health problems continued to plague her family. Her sister developed recurrent endometriosis and Katrina was diagnosed with ovarian cancer at twenty years old.

Katrina initially recovered from her ovarian cancer, only to find three more tumors over the next eight years. One of those tumors was discovered when Katrina was nine weeks pregnant with Cole. At fifteen weeks of pregnancy, Katrina underwent a complicated and miraculous surgery where the physicians were able to remove her tumor but save the baby. During and after the surgery, Katrina was heavily sedated, received antibiotics, and received morphine for nearly a week after the surgery. Katrina carried Cole to term and delivered him via C-section. As is standard for C-sections, Katrina received antibiotics to prevent infections associated with delivery.

After her traumatic battle with cancer and her tumultuous pregnancy with Cole, Katrina developed quite severe environmental allergies and food intolerances. Subsequent to her pregnancy, Katrina became allergic to many foods, including garlic, onions, and other unusual food triggers. At one time, Katrina ended up in the emergency room because exposure to pesticides that had been applied to her lawn caused such a severe reaction that her mouth and throat began to swell and burn.

Katrina senses that whatever happened to her immune system prior to and during her battle with cancer and her pregnancy with Cole, was somehow transferred onto Cole. Although it is not easy to prove, Katrina believes that her family's exposure to the Three Mile Island incident set them up for health problems and these health problems have carried on to the next generation. Fortunately, Cole has been able to recover from his sensitivities to wheat and dairy, and Katrina is now more aware of how food sensitivities, and not just diagnosed IgE allergies can wreak havoc on the body.

Rodger

Unlike Cole, who showed many early signs of immune dysregulation, Rodger was a fairly healthy and typical toddler until he began to show signs of environmental allergies and asthma around three years of age. While he did have eczema (a subtle sign of immune dysregulation) as a baby, there were no other signs that anything was amiss with Rodger as an infant or toddler. Because Rodger's father has known allergies to nuts, they kept highly allergenic foods out of Rodger's diet to protect him from any possible harm. When Rodger entered preschool at three years old, his mother and father, Celia and Rodger Sr., knew they could not control their son's exposure to allergens, so they felt an allergy test was in order. Sure enough, Rodger tested positive on a serum IgE test to shellfish and nuts. Celia and Rodger closely monitored his exposure to these foods from that point on because they knew how dangerous these allergies could be.

During September of his first year at three-year-old preschool, Rodger caught a normal childhood virus and developed a cold with a runny nose, congestion, some wheezing and a persistent cough. Celia took Rodger to the pediatrician, where they were told that Rodger had environmental allergies and asthma, triggered by an infection. Their pediatrician promptly prescribed Zithromax (an antibiotic), Rynatan (an antihistamine), Xopanex (a bronchodialator prescribed for asthma), and prednisolone (a corticosteroid and anti-inflammatory agent). Four medications for Rodger's symptoms seemed like an awful lot at the time, but Celia just wanted her son to get better, so she complied with the physician's recommendations.

About a month later, Rodger developed another cold, with the same symptoms: runny nose, congestion, wheezing and cough. They went back to the pediatrician's office where they were given Xopanex and Rynatan, and this time they were given a new drug, Nasonex (another corticosteroid). That same year, Rodger went back to the pediatrician on several other occasions with the same symptoms and each time he was given more prescriptions. He finally ended up on Singulair, a medication used to treat the symptoms of asthma and allergies. Singulair is a popular, although somewhat controversial, drug as the FDA put out a warning in 2008 because of an increased number of reports of suicidal behaviors among users of Singulair.[1] Celia was told by her pediatrician to give Rodger Singulair every day to prevent symptoms of asthma and allergies. Rodger took Singulair (and some of the other medications intermittently) for nearly two years.

In addition, Rodger's allergist told Celia that Rodger would probably have his allergies and cough for life and that she should consider immunotherapy—a treatment that would require Rodger to get weekly allergy shots for the rest of his life. This suggestion, combined with the overwhelming number of medications that were prescribed to address Rodger's symptoms, began to make Celia feel weary about conventional medicine's approach to allergies and asthma. Celia knew that her son was being drawn into a vicious cycle of pharmaceutical dependency and she was determined to find another way to help him.

It was at this time that one of Celia's coworkers told her how her granddaughter had recovered from celiac disease by going to a BioSET practitioner. Celia liked that BioSET did not require using any drugs, so she found a local practitioner to see if he could help her son. Not long after Rodger began his BioSET treatments, he ate walnuts in a cookie and experienced no allergic reaction, and he was off of all of his asthma and allergy medications with no further symptoms. She made no dietary or other lifestyle changes, and he was able to achieve a full recovery.

Rodger, now seven, has no symptoms of seasonal allergies, asthma, or food allergies. He plays baseball, soccer, golf, tennis, and he loves to swim—all activities that could be difficult for a child with severe environmental allergies or asthma. There is no telling what could have happened to Rodger had Celia kept him on his many medications or had she not found an alternative treatment path for her son. All we know is that Rodger is thriving and living free of allergies, asthma and medications.

Autism: Johnny* and Nate*

Johnny was born in 1997, a year when the word autism was just beginning to make its way into the mainstream media. Johnny was born two weeks early to excited and loving parents, Sarah* and Matt*. Right after Johnny received his hepatitis B vaccine in the hospital, he stopped breathing. Luckily, Johnny recovered from this incident, and after several days in the neonatal intensive care unit, he went home with his parents. Sarah knew right away that something wasn't right with her son. He never made eye contact, and he had chronic acid reflux and would often vomit after nursing. He cried a lot during the first year of his life and always had explosive diarrhea. Sarah took her concerns about her son's physical symptoms and his inability to connect with people to her pediatrician, but because he was gaining weight and hitting certain milestones, her doctor told her not to worry and that he was fine.

There were other signs that something was amiss with Johnny: he didn't like being held or cuddled; he had eczema on his cheeks; he looked pale and sickly; and his hair grew in sparse patches. Although he sat up at seven months, crawled by eight months, and walked at twelve months, Sarah knew that he was not like other kids. He had behaviors that were unusual. He would repeatedly flip pages in a book, or constantly slam doors. Sarah knew at twelve months that her son had autism, but her doctors still said, "Let's wait and see." Because Sarah was persistent in finding out what was wrong with Johnny, she finally got a diagnosis of PDD-NOS (pervasive developmental disorder, not otherwise specified), a subcategory of autism, by the time he was eighteen months old. Highly respected doctors at Cornell University told Sarah and Matt, "I just want to prepare you, your child may never talk." Sarah and Matt were devastated, and secretly, Sarah mourned the life of her son on that very day. It was this same day, however, that this dedicated and tenacious mother also said, "I am not going to accept this!" Thus began the journey into her son's recovery.

Johnny was a very sick toddler; he had chronic ear infections, and by the time he was two years old he had received nearly twenty courses of antibiotics. He just seemed to get sicker and sicker. He had constant postnasal drip that caused a chronic cough and he was eventually diagnosed with asthma. He also had multiple food allergies and was diagnosed with diabetes at two and a half years old. He mostly ate a "white foods" diet, consisting of milk and starches, that is, until Sarah learned about the gluten-free/casein-free diet (GF/CF). Sometime after his second birthday, Sarah began Johnny on the GF/CF diet. Within the first month of the diet he started to talk. He was completely nonverbal prior to the diet, but when he spoke his first words, it came in the form of a ten-word sentence from a familiar book. Sarah felt "like a fog was lifting." The GF/CF diet seemed to benefit Johnny, but he still had severe eczema, wet stools, chronic diaper rash, and other signs of biological impairment. She took him off of soy, and his eczema cleared up, his asthma went away, and his hair started growing in.

It was at this point that Sarah found out about a pediatrician, Dr. Nancy O'Hara, who specializes in treating children with autism through a biomedical (as opposed to therapy-based) approach. Dr. O'Hara was a Defeat Autism Now! doctor, part of the national coalition of clinicians trained to treat autism using a biomedical approach. Sarah immediately took Johnny to see her. Dr. O'Hara ran a number of laboratory tests on Johnny to get a better picture of his many underlying biological problems. The tests revealed that Johnny had severe gut dysbiosis, significant food allergies and sensitivities, and many signs of immune dysregulation. Dr. O'Hara began to address these issues one at a time, hoping to help heal some of Johnny's many dysfunctions.

Several months after Johnny was diagnosed with autism, Sarah gave birth to her second son, Nate. Like his brother before him, Nate showed early signs that something was not right. Sarah describes him as an "expressionless baby." He did not cry, he did not interact; he would just sit and do nothing. By the time he was eight months old, he had flipped to the opposite extreme and would constantly scream and cry, especially when Sarah took him out of the house or around strangers. Nate began to show more classic signs of autism as he got older, like sideways glancing, spinning car wheels and fixating on moving objects like ceiling fans. He also began to show a variety of bizarre behaviors like flipping his eyelids over, and biting the heads off of dolls. He demonstrated significant sensory-seeking behaviors like dragging his head on the carpet or twisting his body into contorted shapes. Sarah knew that she had a second child with autism. Consequently, Sarah sought early intervention services from the state when Nate was only thirteen months old. He was officially diagnosed with PDD-NOS by the physicians at Yale at twenty-two months old.

Because Sarah began the autism biomedical healing journey for both Johnny and Nate at the same time, Nate received many interventions much earlier in his development than Johnny. Nate never ate gluten or casein. Johnny and Nate were both taken off of foods to which they were sensitive or allergic and began a diet known as the Specific Carbohydrate Diet (SCD), developed by Elaine Gottschall. The SCD emphasizes eating specific types of carbohydrates, such as vegetables, rather than grain-based foods like pastas or breads. Sarah also focused on feeding her boys nourishing, organic foods and removed any known toxins from their environment.

When Johnny was four years old and Nate two, Sarah took them to see a homotoxicologist, a practitioner who uses homeopathy to help the body remove toxic and pathogenic influences. In fact, the entire family saw this same practitioner and began treatments aimed at detoxifying the body. Sarah learned that her own body was considered toxic, and stool tests confirmed that she had significant gut dysbiosis. Sarah also had a lot of mercury dental amalgams, which she believes may have contributed to Johnny and Nate's total toxic load. Around the same time that the family began work on detoxification, Dr. O'Hara performed heavy metal tests and found that Johnny, in particular, had high levels of antimony in his body. Antimony is an element used to make children's sleepwear, toys, and mattresses (among other products) flame-retardant. Antimony can be quite toxic if a child's detoxification pathways are in any way impaired, as was the case with Johnny, a boy with significant gut dysbiosis and immune irregularities.

The next intervention that Sarah tried with her boys was aimed at addressing food and environmental allergies and sensitivities with BioSET. When Johnny and Nate began BioSET, they each had many food allergies and sensitivities. One treatment at a time, these allergies and sensitivities were eliminated, and after a few months, the boys could eat foods that once gave them horrible eczema, diarrhea or other symptoms.

Johnny made slow but notable improvements over time, but Sarah saw more significant improvements with Nate. Nate was never as outwardly physically sick as Johnny, but manifested the same intensity of behavior issues. Both boys received therapies like Applied Behavior Analysis (ABA), a comprehensive therapeutic intervention that uses a structured environment to help children learn to modify their behaviors. Sarah believes that ABA was tremendously helpful for both of her boys. The boys continued to follow a healthful diet, free of sugars and processed foods; they took vitamins and other supplements like cod liver oil, folic acid, and probiotics; they continued with behavioral therapies and interventions. Johnny and Nate received many interventions, and the journey was long for Sarah and Matt's family, but no one would dispute that the outcome was well worth the effort.

Nate's autism diagnosis was removed at four and a half years old. Although he was diagnosed with autism before his second birthday, he entered kindergarten as a "normal" boy, and is now a fully recovered, happy, healthy and thriving nine-year-old. He plays football and baseball, has many great friends, and goes to birthday parties all the time. He is very smart and does well in school, particularly in math. Very few people outside of Sarah and Matt's family know that Nate ever had autism. As Sarah says, "He's amazing!"

Like his younger brother, Nate, Johnny's life has been dramatically changed by the many biomedical and behavioral interventions that he has received over his lifetime. Johnny, now eleven years old, is not fully recovered yet, but is considered to have high functioning autism, a term applied to individuals who can function quite normally in many respects but may retain particular traits of autism. Johnny is extremely verbal and is very smart but does have some difficulty with processing speed in school work. He still receives support services in school. He has friends and loves playing computer games online. Many of the physical and neurological problems that plagued Johnny as a young boy are now gone. Johnny was a toe walker and a constant hand-flapper; he had limited speech, significant social and sensory impairments as well as chronic illnesses like ear infections, chronic diarrhea, eczema, asthma and other physical ailments. All of these symptoms are gone. Most people who meet Johnny have no idea how severe his autism was. Rather, many see him as a boy who struggles with learning disabilities and social impairments. He is a friendly, loving, happy boy, still in the process of recovery. At a minimum he will be able to live independently, a dream Sarah never thought he would achieve when he was first diagnosed.

In reflecting on Johnny's recovery, Sarah says, "I never pictured that he would be where he is right now. He is able to do everything for himself, and he constantly wants me to show him how to do more." Johnny's independence and development are far beyond any expectations that Sarah and Matt had for him on the day they were told that he would probably never speak. Nate's recovery is a testament to the fact that full recovery is possible and Johnny gets closer to this reality every day. Sarah and Matt are two dedicated parents who were not willing to accept autism as a lifelong chronic disorder. Because of their commitment to healing and recovery, their boys can now live rich, full, and independent lives.

Autism: Leo*

Upon meeting Leo for the first time, it is difficult to grasp that this friendly, bright-eyed, ten-and-a-half-year-old boy once had autism. Nothing about his demeanor, appearance, or behavior would even suggest that he had any sort of impairment whatsoever. But he did. Leo was diagnosed with autism at two years old by the physicians and researchers at the Yale University Child Study Center. Although it took two years for Leo to get a formal diagnosis, his mother Ashley* knew very early on that something with her baby boy just wasn't right.

After a healthy and normal pregnancy Ashley delivered Leo via C-section. Leo was healthy at birth, with normal APGAR scores and all the signs of being a thriving baby. Ashley began to notice the first signs of something being off with Leo around two months of age; Leo would tremor slightly after nursing. Ashley and her husband took Leo to see a neurologist at the prestigious Mt. Sinai Hospital in New York City, where they were told that the tremors were probably nothing and not to be concerned. Around four months of age, Leo developed severe separation anxiety. "My instinct told me that this was not normal," Ashley recounts, "it was so severe that it just seemed off to me." Despite these early signs, Leo met all of his major development milestones during his first year of life. He rolled over, sat up, crawled and walked—all on time—so Leo's pediatrician did not seem to be concerned that Leo had little to no real verbalization, no babbling or other signs of prelanguage. Ashley began to suspect that her son might have autism after he reached a plateau in development during his second year of life.

Between his first and second year, Leo began to show more signs of autism. He began "stimming" on the wheels of vehicles (obsessively fixating on wheels), he was not developing any speech, and he seemed to be in a fog all the time. Ashley had him evaluated by the state early intervention program where he qualified for speech therapy. After much persistence, Ashley got Leo into the Yale's Child Study Center so that he could be evaluated by top autism experts. When Leo was twenty-four months old, Yale confirmed that, indeed, he was autistic. He had many of the most common characteristics of autism: stimming behavior, social and communication impairments, sensory integration disorder, perseverance (obsessive behaviors), and low frustration point, and he was physically unwell.

With the new diagnosis in hand, Ashley followed the advice of other mothers of autistic children and began Leo on the gluten-free/casein free diet (GF/CF). After only one week with no dairy or wheat, Leo began to talk. He went from no words to many two-word sentences, and Ashley describes it as if a "fog lifted." To be sure, there was much recovery work ahead, but the GF/CF diet gave Ashley the confidence that improvement was possible.

After starting the GF/CF diet, Ashley took Leo to a Defeat Autism Now! doctor and a Defeat Autism Now! dietician who began to treat Leo's biological problems one by one. Leo had many food and environmental allergies, chronic diarrhea, and asthma. Under the advice of her Defeat Autism Now! practitioners, Ashley began to feed Leo a more healthful diet emphasizing organic whole foods and removing allergenic foods that caused inflammation in his body. Ashley felt that the Defeat Autism Now! protocol helped Leo to make incredible gains and that his physical well-being improved substantially. "His eyes, his skin tone, his face looked great." Only six months into the diet changes and biomedical protocol, Leo tested age appropriate for speech. Progress was happening, but his recovery was not complete. Ashley is fond of saying that the biomedical treatment helped to "turn the lights on" in Leo, but it was focused behavioral therapy that corrected his social deficits.

While Leo's biomedical issues were being addressed by the Defeat Autism Now! protocol and diet and environment changes, Ashley began to work intensively on Leo's behavioral training, using techniques that were similar to ABA (Applied Behavioral Analysis). Leo continued to make steady gains from the behavioral therapy, so Ashley sought out highly skilled ABA practitioners to work with Leo. Ashley carefully studied these skilled practitioners as they worked with Leo, and she incorporated ABA into every aspect of their lives. In addition to biomedical and ABA, Leo also worked with a homotoxicologist to detoxify his body, and he saw a BioSET practitioner to address his food and environmental allergies. Ashley also learned homeopathy and used homeopathic remedies to help Leo heal. Ashley believes that biomedical interventions, homeopathy, and energy healing recovered Leo's body so that he could effectively respond to ABA. ABA addressed his social deficits and helped to rewire his brain so that he was able to learn and internalize appropriate behaviors. While ABA and Leo's biomedical treatments resulted in the most immediate and tangible gains, all of the therapies and lifestyle modifications likely played some role in Leo's recovery. Between the ages of two and a half and five and a half, Leo made slow but steady gains, such that he no longer qualified for any special education services.

Before Leo started kindergarten, he officially lost his autism diagnosis. He entered kindergarten without any services or support, and no one, not even his teachers, knew that he was once diagnosed with autism. Today, Leo is a completely "normal" and typical kid. He tests above average on standardized testing and was reevaluated by Yale researchers, who determined that he no longer meets any of the diagnostic criteria for autism. He is very social, friendly, and outgoing. He plays baseball, is a good student, and is popular in school. Ashley knows that her healthy, thriving son would not be anywhere near where he is today had it not been for the many biomedical, healing, and behavioral interventions that he received over his first few years of life.

In fact, Ashley got a second chance to test out these interventions with her second child, Sydney, born just two years after Leo. Like her older brother, Sydney began to show some early signs of autism, including social deficits, sensory integration disorder, food allergies, and other signs of immune dysregulation. A lot more knowledgeable because of her experiences with Leo, Ashley immediately began interventions with Sydney as soon as she saw the familiar signs. Sydney was never vaccinated; she ate the same healthy, organic, whole foods diet as Leo, which included staying gluten-free and casein-free. Despite showing many early signs of autism, Sydney turned a corner toward the end of her first year, and never developed autism. Ashley feels that she saved Sydney from autism.

What caused Leo's autism? Ashley has given this question much thought over the years. Upon reflection, Ashley recalls a number of factors that may have put her son at a high risk for developing autism. These factors include:

- Maternal history of chronic infections:
  - Chronic Lyme—Ashley was diagnosed with chronic Lyme disease years after Leo recovered. Ashley often wonders if the chronic fatigue and chronic colds that she experienced throughout her young adult years might have actually been undiagnosed Lyme disease. It is now believed that Lyme and coinfectors can be transmitted across the placenta from mothers to their babies. Ashley believes that she may have transmitted the Lyme spirochete or Lyme coinfectors (such as babesia) onto her children.
  - Ashley also carries HSV1, the virus responsible for cold sores. HSV1 and other herpes viruses have been found in autistic children in a state of chronic infection.[2]
- Diet—Ashley admits that her family's diet, like that of most American families, was never very good before Leo was diagnosed with autism. As she recalls, "T.V. dinners and McDonalds were staples," but she also grew up in coastal California, where seafood (high likelihood of contamination) was another staple.
- Toxin and pesticide exposure—Ashley grew up in the San Joaquin Valley in California, an important agricultural region. She "routinely saw and smelled pesticide being sprayed" while growing up. She remembers that the tap water that she drank every day growing up had little "flakes" in it, and that it was heavily chlorinated.
- Antibiotic use:
  - Ashley was frequently put on antibiotics during her college years to address minor illnesses, like colds or seasonal allergies.
  - Ashley, like many thousands of women who deliver babies each year, tested positive for group B strep prior to delivery.

Ashley was put on oral antibiotics prior to delivery. The oral antibiotics may have affected her gut flora and predisposed baby Leo to gut dysbiosis and subsequent immune dysregulation.

- Ashley and her husband also believe that their urban lifestyle (with easy access to processed, unhealthy foods, and exposure to many pollutants) may have in some way added to Leo's total toxic burden.

- Years of working in indoor corporate environments prior to Leo's birth may have exposed Ashley and her husband to electromagnetic pollution and indoor air pollution; their careers also keep them cloistered indoors, inhibiting their ability to spend time outdoors in a natural environment.

- Genetic—In Ashley and her husband's family tree you will find a history of allergies and asthma—all illnesses that may indicate some susceptibility to gut dysbiosis, immune dysregulation, or sensitivity to environmental factors.

All of these environmental and genetic factors likely worked in concert to result in a diagnosis of autism for Leo.

Ashley is one of the most dedicated mothers you could ever meet. It was her dedication and love that pulled her children out of the unforgiving grip of autism. Recovering a child from autism is not easy, but it can be done. Ashley can also attest that it is easier to prevent autism in a susceptible child (as with her daughter, Sydney) than it is to recover a child from autism. Ashley recorded her autism recovery journey in an online blog, www.hiddenrecovery.com, so that other parents could benefit from the education she received from her son and his diagnosis. Ashley wants parents to know that there is hope, recovery is possible, and anything can be achieved with love and determination.

For more recovery stories, please go to www.epidemicanswers.org.

chapter 10

What We Can Do to Reverse This Trend

By Victoria Kobliner, MS RD

❧

A NEW FOCUS FOR CHILDREN'S HEALTH

How are we to protect our children from this insidious onslaught of disease? In order to give them the best opportunity for a healthy future, we must look at these chronic illnesses from a new perspective. Instead of focusing on methods of treatment, we must focus on reducing the toxic and inflammatory burden on our children and prevent chronic illness before it begins. We must look outward and take action to limit the toxic overload that is pervasive in our environment. At the same time, we must turn inward and adopt a plan that maximizes the body's ability to heal by supporting optimal digestion, immune function and detoxification.

If such a model of health were implemented in our society, the potential for reducing illnesses would be remarkable. The impact would be far reaching, not only in the tremendous reduction in the burden of healthcare costs but in the increased quality of life for the millions of children and their families affected by these disorders. For such a system to work best, it would require parents and healthcare practitioners to embrace the functional medicine paradigm that has previously been discussed. Since the target is to reduce illness, and consequently the medicalization of our children, through the use of healthy lifestyle principles and good nutrition, it is more appropriate to adopt the term *functional wellness*.

In practical terms, a functional wellness model requires assessing each individual's particular risk factors and then developing appropriate interventions that will address any identified risk factors. Examples of potential risk factors could include a family history of autoimmune disorders, a diet that is high in processed foods, or personal hygiene habits that expose an individual to high levels of chemicals. As mentioned above, the focus must be both outward as well as inward, and as such, an assessment of an individual's risk factors should include:

- Family health history
- Prenatal environmental and occupational exposures (including medication use)
- Current environmental and occupational exposures (of both parents and child)
- Birth and early feeding history
- Current diet
- An individual child's health issues/concerns

Any positive risk factors in these areas should be addressed, either by removing potential problems or by supporting the system to best manage those that cannot be eliminated.

This process will guide many of the daily choices that parents make with regard to the foods their family eats and the household products they use. Potentiating the body's normal biochemical processes by supporting optimal digestion, absorption, immune function and detoxification should be a baseline principle. In all cases, a simple rule of thumb would be that the purer and more natural the item, whether it be food, household cleaner, personal care product or the like, the less toxic it is likely to be.

HOW TO PROTECT OUR CHILDREN

In a society grounded in convenience, technology and consumerism, adopting a functional wellness approach will require some organization and forethought, but is certainly achievable. At the local level, forward thinking parents can spearhead this movement within their own home and neighborhood, by making simple but conscious choices, guided by four important principles. The first two principles concentrate on managing what we take into our bodies, while the second two focus on what we do with those things once they have entered our system:

1. Eat a good clean diet: Consume food and water free of chemicals, pesticides, hormones, antibiotics, artificial colorings, preservatives, flavors, high fructose corn syrup, and other compounds not found in nature.
2. Limit toxins: Although we cannot completely avoid exposure to toxins, we have the power to control some of our exposures. Whether these toxins come from food, water, soil, or air, or whether they are found in furniture, pharmaceuticals, personal care products or large equipment, we can reduce their impact.

3. Promote good bowel function: Taking steps to support good bowel flora (microorganisms), avoiding any food allergies and intolerances, and ensuring appropriate nutrition will enhance gut function.

4. Optimize detoxification: Good bowel support leads to good detoxification. Proper diet supplies the nutrients necessary for normal detoxification to occur. In addition, the use of supportive elements (such as probiotics or other supplements) can further enhance natural detoxification pathways.

It is important to keep in mind that initiating such changes in a family's lifestyle does not have to be undertaken all at once. Small changes still make a difference, and this personal evolution can be achieved with a progression of incremental actions that ultimately lead to much larger changes. Positive changes can be implemented at any time, but can have an especially powerful effect when implemented in the prenatal period. Let us now consider steps that can be taken to provide a nourishing and less toxic environment for a developing baby.

PREPREGNANCY AND PREGNANCY PLANNING

While chronic childhood illnesses are increasing at an alarming rate across the population, segments of the population are at even greater risk for these diseases because of their genetic susceptibility. Any and all concerned parents should establish a plan to potentiate their child's best health, and as mentioned previously, an assessment of individual risk factors will result in the development of a more effective plan.

For the best outcome, this plan must start as early as possible. Even prior to conception, parents should take an active role in the future of their child by assessing their own health status, identifying existing digestive dysfunction, immune dysregulation and noxious environmental burden. The functional wellness principles that are adopted at this stage remain relevant throughout the lifecycle, but the earlier they are adopted, the better.

When we consider the Environmental Working Group's cord blood study referenced earlier,[1] we understand that the placenta cannot, as previously believed, protect the cord blood, and therefore the fetus, from an onslaught of synthetic and potentially life-threatening chemicals. The impact of these chemicals on the unborn child can hardly be imagined. As Congresswoman Nancy Pelosi stated in 2005:

> For years, health experts have told pregnant women not to ingest certain substances, such as alcohol and smoke, that may harm their newborn babies. But today we learn that toxic chemicals in our air and water that are linked to cancer, brain damage, and other birth defects have begun circulating in babies' developing systems even before they have taken their first breath. . . . This new scientific data shows that the developing reproductive, hormonal, and neurological systems of infants are being disrupted by synthetic chemicals that we are exposed to every day.[2]

It is critical, therefore, that we start the process of protecting our children before they are even born, by making sure that their in-utero environment is not setting the stage for long-term problems.

How do we protect children before they are born? First, examine the family history. The existence of digestive disorders, food allergies, eczema, autoimmune disorders, or psychiatric disorders in family members increases the risk of related disorders in genetically vulnerable children.[3] When these risks are known, appropriate steps can be taken to reduce or counteract any potential harm.

Second, assess the mother's current health status, taking into account the following important factors: existence of current illnesses, gastrointestinal health, nutritional quality of diet, past and current exposure to environmental toxins, use of medications or supplements, any existing abnormal laboratory markers, and stress. Many of these factors will be discussed in further detail later in the chapter.

Third, we cannot ignore the impact that fathers have on the health of their offspring. Studies underscore an increased risk of childhood cancer in children whose fathers work in heavy industry and an association between paternal occupational exposure to organic solvents and congenital malformations in their offspring.[4]

Finally, consider any siblings with health concerns as this child can be considered a marker for genetic susceptibility combined with environmental exposure. Siblings share much of the same environment, diet, air quality and other risk factors. If one child is already compromised, a new baby has the potential to suffer from a related or similar disorder, and early action should be taken to limit environmental insults. Once a full assessment has been completed parents can initiate an appropriate plan. Such a plan will remove potential toxins, provide supportive nutrients for fetal development and mitigate the influences that lead to chronic illness.

Following is a detailed discussion of the most important things to include or remove from your lifestyle before becoming pregnant and during pregnancy. If you have children already, these same guidelines can be applied (minus pregnancy-specific nutrients) to help keep your children healthy and ward off chronic illnesses.

Remove Known and Potentially Toxic Substances

Before conception is the best time to clean up the environment in which the family lives, reducing potential exposure to toxins. Conduct a thorough review of the home environment, both inside and out. Personal care products, household cleaners, lawn care products and potential allergens produced from these contaminants should be eliminated. Substitute products that are natural, free of chemicals, pesticides, synthetic dyes, heavy metals and other health risks. Some examples include replacing aluminum-containing items such as deodorant with more natural options, since aluminum is a potent neurotoxin implicated in the development of Alzheimer's and autoimmune disorders.[5]

Fluoride, another neurotoxin, is toxic to children at low doses and should not be ingested via toothpaste, water, or any other means.[6]

Since the public water supply is highly fluoridated in most of the United States, and this water is used for home food preparation as well as industrial food processing and as a source for many bottled waters, there is no way to quantify the true amount of fluoride that an individual ingests. This compound is known to impair fertility in rats and has been implicated in a decrease in birth rates in areas where water is highly fluoridated.[7] A strong association exists between low IQ and highly fluoridated areas[8] and it has also been found in rat brain tissue, complexed with aluminum.[9] The synergistic effects of aluminum and fluoride on brain development are as of yet unknown. These neurotoxins are only two of a long list of seemingly harmless or even supposedly beneficial compounds that we passively accept in our lives.

Since the skin is a large absorptive surface, body washes, shampoos, creams and lotions should be pure as well. In 2004, The Environmental Working Group reported that only 28 of 7500 cosmetic product ingredients had ever been tested for safety by a cosmetics review panel, and the rest had never undergone a public safety review.[10] In addition, although the FDA permits their use in small quantities, there is no data that analyzes the impact of the cumulative use of the substances over time, or the potential impact of them in combination.

Some common but suspect ingredients include triclosan and BHA, to name only two. Triclosan, the agent used in many antibacterial soaps and lotions, has been found in human breast milk[11] and is a possible thyroid hormone disruptor,[12] an immune system toxicant,[13] and an endocrine disruptor[14] that complexes with chlorinated water to form carcinogens.[15] BHA is a ubiquitous preservative that has been implicated in immune system toxicity, is a possible carcinogen, and has been shown to initiate liver damage in rats.[16]

Paint, flame retardant textiles, and detergents are a few of the common household items that often contain known health hazards. Toluene for example, is found in paints, nail polish, aerosols and adhesives. California's Office of Environmental Health Hazard Assessment's Chronic Toxicity Summary of Toluene cites multiple studies of this compound's detrimental effects as both a reproductive toxin and a neurotoxin.[17] Ethoxylated nonyl phenols (NPEs) are a group of endocrine disrupting chemicals commonly found in detergents and in some pesticides. In the European Union they have been removed from laundry cleaners because they have been shown to cause abnormal sexual development in water dwelling organisms and are considered toxic by the Canadian Environmental Protection Act.[18] Another example, Perchloroethylene (PERC), is commonly used in dry cleaning.[19] It is also found in adhesives, inks, lubricants and aerosol products. Short-term exposure can affect the central nervous system, and PERC is "reasonably anticipated to be a human carcinogen."[20] Long-term exposure may also damage liver and kidneys, impair memory and may damage a developing fetus.[21] These are just three examples of numerous compounds that we are unwittingly exposed to in our everyday lives. It must be remembered that these compounds are studied in isolation, not in combination, and research involving infants and children is understandably lacking. The magnitude of the synergistic effect of a multitude of neurological, reproductive and carcinogenic substances on a developing fetus is completely unknown. In addition, the levels of these contaminants continue to rise in our environment, creating a greater burden on our children's detoxification systems than we experienced in our youth.

Include Good Clean Water

Depending upon age and body composition, the human body contains 55-78 percent water. We can live longer without food than when deprived of this important substance. Among a myriad of other roles, water keeps our blood flowing, and is essential for detoxification. It should be obvious that the quality of the water we drink will have a direct impact on our health. Our drinking water must be clean and contaminant free. Unfortunately, while we are led to believe that municipal water supplies provide us with a source of safe drinking water, the truth is quite different.

Wastewater purification policies and strategies are designed to remove sewage sludge, pathogenic microorganisms and some heavy metals from our public water supply. While on the whole, these procedures are effective, there are two problems with the system as it exists. The first problem is that the systems are not designed to remove the increasing load of new or unknown chemicals entering our water supplies. An assessment of water quality by the US Geological Survey and Centers for Disease Control and Prevention found posttreatment evidence of prescription medications and industrial chemicals in local water, which these protocols did not adequately remove.[22] Second, some of the very compounds added to our water can also be toxic to our cells. Chlorine is the predominant disinfectant used in water treatment facilities and its byproducts are of great concern in this regard. There is evidence for its relationship to bladder cancer[23] as well as a link between preterm delivery, low birth weight infants, birth defects, and newborns that are small for gestational age.[24] As previously mentioned, fluoride, also purposely added to the water supply, is another potent neurotoxin. Well water may be no safer, as its purity is dependent upon the often contaminated soil that surrounds it.

It is critical to factor in the quality of the water used not only for drinking but for bath and shower. Because of the high absorptive capacity of the skin, toxins in our water supply will be absorbed rapidly. According to one study that examined the rates of chloroform exposure in water, although ingestion is believed to be the primary source of chloroform from tap water, "inhalation and skin absorption exposure were found to be even higher."[25] In addition to chlorinated byproducts, our water supply contains the aforementioned fluoride as well as the residue of industrial waste and prescription medications that have been flushed down toilets.[26] To complicate matters further, once this water reaches the home, the quality of the pipes that transport it throughout the house will also affect its purity. Pipes may leach lead or copper into the water that comes out of the tap. Testing the water can identify what contaminants are present and help guide the choice of filters. In most cases, a whole house filter is appropriate and in some cases should be combined with point of entry filters that remove contaminants from the pipes. Reverse osmosis systems are most effective at removing the largest number of contaminants, but even a carbon filter will make a considerable difference in water quality.

Include Nourishing and Uncontaminated Food

The food we eat is one of the most powerful resources at our disposal in our quest for optimal health. We have the ability to choose the types and quality of what we put in our mouths and the mouths of our children, positively impacting their health at the most basic level. We know that our digestive system is the first line of defense against toxins, and much of the assault on our digestive system comes directly from the foods we eat. Reducing this body burden will provide a safer environment for a developing fetus. Not only do we remove toxins by providing clean food, but the interplay of vitamins, minerals, antioxidants, phytochemicals, healthy fats, proteins, fiber and complex carbohydrates found in whole foods provide the very source of health itself. Parents have the power of nutrition at their disposal. A few simple guidelines will help parents make good food choices.

1. Choose whole, fresh, unprocessed, organic foods with an appropriate balance of nutrients, including:
    a. Good Quality Protein—meat, poultry, fish and dairy (for those who tolerate it). Nuts, legumes and seeds also provide essential protein.
    b. Fresh Fruits and Vegetables—7-9 daily servings of brightly colored fruits and vegetables are ideal.
    c. Complex, High Fiber Carbohydrates—including less well-known grains like quinoa or millet to supply energy, vitamins and fiber.
    d. Good Fats—Enjoy good fats, such as olive oil and omega-3 fats, (but avoid trans fats) for healthy brain and body cells.
2. Avoid refined and processed foods, including any artificial ingredients, preservatives, colorings, dyes, additives, etc; avoid processed sugars, high fructose corn syrup, and highly refined grains and flours.

Adopting a healthy diet requires an understanding of two different concepts regarding food choice. First, a good balance of foods from different food groups must be achieved. Foods are classified into groups based on the types of nutrients they offer. We eat animal flesh, nuts, seeds and beans for protein and iron (as well as other nutrients), while fruits and vegetables provide fiber, vitamins and minerals. Fats are carriers for fat-soluble vitamins, such as A and D. Without a balance of foods from all these categories, true wellness is difficult to achieve. Be advised that following the USDA Food Pyramid guidelines will not achieve a truly healthy balance.

Many people use the Food Guide Pyramid and the newer My Pyramid to inform them about the appropriate balance of foods in the diet, but in truth, as we've seen before, what we are led to believe is in our best interest is not always based on sound scientific principles. Since 1994, when the first Food Guide Pyramid was launched, and again with the introduction of the 2005 My Pyramid recommendations, many nutrition experts have taken these pyramids to task for being scientifically unsound, politically biased, and unclear. Following are listed a few of the shortcomings inherent in these guidelines:

1) They do not distinguish between healthy and unhealthy fats and recommend limiting all fats with no explanation of the importance of fats such as omega-3s.
2) Within the grain group, there is no distinction between nutritionally vacant, refined, processed carbohydrates and more desirable whole grains.
3) The vegetables group includes both brightly colored non-starchy vegetables and white potatoes within the same category despite vastly different nutrient composition.
4) Grains are touted as the foundation of the diet despite the fact that humans have no dietary requirement for them.
5) Portion size guidelines result in a diet that has less protein and more carbohydrates than is truly healthful.

What is even more troubling is that the very organization that developed these guidelines, the USDA, is also responsible for representing the agricultural interests of farmers trying to sell the very foods that are recommended in the pyramid but are implicated in poor health outcomes. Potato, cattle and dairy lobbies, representing their individual agendas, are but a few of the special interests that played a role in influencing the final design of the pyramid, as well as the wording that supported it. A good balance of foods across the various food groups is important, but the pyramids are not the place to look for guidance.

We can, however, still use the principles of food groups to make meal planning easier. Foods can be grouped into categories based on the nutrients they provide, and then a variety of foods can be selected from within each group. Protein should be eaten at every meal, and good quality protein comes from meat, poultry, and fish; nuts, legumes and seeds also provide essential protein, as well as some carbohydrates and fiber. Protein is also found in dairy products, which also contain calcium and fat soluble vitamins not found in meats. For those that tolerate it, dairy can be a good source of these nutrients.

Fresh fruits and vegetables are an ideal source of energy, antioxidants, fiber and a host of vitamins and minerals. Seven to nine servings daily of brightly colored fruits and vegetables are ideal. Complex, high fiber carbohydrates provide energy, fiber, B vitamins and some minerals. Some less well known grains like quinoa and amaranth are also excellent sources of high quality protein. Finally, the importance of good fats cannot be underestimated, despite the low fat dogma that is so pervasive in our culture. Eat olive oil and omega-3 fats, and avoid trans fats, for healthy brain and body cells.

Not only is the balance of foods important to overall health, but the purity of the food is critical. In the same way that household products and water can be either clean or contaminated, our food supplies run the gamut from factory produced synthetic creations to wholesome gems. Optimally, all food should be organic. Organic food contains less pesticides, chemicals, antibiotics and hormones than its conventional counterparts.[27] As an added benefit, a small group of studies indicate that organic food contains increased levels of nutrients as well.[28] A study by the Environmental Working Group found that people who eat the twelve most contaminated conventionally grown fruits and vegetables consume an average of ten pesticides daily. If it is not possible to eat only organic food, the EWG provides a list of their Dirty Dozen, the most contaminated fruits and vegetables. These include peaches, apples, bell peppers, celery, nectarines, strawberries, cherries, kale, lettuce, grapes, carrots and pears—these foods should be eaten only when organic. In addition, meat, poultry, milk and eggs should be organic in order to avoid the antibiotics and hormones prevalent in the conventional food supply.

Availability of organic food is much greater today than in the past. This can be both a benefit and a challenge to the consumer. On one hand, organic food is more accessible physically and financially as availability increases and price differences between organic and conventional foods diminish. Conversely, as the organic food industry becomes more commercial, small farms and suppliers are being bought out by large conglomerates that stretch the boundaries of organic labeling laws and the basic principles of naturally grown foodstuffs. One has only to look at the practices regarding livestock to see this change. The image of conventional cattle farms often brings to mind visions of sick animals crowded into pens, fed unnatural diets laced with antibiotics, growth hormones, and pesticides and barred from roaming free. On the opposite side, we imagine organic cattle allowed to roam free, happily grazing on fields of grass, calm and stress-free before a humane slaughter. In truth, with the influx of big agri-businesses into the organic industry, we now find organic farms where the cattle are penned for long periods, and are fed an organic yet species inappropriate diet comprised of corn, soy and other grains. Although the avoidance of hormones, pesticides and chemicals is preferable to of the way conventional livestock is fed, we must recognize that cows were not meant to eat soy and corn, and the quality of the meat that comes from these animals will still be subpar when compared to truly free living animals.

Chickens that are housed indoors and fed a diet of grain and soy produce eggs and meat that are as much as ten times lower in omega-3 fatty acids than pasture fed birds.[29] Free-range chickens also provide more than their caged counterparts of several nutrients essential for normal detoxification pathways, including folic acid and vitamin B12, as well as vitamin E and beta-carotene, two important antioxidants.[30] Eggs are also a good source of choline, an important nutrient required for normal neurotransmitter function.

Grass-fed beef is also better for human health than its grain-fed counterparts along a number of nutritional parameters. It is lower in fat, has a more balanced ratio of omega-3 to omega-6 fatty acids, and it has more total anti-inflammatory omega-3s. Grass-fed beef also contains more calcium, magnesium, and potassium, B vitamins, vitamin E, and beta-carotene.[31] Grass-fed beef also contains more Conjugated Linoleic Acid (CLA), another important fat that may have cancer-fighting activity.[32] Although research results on human subjects are mixed, CLA has also been shown to reduce obesity and beneficially increase bone mass in animal studies.[33] Cattle fed on grass provide meat that is 3-5 times higher in CLA than conventionally farmed cattle.[34]

Farmed salmon also pales in comparison to wild caught varieties when toxin levels are assessed. In a 2004 study of more than two metric tons of fish, the farmed salmon had significantly higher levels of thirteen out of fourteen organochlorine toxins than the wild variety.[35] Fishmeal fed to farmed salmon is often contaminated with PCBs, which are then deposited in the fatty tissue. Since farm raised fish generally contain more fat than wild salmon, the retention of PCBs is magnified. In sum, those seeking the healthiest and most nutritious animal protein should choose grass-fed meats, meat and eggs from free-range poultry, and wild fish.

The importance and quality of the milk in the human diet is a subject of great debate. On one hand, milk is a staple of American diets and has been consumed in one form or another by traditional cultures throughout history. Whole milk naturally provides needed nutrients, such as calcium and vitamins A and D. We are inculcated with messages that milk "does a body good," yet the story is more complex than it appears. Milk's detractors point out that humans are the only mammals that continue to drink milk after weaning, and that the milk of animals is an appropriate source of nourishment only for baby animals. In addition, the milk sugar lactose, which enhances the absorption of calcium, magnesium and zinc from milk, requires the lactase enzyme for digestion. Yet the loss of lactase activity in the intestine is genetically programmed in humans and its incidence ranges from 5 to 70 percent of the population from country to country.

From a different perspective, milk's opponents cite not only the evolutionary contraindications for milk drinking, but also point to the adulteration of milk through pasteurization that some believe has rendered it a possible health hazard. Pasteurization is the process of heating milk to a temperature high enough to kill potential pathogens. Its purpose was to prevent diseases caused by the transfer of pathogens from cow's milk to humans. As today's milk suppliers transport milk all over the country, it has become increasingly common to ultrapasteurize the milk at even higher temperatures so that it can remain stable, even at room temperature for long periods. This heating of milk destroys live enzymes required for optimal absorption of milk's nutrients and kills desirable bacteria. It also denatures (alters the shape of) the whey proteins[36] in milk, which are poorly digested and then perceived (in their unnatural shape) as foreigners by the immune system. This can result in food allergy or intolerance, which can lead to chronic inflammation.

Although conventional milk, replete with undesirable hormones and antibiotics, should be avoided in any healthy diet, even organic milk is pasteurized and its nutritional quality is questionable. Milk consumption has been implicated in the development of diabetes[37] and cancer,[38] and is one of the eight most common food allergens.[39] To further complicate the issue, some followers of traditional foodways support the use of raw, unpasteurized milk, citing its long history of traditional use and the availability of important nutrients. In the majority of cases, the milk is fermented into natural yogurt or kefir (a fermented dairy beverage), which allows for the growth of desirable bacteria, reduces pathogens, and results in a more readily digestible source of nutrients. If dairy is consumed while pregnant, fermented forms, such as yogurt or kefir, are the best choice.

Include the Right Type of Carbohydrates

The word *carbohydrate* has become almost synonymous with evil in the public eye, and low carbohydrate diet manuals remain a mainstay on the weight loss shelves in bookstores. What seems to get lost in the carbohydrate-bashing frenzy is a true understanding of the varied forms of carbohydrates in a typical diet and the role they play in overall wellness. Carbohydrates are often equated only with processed, refined, sugary starches, such as cereal, pasta, bread, cakes, crackers and the like, yet fruits and vegetables contain carbohydrates as well. Beans, whole grains, nuts and seeds are also healthful carbohydrate sources. These foods provide energy for the brain, fiber for normal digestive function, immune boosting phytonutrients and a host of vitamins and minerals not found in animal-based foods.

The typical American diet is far too heavily weighed down by large portions of starches from processed white flour, and refined sugars and these carbohydrates should be removed from the diet. These nutrient-bereft choices are the source of a sugar overload implicated in the development of mood swings, obesity, cancer, diabetes, heart disease, Alzheimer's and chronic inflammation. To make matters worse, these white flours and refined sugars often come in a package replete with artificial colors, preservatives and other additives that further sicken us. These are the carbohydrates that should be replaced with a cornucopia of nonstarchy vegetables and fruits, and smaller amounts of whole grains, beans, nuts and seeds. Seven to nine half-cup servings of a variety of brightly colored fruits and vegetables in an array of red, green, orange, yellow and purple are truly the best medicine.

When we consume grain-based foods, they should be whole grains, minimally processed and rarely white. In addition to whole wheat (for those who tolerate gluten) and brown rice, many healthy grains are available for our consumption that are used in other cultures but are relatively unknown in the United States. Quinoa, amaranth, millet and buckwheat are just a few alternative grains that have a better nutritional profile and can provide variety to the daily menu. Quinoa (keen-wa) is neither a grain nor a grass, but is a pseudo-grain with a high protein content. It is a good source of fiber, phosphorous, magnesium and iron. It is gluten-free and easily digestible. Amaranth, another gluten-free pseudo-grain, was the source of nutrition for Mayan and Incan civilizations for thousands of years. It is another high protein grain, especially rich in L-lysine, an amino acid usually low in cereal grains, and especially nutritious. Cream of buckwheat makes a tasty breakfast cereal and millet breads and crackers have a pleasing nutty flavor. Starchy vegetables, such as corn and potato, are part of this category as well.

Include Fat, But Good Kinds of Fat

Fats are necessary. Fats are important. Fats make up the biggest part of our brains, are required for hormone production and insulation, and they carry certain vitamins to the cells. They provide energy, and the right fats even decrease inflammation. We need fat in our diets, just not too much, and in the correct proportion. Choosing the right fats can be extremely confusing as supposedly expert recommendations have flip-flopped in the last decade. We have been taught that vegetable oils are healthful, and saturated fats cause disease. Yet vegetable oils are high in omega-6 fatty acids, and in excess these promote inflammation. Omega-6 and omega-3 fatty acids are essential in the human diet since we cannot manufacture them ourselves, and a healthy balance of omega-6 to omega-3 is believed to be 1:1 to 4:1.[40] As previously noted, the ratio in the typical American diet is approximately 25:1! In addition to the imbalance in the anti-inflammatory omega-3s and proinflammatory omega-6s, margarine and other hydrogenated and partially hydrogenated oils contain trans fats, which have been shown to cause heart disease and increase inflammation.[41] This type of fat is used in a plethora of processed foods, and although once lauded as the healthier choice, its disease promoting power is so great that municipalities are even banning trans fats in restaurants and food supplies.[42]

Margarines with minimal trans fats are now on the market, but a decade from now we may find them as dangerous as the partially hy-drogenated fats we used to trust. Once again, a food not found in na-ture has stressed our normal biochemistry. The best fats come from natural sources, such as olive oil, organic butter, coconut oil, rice bran oil, avocado, nuts and seeds. Despite the coconut's categorization as a saturated fat, it is actually quite healthy. The saturated fat in co-conuts is mostly composed of something called medium chain triglyc-erides (MCT) which have antimicrobial qualities,[43] and are easily digested as an added benefit to their delicious taste. Fats are delicate and many become rancid when heated, producing disease-promoting free radicals. Nut and olive oil do not tolerate heat well, while coconut and rice bran oil are appropriate for high heat cooking.

While making these sorts of changes to your diet may seem finan-cially prohibitive, it is possible to embrace a whole foods diet in an economical way. By its very nature, a whole foods diet reduces re-liance on processed foods. Although organic snacks, cookies, cereals and the like fill the shelves of whole foods markets, even in organic form these items should not comprise the bulk of the diet. In fact, as Mark Hyman MD recommends in *The UltraMind Solution*, avoid "any food in a box, can or package: in other words, if it has a label, don't eat it."[44] The end result is more homemade food, which is often less expensive. Buying food in bulk, from organic co-ops and Com-munity Supported Agriculture (CSAs) organizations, cuts out the mid-dleman and gets fresh food from farm to your table more quickly and with less expense. Incorporating beans into the menu more often will also increase the nutritive value of the meal while limiting costs.

Include Pregnancy-Specific Nutrients

During the perinatal period, the need for certain nutrients increases. With the exception of an additional 100-300 calories during preg-nancy that are not necessary during the prepregnancy phase, the same nutritional support is appropriate during preconception, pregnancy and breast-feeding.

Calcium requirements increase to 1300mg daily during pregnancy to provide the foundation for bone and tooth development in the fetus. If the maternal diet is deficient in calcium, the baby will deplete the mother's stores as the skeleton matures. Calcium is not only necessary for the bone matrix but is required for regulation of heart rhythm, blood pressure, blood clotting, and other biochemical processes. The formation of bones requires not only calcium but also magnesium, zinc and phosphorous, while absorption is facilitated by Vitamin D.[45] Balanced magnesium and calcium ratios are also necessary for normal heart rhythm. Any discussion of calcium must take into account the use of milk and dairy sources.

As previously described, pasteurized milk is not the nutritional powerhouse we are led to believe. Not only are the nutrients from pasteurized milk less bioavailable, but milk contains calcium without the supportive magnesium and zinc. Other sources of calcium that have a better balance of magnesium and zinc, such as leafy greens, almonds, and beans, should be included in the diet. One caveat: nuts and beans contain inhibitors that impair the uptake of minerals from the foods and will not supply the needed nutrients unless the nuts and beans are soaked first. Soaking is a simple process that can easily be done at home.

Calcium supplements can bridge any difference between dietary quantities and nutritional recommendations, but here too, the variety and quality of supplemental calcium varies greatly. Carbonate forms of calcium are not well absorbed but require fewer pills, improving compliance. Citrate-malate formulations are better utilized, but require more pills since the compound is larger.[46] Oyster shell should not be used as a calcium source since it may be contaminated with lead.[47] Regardless of the source, one should choose a supplement based on the amount of elemental calcium in the dosage. No more than 500mg elemental calcium should be taken at one time since more than this is poorly absorbed, and calcium should be taken with meals where acid production in the stomach enhances absorption.

As noted above, vitamin D is necessary for calcium absorption, and it plays many other important roles as well. It is not truly a vitamin, but a hormone precursor that can be supplied by food, but it is also produced naturally when the body is exposed to sunlight. Americans have been advised to protect themselves from skin cancer by judiciously avoiding sunlight and always applying sunscreen. An unfortunate outgrowth of this trend is an increase in vitamin D deficiency throughout the population. Since low vitamin D is linked to cancer, obesity, autoimmune disorders and depression, this deficiency has far reaching consequences. A review published in *Nutrition Reviews* looked at the impact of vitamin D on maternal, fetal, and infant health. It reported that vitamin D contributes to improving pregnancy outcomes, such as decreasing the risk of preeclampsia, and improving length of gestation, birth weight, and infant bone mineralization. There is also evidence that adequate vitamin D in infancy may be protective against development of future diseases such schizophrenia, brain tumors, asthma, multiple sclerosis, and autoimmune diseases.[48] Current recommendations of 200IU (5mcg) per day of vitamin D are believed by many researchers to be inadequate and there is debate as to what amount of vitamin D is optimal. For individuals, vitamin D levels can be checked with a simple blood test, and supported with adequate sunlight and a teaspoon of cod liver oil daily.

Additional iron is also required during pregnancy. Your body produces 60 percent more blood during pregnancy to facilitate the transport of oxygen and other nutrients to the developing baby. Increased iron is necessary for the manufacture of red blood cells and also allows the fetus to store iron needed during the first six months of life. Since breast milk is a poor source of iron, but is the sole source of nutrition during the first half year of life, the baby must develop its own iron reserves prior to delivery to carry it through those early months. Animal protein, kidney beans, chickpeas and black strap molasses are iron rich. The best-absorbed iron comes from animal protein, while plant-based iron is less well absorbed. The addition of vitamin-C-rich foods will increase iron absorption from meat or plants. Citrus fruits, broccoli, strawberries, papaya, mango, kiwi and even white potatoes are good food sources of vitamin C, so pairing the iron rich foods with a vitamin C source maximizes absorption.

Acidic foods cooked in a cast iron pan will also provide dietary iron, while certain foods, such as spinach, coffee, tea and bran, will block iron absorption, as will calcium. Calcium supplements are best taken separately from iron. If supplemental iron is required, as with calcium, the form of the supplement does matter. Ferrous iron is better absorbed than ferric forms, but within the ferrous category, ferrous sulphate can cause constipation and bloating, while the gluconate, fumarate and glycinate forms are readily absorbed with fewer side effects.[49] Excess iron can cause adverse side effects and extra iron should be taken only under the advice of a physician.

Folic acid is another nutrient that is of special importance during pregnancy since deficiencies of folic acid are implicated in the development of neural tube defects. Since pregnancy can precipitate a deficiency of folic acid, pregnancy requirements are 800mcg daily from all sources, of which 400mcg from supplemental folate is recommended. The FDA has mandated the addition of folate to grain products to avoid deficiency, but the amount added may not provide optimal levels of folate. Allergies that curtail the use of typical grains, such as celiac disease or wheat allergies, will eliminate this source of folate from the diet. Surprisingly, supplemental folate (folic acid) is better absorbed than food folate, but here again, a choice needs to be made. Some people have a genetic defect in a gene required to process folic acid, called methylenetetrahydrofolate reductase (MTHFR). The MTHFR mutation can increase homocysteine in the blood and is linked to recurrent pregnancy loss, chromosomal abnormalities and preeclampsia.[50] It inhibits the absorption of folic acid and can impair normal detoxification pathways since folate is a necessary cofactor in detoxification processes. A simple blood test can detect this polymorphism, and if found, other forms of folic acid, which are farther along the metabolic pathway, such as folinic acid or 5-methytetrahydrofolate, can be utilized to support folate processes.

Vitamin A is a fat-soluble vitamin found in fish oil and dairy products. A 1995 study in the *New England Journal of Medicine* linked supplementation with more than 10,000IU of vitamin A with an increased risk of birth defects.[51] Since that time, pregnant women have been counseled to avoid excesses of vitamin A while pregnant. However, a more recent study of several hundred women with a vitamin A intake ranging from 10,000 to 300,000IU per day found an increased risk in those women consuming between 10,000 and 40,000IU daily, but paradoxically, intake above 50,000IU daily resulted in a decrease in birth defects.[52] Vitamin A is found in prenatal vitamins as well as cod liver oil, butter, liver, eggs and whole milk. Orange fruits and green and orange vegetables supply beta-carotene. Beta-carotene, the preformed version of vitamin A found in many orange vegetables, does not contribute to the risk, but at this time, more than 10,000IU vitamin A daily should not be consumed without medical supervision. If you are concerned that you are not receiving adequate levels of vitamin A from your diet, consult with a functional nutritionist to help make the appropriate decision for you.

Choline is an essential nutrient found in egg yolks, wheat germ, and meat, and is important for brain development. The availability of choline in the prenatal period influences neural and cognitive development. When dietary recommendations to limit egg yolks and meat are adopted, choline levels can fall. In a Duke University study, rats born to mothers supplemented with choline were faster learners with better memories and larger brain cells than those who were not supplemented.[53] In addition, a recent Stanford University study found that choline levels are inversely related to the risk of certain neural tube defects.[54] Of thirteen nutrients studied, only choline deficiency was linked to increased risk of spina bifida. Although an optimal dose during pregnancy has not been determined, general recommendations range from 450mg to 850mg daily.

Although the essential omega-3 fatty acids are underrepresented in typical American diets and important for everyone at every age, they are an especially critical component of a healthy pre- and postpregnancy nutrition protocol. The American diet is woefully deficient in omega-3s and the importance of these essential fatty acids cannot be overstated. Here again we are presented with a challenge as to how to get enough brain building and immune modulating DHA and EPA without ingesting fish laden with toxins. In our diet, grass-fed beef, wild fish and free-range eggs are healthy sources of these nutrients, as are walnuts and baked winter squash. Flax seeds also provide omega-3s but require more biochemical processing to make the fatty acids available to the body.

A 2002 study published in *Journal of the American College of Nutrition* noted that the omega-3 fatty acids in fish oil "are more biologically potent than alpha-linolenic acid" or ALA found in flaxseed, primrose and borage oil.[55] Essential fatty acid intake can also be boosted with a fish oil supplement. Once again, quality and concentration vary with the manufacturer. A good quality essential fatty acid supplement will be tested for PCBs, dioxins, heavy metals and other contaminants in parts per trillion. The supplement manufacturer should list the fish source (salmon, sardines, cod, tuna and anchovy are preferred), and specifically list the concentration of DHA and EPA. During and prior to pregnancy a product with higher levels of DHA are desirable as DHA is the fatty acid that is found predominantly in the brain, and supports healthy brain development in the pre- and postnatal period. As children get older, a higher EPA supplement will promote good immune function and reduce inflammation.

A well-planned diet will provide many of the needed nutrients, but the addition of a natural multivitamin will provide extra insurance that increased nutritional needs are met. A good quality prenatal multivitamin is a must for any woman preparing for pregnancy, and this supplement should contain increased levels of calcium, folic acid and other important nutrients mentioned above. Just as important is the absence of unnecessary artificial ingredients, allergens and excipients that are not recognized or processed by the body. Many natural prenatal vitamins will also include herbs that help support digestion, such as red raspberry, nettles, ginger and chamomile, and may include choline for brain development. A hypoallergenic multivitamin with supportive herbs can increase a mother's tolerance and limit any nausea or GI discomfort often associated with prenatals.

Include Support for Good Bowel Function

Providing needed nutrients by consuming the right balance of foods in the healthiest form is only as effective as the digestive system's ability to process and absorb them. The digestive process cannot work effectively without adequate probiotic support.[56] As such it is critical that these essential microorganisms are allowed to flourish in the gut and do their vital work. The flora that baby is exposed to upon passing through the birth canal and then ingests via his mother's breast milk supplies the foundation upon which to build his microbial intestinal barrier. Healthy levels of beneficial flora in a mother's intestine and vaginal tract will promote proper development of the baby's gastrointestinal and immune systems. Bottle-feeding and delivery by cesarean section may compromise an infant's ability to establish his own healthy flora. Before and during pregnancy, a mother's flora can be affected by a variety of factors. Stress, infection, poor diet, and use of antibiotics or other medications can all compromise a mother's normal gut milieu.

Remove Unnecessary Pharmaceuticals That Harm Gut Ecology

The casual use of antibiotics must be avoided so that the beneficial flora is not needlessly eradicated, but it is not only antibiotics that deplete the good gut flora. Birth control pills, antacids, heartburn medications, chlorinated water and oral steroids (including some asthma medications) all have detrimental effects on normal microbial balance and should likewise be avoided both preconception and during pregnancy, unless medically necessary. If probiotics are compromised, the good bacteria absolutely must be replaced via probiotic supplements, lacto-fermented foods and preferably a combination of both.

Include Good Probiotics

As the benefits of probiotics become well known to the public, market forces have come in to play. A dizzying array of probiotic supplements is now available not only in health food stores but also in local pharmacies and even in some grocery stores. Not all of these provide the same level of therapeutic activity, as the concentration, viability, and efficacy of different brands are extremely variable and each provides a different combination of bacterial strains. A good probiotic supplement will contain a broad spectrum of live bacterial strains numbering in the billions of colony forming units (CFUs), and must be able to survive the acidic stomach environment and successfully reach the intestinal tract where it can begin to colonize. Since undesirable yeast and bacteria thrive on sugar and crowd out the desirable flora in the gut, the plethora of highly sweetened conventional yogurts on grocery shelves are not a good source of probiotic support, despite great marketing campaigns to the contrary.

Good food sources of beneficial flora do exist although they are not part of the standard American diet. Korean kimchi, Japanese umeboshi, and Europe's naturally fermented sauerkraut are all examples of lacto-fermentation. Lacto-fermentation is a traditional way of preserving foods that induces the growth of good bacteria and increases the bioavailability of nutrients such as B vitamins. The process of lacto-fermentation does require sugar to set it in motion, as the desirable bacteria will feast on this sugar in order to grow. As the good bacteria increases, the sugar levels decline, beneficial enzymes and vitamins are produced by the bacteria and a health-giving food is made. Naturally fermented yogurts, without excess sweeteners and dairy or coconut-based kefir beverages also provide a rich source of good quality bacteria that does not come in a compromised package. Traditional societies throughout the world have historically included lacto-fermented foods in their diet, but their inclusion in the American menu has decreased with industrialization. The few cultured foods that we are familiar with, such as conventional sauerkraut, are usually pasteurized at a temperature high enough to kill any of the beneficial microorganisms that may have existed, and are of little therapeutic benefit.

Remove Allergens

In addition to an abundance of good bacteria in the gut, the avoidance of existing food allergies, or those that may cause food allergy or sensitivity, will avoid inflammation and promote good digestion. Environmental allergies should be considered here as well, since a body prone to allergies may develop either food or environmental allergies. The top eight food allergens are wheat, milk, soy, peanut, egg, tree nut, shellfish and fish. As previously mentioned, celiac disease (an intolerance to gluten) is estimated to occur in one out of every 133 people in the Untied States. Patients with celiac disease follow a diet of 100 percent gluten avoidance, and this disorder is believed to be heritable. Recent studies do not support the use of a maternal restricted diet in the prevention of atopic disease, but preventive measures include the reduction of allergen exposure through food and inhalation as well as the introduction of immune modulators, such as essential fatty acids.[57]

Smoking avoidance and exclusive breastfeeding after birth are two of the most effective interventions for allergy avoidance.[58] For those who cannot breastfeed, a protein hydrolysate formula (one in which the proteins are more fully broken down before ingestion) has shown benefit in reducing the onset of allergies.[59] In addition, the avoidance of indoor allergens, such as dust mites, mold, and animal dander, is protective as well.[60] The typical window to introduce solids used to be between four to six months, but many organizations, such as the World Health Organization and American Academy of Pediatrics, have updated their recommendations, since newer research indicates that deferring the introduction of solids until six months of age is also protective. Of note, a Helsinki Skin and Allergy Hospital Study has shown that exclusive breastfeeding without solids past nine months may actually increase allergies, so it appears that introduction of hypoallergenic solids shortly after six months is ideal.[61]

Remove Food Toxins

It is impossible to detail the extent of damage that the myriad chemicals that lace our food supply can inflict upon the body, but two ingredients provide a cautionary example. Monosodium glutamate (MSG) and aspartame are excitotoxins linked to a host of maladies.

Adverse side effects of MSG include headache, dizziness, brain fog, brain cell death, and ailments involving the immune system and neurologic system, yet it is pervasive in the food supply. Part of the challenge for those trying to avoid MSG is learning the ingredient names that hide MSG. A small sampling of names that may signify MSG include glutamate, vegetable protein extract, autolyzed plant protein, yeast, and meat tenderizer, and there are many others.

The FDA has received reports of ninety-two different types of maladies attributed to aspartame by the public, and symptoms of fibromyalgia have been shown to improve with the removal of aspartame from the sufferer's diet.[62] It has also been implicated in the development of cancer in rats.[63] A *New York Times* article that reported on the cancer study also discussed an analysis of aspartame research by Ralph Walton, MD that found that of ninety nonindustry aspartame studies, 83 percent positively identified adverse effects. Conversely, of seventy-four industry-sponsored research studies, all seventy-four found no problems with aspartame. It is these seventy-four studies that are often quoted in the media to support the safety of aspartame.[64]

In 2007, Asda, the United Kingdom subsidiary of American Wal-Mart, removed all artificial ingredients from its private label food products in an effort to address the desires of their customers. Shouldn't it be possible for American Wal-Mart to do the same? Surely, if such an influential market force made a move like this, others retailers would quickly follow suit.

Include Effective Detoxification Support

A healthy body is naturally able to detoxify the compounds it comes in contact with on a daily basis, but when the system is overloaded with increasing environmental insults and devoid of the nutrients it needs to support normal detoxification pathways, the process breaks down. The importance of this balance cannot be overemphasized. Limiting the food and environmental toxins that we can control is one step, but maintaining that ever-critical microbial balance is another.

In addition, providing the right foods will allow for the production of essential detoxification compounds.

Normal detoxification in our bodies occurs in two steps, called Phase I and Phase II, both of which occur in the liver. In Phase I detoxification, undesirable compounds are given a "handle" that makes them less harmful and allows the "garbage men" in Phase II to carry them out of the body. Phase I produces free radicals that must be quenched by antioxidants and phytochemicals, while sulfur compounds (particularly an antioxidant called glutathione) are necessary for the two phases to proceed successfully. Foods that support the liver and supply antioxidants, phytonutrients, B vitamins including folic acid, sulfur and the building blocks of glutathione provide support for natural detoxification.

Antioxidants, such as vitamins C, E, and selenium, are found in fruits, vegetables and some whole grains. Unfortunately, selenium levels in fruits and vegetables are dependent upon the selenium levels of the soil in which they are grown, so vegetables from high and low selenium areas will contain widely different quantities of the antioxidant. Sulfur is the compound that causes rotten eggs to smell, and sulfur-containing foods often have an interesting odor. Broccoli, cabbage, Brussels sprouts, onion, and garlic supply sulfur. Asparagus, avocado, eggs, and garlic supply glutathione, while animal protein contains all the amino acid building blocks needed to produce glutathione. Once again, we see that eating clean foods from across the food groups supplies a variety of needed nutrients. Eating right allows us to produce glutathione. Remember, glutathione can be depleted by medications such as acetaminophen (Tylenol), pollution, stress, heavy metals, excess dietary fat, deficiencies in the amino acids that comprise it, as well as by deficiencies in the B vitamins, which are cofactors in glutathione production. Good dietary practices and toxin avoidance help ensure adequate glutathione levels.

If parents have been exposed to high levels of environmental toxins in the past, laboratory tests can assess their current level of toxic burden, and diet and supplements can be used to strengthen the normal detoxification processes. It is important never to aggressively attempt to remove the body's toxins during pregnancy, however, as this can be too stressful for the baby.

Remove Mercury and Other Heavy Metals

Toxicity from mercury and other heavy metals is a subject of ongoing heated debate. Mercury has been associated with the onset of autism, autoimmune disorders, and a host of chronic diseases.[65] Arsenic and aluminum are only two of a host of other heavy metals that are omnipresent in our food, air, and water supply and may cause serious harm.[66] Mercury has been shown to migrate from amalgams across the placenta to the fetus as well as into breast milk.[67] A study published in the *American Journal of Physiology* demonstrated that mercury vapor is continuously released from dental amalgams for prolonged periods after chewing, and the study's investigators caution that the placement of dental amalgams during pregnancy and in children should be reconsidered.[68] In addition, women with more than six dental amalgams in place during pregnancy have been shown to have a 3.2 times higher likelihood of having a child diagnosed with severe autism.[69] Women of childbearing age who have mercury-containing dental amalgams in place should consider having them removed well in advance of conception. The International Academy of Oral Medicine and Toxicology provides a protocol for the safe removal of amalgams, but once the amalgams are removed, additional protocols exist to help the body eliminate any toxins that have been stimulated during the removal process. If it is not possible to remove amalgams at least a year before conception, they should not be disturbed, as this will cause more harm than good.

Arsenic is another heavy metal found in surprising places. It has antibacterial properties and is routinely used in nonorganic chicken feed to prevent bacterial degradation of the feed. Nonorganic rice is often contaminated with arsenic. For years, pressure-treated wood was sprayed with arsenic-containing compounds to prevent bacterial overgrowth, and research has shown that children absorb arsenic from playground equipment and decks constructed from this wood.

Arsenic and mercury are only two of the toxic metals to which we are routinely exposed. Despite the removal of lead from paints and gasoline, we continue to be exposed unknowingly to toxic lead from soil, groundwater, and air. In addition, toys and other products imported from China have been found to be contaminated with lead. Since these items often find their way into children's mouths, they are of particular concern. Since heavy metals that cannot be excreted by a healthy detoxification system are quickly moved from blood into fatty tissue, a routine blood test for lead will provide false assurance that an adult or child has not been exposed to harmful amounts of these toxins.

Although it can be difficult to stay abreast of current information on environmental toxins and heavy metals, the use of naturally produced products and clean water and food will greatly reduce our body burden. In addition, resources such as the Environmental Working Group, www.ewg.org; and Healthy Child, Healthy World, www.healthychild .org; provide information on optimal product choices.

HOW TO HELP CHILDREN WITH CHRONIC ILLNESSES NOW

While making these changes in the prenatal period can have great benefit in improving long-term health outcomes in our children, there are advantages to applying the same concepts during all stages of life. For children who are already suffering from chronic health issues, the same underlying principles apply:

- Eat nourishing clean food.
  - Eliminate processed foods and artificial ingredients.
  - Limit refined sugars.
  - Use whole foods, including a variety across all food groups.
- Support good bowel function with probiotics.
- Determine any possible food or environmental allergens and eliminate exposure to them.
- Remove toxic exposures, whether from food, water, the environment or household products.

- Approach the use of pharmaceutical products in children cautiously (including antibiotics, pain medications such as Tylenol, and vaccines).

In addition, seek a healthcare practitioner experienced in recovering children with chronic illnesses. Not all physicians or dietitians are well versed in the principles of functional medicine. At the same time, the term *nutritionist* is not regulated by any agency, and individuals with vastly different levels of expertise may use the term. To find a qualified individual, consider using the following resources as a guide.

Medical Practitioner Provider Directories:
- Institute of Functional Medicine — www.functionalmedicine.org
- Center for Mind Body Medicine — www.cmbm.org
- American Association of Naturopathic Physicians — www.naturopathic.org

Registered Dietitian and Nutritionist Directories:
- Nutritionists Complementary Care — www.complementarynutrition.org (registered dietitians with experience in functional nutrition)
- IAACN — www.iaacn.org (nutritionists with functional nutrition training)

Environmental Resources:
- Environmental Working Group — www.ewg.org
- Healthy Child, Healthy World — www.healthychild.org
- Deirdre Imus Environmental Center for Pediatric Oncology — www.dienviro.com

Nutrition Resources:
- Marion Nestles Food Blog — www.foodpolitics.com

- Local foods, CSAs and Farmers Markets —
  www.localharvest.org

Alternative Healing Resources:
- BioSET (Bioenergetic Sensitivity and Enyzme Therapy) —
  www.drellencutler.com
- NAET (Nambudripad's Allergy Elimination Techniques) —
  www.naet.com
- National Certification Commission for Acupuncture and
  Oriental Medicine — www.nccaom.org
- North American Society of Homeopaths —
  www.homeopathy.org
- The American Chiropractic Association —
  www.acatoday.org
- International Chiropractic Pediatric Association —
  icpa4kids.com

Spreading the Message

We, as individuals, have the capacity to positively impact our own children's health today, but it will require a change in some of our cultural beliefs before we see these principles in action across society. As parents implement these practices locally, they will clearly want to disseminate their actions and information to the larger population. Institutions and organizations are already trying to take this message to a wider audience. The Environmental Working Group, Healthy Child.org, The Deirdre Imus Environmental Center for Pediatric Oncology, Clean Eating Magazine, SOKHOP (Saving Our Kids, Healing Our Planet), Parents Ending America's Childhood Epidemic, and the Holistic Moms Network are just some of the resources available to parents, and these organizations should be utilized and supported. While these organizations are providing information and ideas and spreading the word to interested parties, much work is still left to be done.

Our children spend hours every day in schools and daycare facilities where a menu of processed, chemical laden food and snacks of cheese crackers, pretzels, and other processed grains is the norm. The facilities are cleaned with toxic chemicals that our children inhale and ingest every day. When they go out on the playground they are exposed to disease-inducing pesticide residues. The child who goes to school with a synthetic-free lunch in a chemical-free lunch box is an outlier. A huge opportunity for change lies here in these facilities.

The Deirdre Imus Environmental Center for Pediatric Oncology has as its mission to identify, control, and ultimately prevent exposures to environmental toxins in children and adults. The center has developed a Greening the Cleaning® program, which has been implemented at Hackensack University Medical Center as well as a number of area schools. They provide a resource packet to help schools adopt the Greening the Cleaning® program, and have shown the products to be cost effective and of good quality. Taking this message to local schools and daycare facilities is an important step in lessening our children's exposure to environmental insults.

The Organic School Project is a Chicago-based nonprofit organization, whose mission is to combat childhood obesity and related health epidemics through a program called Grow Teach Feed (GTF). GTF reconnects children to their food sources through community gardens, and supplies More Positive Food, local when possible, mostly organic made-from-scratch meals. Some local Chicago schools have adopted the program, and these efforts can be duplicated in schools throughout the nation. The Wisconsin Homegrown Lunch program has a mission to bring local and sustainably grown foods into the Wisconsin school system. Although organic criteria are not included in this program, the push for local food, minimally processed, with an emphasis on fresh produce, is certainly better than the standard school meal. At the very least, schools can remove the candy and soda vending machines that remain a siren's song to students of all ages.

Our children's desire for junk in the guise of food will not end until they are no longer bombarded with a visual diet of advertising as devoid of quality as the very "foods" they attempt to sell. In 2008 the Federal Trade Commission released the results of a study on food marketing to children and adolescents that found that forty-four major food and beverage retailers spent over $1.6 billion marketing products to children age seventeen and under.[70] These promotions are a complex web of advertising, packaging, internet links, and licensing and cross promotion with movies and television shows. The foods they promote are usually highly processed and filled with artificial additives. Michael Jacobson, the executive director of Center for Science in the Public Interest, has been quoted in regard to marketing junk food to children:

> No parent would allow a door-to-door salesman to come into the house and spend a few unsupervised minutes with their kids, yet junk-food manufacturers have similar unfettered access to kids' impressionable minds via advertising and marketing. Food manufacturers like to put all the blame on parents, but these companies go right around parents' backs, directly to kids—and sometimes directly to toddlers—with sales pitches for unhealthful foods.[71]

The United States medical model, with its emphasis on treating instead of preventing disease, is another broken piece of the wellness machine. Barbara Starfield *et al.*, in the *Journal of Epidemiology and Community Health*, noted that while in the 1960s the medical perception of prevention used to mean averting the development of a pathological state, by 1998 the concept of disease prevention had shifted to mean identifying diseases or risk factors early and taking steps to arrest their progression.[72] This change in focus from lifestyles that avoid disease to earlier detection and early medical treatment misses the point. Gilbert Welch, in a *New York Times* essay about health care reform, had this to say:

> The term "preventive medicine" no longer means what it used to: keeping people well by promoting healthy habits, like exercising, eating a balanced diet and not smoking. . . . But the medical model for prevention has become less about health promotion and more

about early diagnosis. . . . And that approach doesn't save money; it costs money.[73]

Our physicians are trained to value early detection and treatment of disease, but do not have the resources to support true preventive efforts. Insurance companies do not allow them the luxury of time to explain preventive measures, nor do they value the role of the registered dietitian to provide comprehensive nutrition counseling unrelated to an existing disease state. Reimbursement for dietitians' services is included in some insurance plans, but only for specific disorders, such as high cholesterol or diabetes. Once again, the disease must develop before it can be treated, and an individual seeking to prevent illness is left to pay out of pocket. Our health care costs continue to rise as we wait for disease to develop, and while food companies spend billions of dollars marketing toxic food to children and adults. As a nation we bemoan the toll that healthcare spending takes on society, yet we perpetuate the progression of chronic disease through the institutional and lifestyle choices we make.

America's children do not have to be consigned to a life of chronic illness, so long as caring parents take action to limit toxic overload and return to good, clean, nourishing food. By making these conscious choices well before pregnancy and throughout the life cycle, parents have the power to impact their children's lives and our future. Parents: recognize your power, accept the challenge, and change the future.

Conclusion

If you tune in to the news media, you will likely hear many mixed messages regarding the epidemic of chronic childhood illness in America. There are those who believe that there is no autism epidemic, and those who believe that the autism epidemic is only the tip of the iceberg. There are those who believe that autism is a disorder rooted in neurobiology and genetics, and those who believe that autism is an environmentally derived disorder that affects many biological systems in the body. The aim of this book is to present enough evidence so that we can begin to move beyond these debates and toward healing our children. As the evidence supporting the existence of an epidemic grows, so does the number of children affected. Can we afford to wait for public health organizations to acknowledge the enormity of this epidemic?

It might have been appropriate to have these debates two decades ago, before we had any epidemiological or scientific data to analyze concerning the epidemic. But we are well into the second decade of an epidemic of chronic illnesses striking American children in their prime. The debate needs to move forward. Our children are chronically ill, and we need to take action today, before it is too late.

Yet public health and professional medical organizations like the Centers for Disease Control and the American Academy of Pediatrics continue to assure us that all is well with our children and that any problems our children have are largely due to genetics. Are the leaders of these organizations simply out of touch with the evidence? Are they ignoring the science, or just waiting for "better" or "more conclusive" data? Are they subverting the truth? Avoiding the problem? Why does it seem like members of these organizations have their heads in the sand?

For years, doctors and researchers within the autism community, like Dr. Natasha Campbell-McBride, Dr. Bryan Jepson, Dr. Sydney Baker, Dr. Andrew Wakefield, Dr. Elizabeth Mumper and many others, have asked the medical establishment to recognize that autism is not purely a genetic disease and that we must look into the environmental factors contributing to this epidemic. New scientific discoveries coming out of autism research reveal that children with autism, ADHD, allergies, and many other chronic illnesses are deeply impacted by their environment. Why isn't the medical establishment listening to the autism experts?

Orthodox medicine, that which is represented by highly respected medical organizations like the American Academy of Pediatrics (AAP), can be a slow moving and stubborn animal. Sometimes, the medical establishment will not embrace new discoveries until they are pressured to do so or until the data becomes so irrefutable that it would seem foolish not to embrace it. It is a well-known fact that many new scientific discoveries take at least twenty years to penetrate the established medical community, especially if there are particular industries or interests that will be hurt by the new discoveries. Following are a few historical examples that illustrate how the established medical community is slow in accepting new scientific discoveries.

EXAMPLE A

Scientific Discovery: A Bacteria Causes Stomach Ulcers

Length of Time Before Embraced by American Medical Community: Nearly twenty years

In 1982, it was discovered that an overgrowth of *H. pylori*, a bacteria in the stomach (and not spicy food and stress as was previously believed), was the cause of some stomach ulcers. Furthermore, researchers determined that stomach ulcers could be cured with a course of oral antibiotics. For years, the medical community insisted that there was no cure for stomach ulcers and that antibiotic therapy was just too simple. It took until 1994 for the NIH to acknowledge that it was indeed *H. pylori* that caused stomach ulcers, and it took several more years beyond that before this information (and associated antibiotic treatment protocols) penetrated the mainstream medical community. In 2005, the two researchers who made this medical discovery were awarded the Nobel Prize in Medicine. It took over twenty years for their initially controversial study to be widely embraced.

EXAMPLE B

Scientific Discovery: Epidemic of Pellagra Caused by Nutritional Deficiency

Length of Time Before Embraced by American Medical Community: Over twenty years

In the early twentieth century, an epidemic of pellagra swept through the American South, killing a hundred thousand and making millions more sick.[1] Pellagra, called the 3-D disease for its primary symptoms of dermatitis, diarrhea, and dementia, mainly affected sharecroppers, tenant farmers, and urban millworkers. The American medical community believed for years that pellagra was caused by an infectious agent like a bacteria or worm or even a toxic mold, but none of these hypotheses were helpful in controlling the epidemic.

In 1914, Dr. Joseph Goldberger, a renowned epidemiologist, began to investigate the epidemic. After spending several years traveling throughout the South learning about the epidemic and the people it affected, Goldberger concluded that the affliction was the result of widespread nutrient deficiency rather than an infectious agent. Many of those who were affected by pellagra subsisted primarily on a diet of corn. Despite a convincing clinical study that Goldberger conducted on inmates that demonstrated that otherwise healthy men developed pellagra when fed a "poverty diet," consisting mainly of corn, the established medical community refused to listen to Goldberger's theory.

At the time, corn was America's biggest crop and corn growers were appalled at the notion that a diet of corn could lead to nutritional deficiency, thus they pressured the medical establishment to consider other possible etiologies, such as infectious agents, heredity and even race-based etiologies. And some southerners, concerned about the South's reputation for being backward or unsophisticated, denied that the epidemic existed at all. It was not until 1939, two years after Dr. Goldberger's death and over twenty years after his initial discovery, that researchers finally concluded that it was indeed nutritional deficiency, a deficiency in niacin (a B vitamin), which was responsible for the epidemic.

EXAMPLE C

Scientific Discovery: Smoking Causes Cancer

Length of Time Before Embraced by American Medical Community: More than thirty years

In the early 1950s, researchers by the names of Wynder, Graham, and Croninger repeatedly demonstrated in the laboratory that cigarettes were carcinogenic (cancer causing). The tobacco industry kicked into high gear with an advertising and media blitz designed to assuage the public's fears about cancer and gloss over the science that had demonstrated the link. In fact, the tobacco industry crafted authoritative-looking scientific documents that concluded that there was "no proof establishing that cigarette smoking is a cause of lung cancer," and these documents were distributed to hundreds of thousands of doctors, and the information within these documents was treated as established fact by reputable media such as the *New York Times* and the *Wall Street Journal.*

As more and more conclusive data against cigarette smoking accumulated over the remainder of the decade, the U.S. Surgeon General finally took a stand. In 1964, the Surgeon General issued a report on smoking and health that concluded that smoking tobacco caused lung cancer. Yet, according to author Devra Davis, ties between the tobacco industry and the American Medical Association (AMA) and the American Cancer Society (ACS) kept these organizations silent on the matter, when they should have been loudly denouncing cigarette smoking.

Well into the 1970s, the AMA continued to accept funding from the tobacco industry and collude in a conspiracy of silence. It wasn't until 1979 that the AMA acknowledged that smoking was bad for the lungs, but even then they did not concede that it caused cancer. It took more than thirty years for the mainstream medical establishment to embrace the scientific fact that smoking causes cancer.[2] In this case, industry worked aggressively to suppress the science because the science would jeopardize profits.

These historical examples serve as powerful reminders of two key facts:

1. It often takes a long time for new scientific information and discoveries to be adopted by the medical establishment. It may take twenty years or longer for new science to be incorporated

into public health policy or to make its way into the physician's office.

2.   Public health organizations (such as the CDC or the NIH)
     and professional medical organizations (such as the AMA or
     the AAP) do not always act in the interest of the public, despite
     claims otherwise. The influence of industry is insidious and
     powerful. We may not immediately see the influence, but that
     does not mean it is not there.

In light of these facts, we must scrutinize how public health organizations and professional medical organizations are currently responding both to the epidemic of chronic illness in children and to the
proposed reasons for the epidemic.

A tremendous amount of evidence shows that children with autism,
asthma, ADHD, allergies and other chronic illnesses are suffering
from gut dysbiosis and immune dysregulation. This is science that is
circulating, being discussed at professional conferences, and being applied in the offices of progressive integrative practitioners. Hundreds
of scientists and physicians across the country are well aware that these
illnesses are largely driven by external environmental factors—factors
like the overuse of pharmaceuticals, excessive vaccination, and environmental pollution.

And still, despite reams of evidence that support these facts, the
American Academy of Pediatrics will not concede that we are experiencing an epidemic, nor will they entertain the notion that environmental factors may be central to the etiology of autism. In fact, it
seems as if the AAP is spreading disinformation about the epidemic
of autism. In late July 2009, *Pediatrics* (the journal of the American
Academy of Pediatrics) announced the publication of a study claiming
that children with autism do not have a higher incidence of gastrointestinal problems than other children.[3] Partly because of press releases
pushed by the AAP, the news media immediately picked up on this
story and blasted out the following headlines:

- *The New York Times*: "Study Finds Diet Has No Effect on Autism" and "With Autism, Diet Restrictions May Do More Harm Than Good; Study finds no increase in gastrointestinal problems in kids with the disorder"
- *The Chicago Tribune*: "Mayo Clinic Doubts Autism-Digestion Link"
- *NBC The Today Show*: "Study proves there's no link between gastrointestinal disease and autism."
- *AAP News Release*: "Gastrointestinal Disorders are Not Linked to Autism, A Study Finds."

Any person watching a news report or reading a newspaper with these headlines might think that scientists definitely proved that there is no connection between the gut and autism. *This is simply not true.* The news media reported on a fairly weak scientific study that never should have made news in the first place. In this sound-bite-driven society, however, people walk away believing that there is no connection between autism and the gut because this is what they read, saw or heard from the mainstream news media.

By most scientific standards, the study published in *Pediatrics* was a weak study with unimpressive and virtually meaningless results. Yet the media portrayed this study as if it was somehow conclusive and *proved* that there is no link between autism and the gut. The medical editor for NBC's *The Today Show* reported:

> . . . the findings [of the Mayo Clinic study] are important because they really dismiss the link between the gut and these neurological problems that we see in autism, and primarily they were looking for problems like malabsorption and inflammation. 124 children were followed, matched with otherwise normal children, and these findings are really conclusive. *There is no link between illness in the gut and the signs and symptoms in what we see in autism.* . . . This is a really important study for parents, because it means that if you are

putting your child on a restrictive diet or you are doing colonics . . .
if you are using extra vitamins or nutrients, and you're spending a
lot of money and putting your child through that, there is no reason
to; there is no link between the gut and the signs and symptoms that
we see in autism.[4]

The medical editor offers a very conclusive statement dismissing
the link between autism and the gut. She is very convincing. A person
with no other knowledge of autism or no way to access this study might
begin to feel fairly certain that there is no connection between the
brain and the gut. A closer examination of the actual study tells a different story.

The study in question simplified exceedingly complex issues and
irresponsibly drew sweeping conclusions about autism and autism
treatment protocols based on their "data." The study found that of the
124 autistic patients whose medical records were examined over eighteen years, 77 percent had diagnosed gastrointestinal disorders. Of the
age and gender-matched controls, 72 percent had diagnosed gastrointestinal disorders. The way the investigators tracked the incidence of
gastrointestinal disorders was deeply flawed. The study used nothing
other than medical records (no laboratory tests, no surveys, no endoscopy, no physical examinations) to determine if children had gastrointestinal disorders. This means that if a child had chronic
constipation or acid reflux but never complained to the doctor about
it, then that child's gastrointestinal disorder was not recorded. If the
parents of an autistic child with chronic diarrhea complained to the
doctor about it only once, then it was counted as only one incident
and was considered to be equal to a short-term case of viral diarrhea
in a normally developing child.[5]

All that this study really reveals is that over 70 percent of both autistic and normally developing children complain of gastrointestinal
problems at some point during their childhood. That's it. It does not
conclusively prove that there is no link between the gut and autism,
and it certainly does not prove that special diets are harmful to chil-

dren with autism. Analysis of the therapeutic benefit of special diets was not even a part of the study. The media needs to be careful about how it portrays scientific studies, especially when dealing with a topic as complex and controversial as autism.

So why did the AAP put out a press release to publicize such a weak study? Why did the news media pick it up and distort it? Could the pharmaceutical and vaccine industry be influencing decision makers at governmental and professional medical organizations and the news media in an effort to obscure the science that implicates pharmaceuticals and vaccines in an epidemic of chronic childhood illnesses? This seems awfully conspiratorial, yet history tells us that this sort of unsavory alliance between industry and public health and professional medical organizations does occur.

In the spring of 2009, the *New York Times* reported on a growing movement among Harvard medical students "intent on exposing and curtailing the [pharmaceutical] industry influence in their classrooms and laboratories, as well as in Harvard's 17 affiliated teaching hospitals and institutes."[6] Investigations prompted by this group of Harvard students revealed that one Harvard professor had forty-seven corporate affiliations. In addition, there were 149 professors that had financial ties to Pfizer, and 130 professors who had ties to Merck.[7]

Of course the pharmaceutical industry is involved in academia, public health organizations and professional medical organizations. Often, people who used to work for pharmaceutical companies, for instance, end up working in public or private health organizations, and many academic professors require funding from private sources (such as pharmaceutical companies) to conduct their very expensive research. That the pharmaceutical companies are financially tied to these public organizations does not necessarily mean that there are unethical dealings between the two. The resistance movement organized by Harvard's medical students, however, serves to remind us that the ethics of these liaisons are not always pure, and we cannot always assume that noncorporate entities (like Harvard, the AAP, or the CDC) are acting ethically or in the interest of the public.

You do not have to be conspiratorial to understand that many different and powerful interests would be negatively impacted by the public revelation that man-made environmental factors are causing an entire generation of children to become chronically ill. Let's examine who stands to lose from this sort of revelation. If you look at all the factors that may be contributing to the epidemic of chronic illnesses in children, you see that many corporations produce products that may be harmful to children, including pharmaceutical companies, vaccine manufacturers, many consumer products companies, chemical companies, telecommunications companies, technology companies, the food industry, agribusiness, the energy industry, retailers, and many others. This information will not be taken lightly by any of these interests.

On some level, the professional medical and public health organizations also stand to lose if this information becomes widely known. The preliminary research documented in this book that links well-established standards of care in the pediatrician's office (such as antibiotic use and vaccination) to the increased prevalence of autism, ADHD, learning disorders and other illnesses puts the American Academy of Pediatrics, the Centers for Disease Control, and the Food and Drug Administration in an awkward position. What if the current childhood immunization program and lax pharmaceutical use (especially in the pediatric population) are indeed partly responsible for the epidemic of chronic childhood illnesses? What are the AAP, the CDC, and the FDA to do then? Can they admit that the practices that they have been advocating over recent decades were flawed, in error, or perhaps even harmful to children? In the case of childhood immunizations, to admit that they are in any way harmful to even a portion of children would require them to undertake a massive reevaluation of the existing infectious disease management program, a program that does not have a plan B. It is no wonder that the science demonstrating the gut-immune-brain connection is being met with fierce resistance.

This resistance goes beyond the established medical community. If vaccines, pharmaceuticals, toxins, electromagnetic pollution, consumer products, and the standard American diet are to blame for the epidemic of chronic childhood illness in this country, then our culture and our very way of life come under close scrutiny. Does this mean that we can no longer enjoy our fast food meals, play with our technological gadgets, or rely on fast pharmaceutical interventions every time we have a headache or upset stomach? Do we need to change how we live? None of us wants to change our life, but we do not want our children to be sick either. There are many ways that we can make small changes that will both benefit our children and enable us to still enjoy our way of life. The problem then becomes: Where do we get guidance about the right choices to make for our children's health? How do we begin to make the incremental changes necessary to protect our children from further harm?

It is likely that we cannot wait for the American medical establishment to take the lead in addressing this crisis. If we decide to wait for organizations like the CDC, the NIH or the AAP to take the lead, it could be a long time coming, and many more children will suffer needlessly. Right now, the governing medical organizations are telling us that current pharmaceutical and vaccines protocols are perfectly safe for children and they also endorse the use of certain consumer products (e.g., sunscreen) that may be unhealthy for our children. Is it wise for us to continue to follow the advice of the orthodox medical community when it does not seem to be providing us with any answers and may even be giving us advice that is harmful to our children?

We do have choices and we do have the power to end this epidemic. We can each take steps in our own lives to heal our children and prevent others from getting sick. As individuals we can make small changes that will lessen the impact of harmful environmental factors on our children. There are larger problems that we cannot address alone, but collectively we can organize ourselves to pressure public health organizations to conduct more research and to discover new ways to tackle the bigger issues.

One of these issues is how to develop a national childhood infectious disease management program that does not in any way contribute

to chronic illnesses. This is likely to be the most controversial and difficult part of ending the epidemic. Public health and professional
medical organizations tend to see the vaccine question in very black
and white terms. We either continue to implement the childhood immunization protocol as it is, or else we risk the resurgence of dangerous infectious diseases. Yet, there is middle ground to be had.

We need to aggressively research and precisely define the factors
that predispose a particular child to vaccine-induced immune dysregulation. Perhaps we can prescreen children according to a variety of
risk factors before they are vaccinated. For instance, blood tests that
measure immune function (levels of natural killer cells, immunoglobulins, or other immune factors) can be used to evaluate a particular
child's immunocompetence prior to vaccination. We could also
screen infants for glutathione deficiency or mitochondrial disorders
to evaluate their ability to tolerate vaccines. A cheaper solution would
be to use clinical evaluation and specific clinical criteria to determine
a child's relative risk. For example, if a child has a history of heavy antibiotic use, a family history of autoimmune disorders or gastrointestinal disorders, mitochondrial disease, or other factors that would
indicate a particular predisposition to immune dysregulation, then the
parents and the child's pediatrician can make an informed decision
about the level of risk that such a child faces being immunized.

Another alternative is to evaluate the necessity of the current full
childhood immunization program. Just thirty years ago, most children
were vaccinated against seven diseases: measles, mumps, rubella,
polio, diphtheria, tetanus, and pertussis. Do we really need to vaccinate all newborn babies against hepatitis B, a disease transmitted sexually or through the use of dirty hypodermic needles? Surely, better,
less expensive, and less risky public health initiatives can be taken to
control hepatitis B. Similarly, the chicken pox vaccine is unpopular
with many parents as many consider it an unnecessary vaccination
that may not be providing adequate protection in the first place. We
can protect the vulnerable from complications associated with infectious diseases like chicken pox in other ways, such as focusing on im-

proving nutrition and immune function in mothers and children. Let us think outside of the immunization box. We can develop other ways besides immunization to manage some, but maybe not all, infectious diseases.

Similarly, we need to reevaluate how we as a society use pharmaceutical medications, especially antibiotics (which damage microflora), reflux medications (which alter gastrointestinal ecology), and steroid-based drugs (which suppress and alter immune function). These are important drugs that can help many people, but perhaps we are using them too aggressively in certain patient populations. In particular, we need to take great care when we use these medications in children and women of childbearing years. We can develop specific therapeutic protocols so that when drugs like antibiotics are used, they are prescribed concurrently with prophylactic supplements like probiotics. Many knowledgeable and progressive physicians are already doing this in their practices.

We also need to take a long hard look at the toxic world that we live in. The environmental pollution that we are all subjected to on a daily basis may not affect those of us with exceptionally strong immune systems, but children are being affected, and our chemically laden way of life cannot be sustained through another generation. We need to green our consumer products, our industries, our new technologies and our entire way of life. We need to learn how to eat real whole foods, rather than toxic, processed and nutrient-depleted food. These are changes that we can make, but not without commitment and effort.

It is human nature to cling to old ideas and to fear new ones. Galileo, Copernicus, Darwin and other scientific contrarians all had intimate knowledge of this fact. It is never easy to challenge prevailing scientific or social opinion with new, controversial ideas. Yet human progress depends on our very ability to do this. We cannot advance knowledge without challenging conventional ideas and testing new and innovative ones. Scientists in the autism and functional medicine communities who have discovered the epidemic of chronic illness in children are doing just this. They are courageously challenging the status quo and asking us to consider new scientific explanations for all of these disorders in our children.

Unfortunately, we do not have the requisite twenty years it takes for mainstream medicine to catch up or to embrace new scientific theories about the causes behind this epidemic. Children are suffering today, and we desperately need parents and the American medical and scientific community to begin aggressively pursuing solutions. If this epidemic continues at the rate we have seen over the last few decades, our society will begin to buckle under the tremendous economic and social burden. The rate of autism diagnoses is believed to be growing at 10-17 percent per year.[8] Do we need to wait until autism affects one in fifty or one in thirty children before we take action? Nearly one in five African American children has asthma. Do we wait until that number is one in three? One in two? At what point do we seriously address this epidemic?

Parents: it is within your power to protect the health of your children. Pay attention to your children's symptoms. Listen when your gut tells you that something is not right with your child. Get educated. Find a healthcare provider who can help you get to the bottom of your child's illness or who will listen to your concerns about preventing chronic illness. Thousands of parents across this country have recovered their children from chronic illnesses and many thousands more are working tirelessly to keep their children safe and healthy. You can too.

For more information about how to get help for your child, or to connect with other parents dealing with their children's chronic illnesses, go to www.epidemicanswers.org.

NOTES

CHAPTER ONE

1. The Centers for Disease Control and Prevention, "Obesity Prevalence," The CDC, www.cdc.gov/nccdphp/dnpa/obesity/childhood/prevalence.html (accessed January 10, 2009).

2. Mary Jo Stanley, RN MS, "Assessing Prevalence of Emotional and Behavioral Problems in Suspended Middle School Students," *The Journal of School Nursing* 22 (2006): 40-47; "Rx for Behavior Problems in Pre-K," *Preschool Matters, A publication of the National Institute for Early Education Research* 5 (November/December 2007); Walter S. Gilliam, PhD, "Prekindergarteners Left Behind: Expulsion Rates in State Prekindergarten Programs," *Foundation for Child Development Policy Brief*, Series No. 3 (May 2005).

3. Cathy Huanqing Qi et al., "Behavior Problems of Preschool Children From Low-Income Families: Review of the Literature," *Topics in Early Childhood Special Education* 162 (June 2005).

4. Kenneth Bock, M.D, *Healing the New Childhood Epidemics: Autism, ADHD, Asthma, and Allergies* (New York: Ballantine Books, 2007).

5. National Center for Health Statistics 2006, The CDC, www.cdc.gov/nchs/fastats/asthma.htm (accessed January 10, 2009); American Academy of Asthma, Allergy and Immunology, www.aaai.org (accessed January 10, 2009).

6. National Center For Health Statistics, The CDC, www.cdc.gov/nchs/fastats/asthma.htm (accessed January 10, 2009).

7. The American College of Allergy, Asthma, & Immunology, "Asthma Uncontrolled in 85 percent of Inner City Students," *American College of Allergy,*

Asthma, & Immunology Online (July 10, 2006) www.acaai.org/public/
linkpages/AsthmaInnerCity.htm (accessed August 15, 2009).

8. The Centers for Disease Control, *NCHS Data Brief No. 10,*by Amy M.
Branum et al., The CDC, National Center for Health Statistics (October 2007).

9. Elizabeth Lipski, *Digestive Wellness* (New York: McGraw Hill, 2004) 90.

10. National Institute of Allergy and Infectious Diseases, "Food Allergy: Report of the NIH Expert Panel on Food Allergy Research," NIH,
www3.niaid.nih.gov/topics/foodAllergy/research/ReportFoodAllergy.htp (accessed August 3, 2009).

11. Ibid.

12. Mark Jackson, *Allergy: The History of a Modern Malady* (London: Reaktion Books, 2006) 58.

13. The Centers for Disease Control, *NCHS Data Brief No. 10,*by Amy M.
Branum et al., The CDC, National Center for Health Statistics (October
2007).

14. Phil Lieberman, MD and John A. Anderson, MD, *Allergic Diseases* (To-
towa, NJ: Human Press, 2007), 272.

15. Dr. William Walsh, interview with author, February, 2009.

16. The Centers for Disease Control, "QuickStats: Percentage of Children
Aged 5-17 Years Ever Having Diagnoses of Attention Deficit/Hyperactivity Disorder (ADHD) or Learning Disability (LD) by Sex and Diagnosis," *Morbidity
and Mortality Weekly* 54, no. 43(November 2005): 1107, www.cdc.gov/mmwr/
preview/mmwrhtml/mm5443a8.htm (accessed September 9, 2009).

17. Lynn Waterhouse, "Autism Overflows: Increasing Prevalence and Proliferating Theories," *Neuropsychology Review* 18 (2008) 273-286.

18. Sue Reid, "One child in 60 'suffers from a form of autism,'" *The Daily
Mail Online,* www.dailymail.co.uk/news/article-1163606/One-child-60-suffers
-form-autism.html (accessed August 3, 2009).

19. Autism Research Institute, "Recently Released Data from the National
Survey of Children's Health Reports that Autism Now Affects 1 percent of Children and is More Common Than Children's Cancer, Diabetes, and AIDS
combined," *Reuters,* August 3, 2009 (accessed August 3, 2009).

20. Autism Research Institute, *ARI Calls for Immediate Federal Response to
New Autism Figures - Oct. '09* (October 2009) www.autism.com (accessed October 6, 2009).

21. National Institutes of Mental Health, *ADHD Booklet* (2003) www.nimh
.nih.gov/health/publications/attention-deficit-hyperactivity-disorder/
adhd_booklet.pdf (accessed March 11, 2009); William E. Pelham PhD, et al.,
"The Economic Impact of Attention-Deficit/Hyperactivity Disorder in Children and Adolescents," *Ambulatory Pediatrics* (January/February 2007): 1.

22. Melissa A Brotman et al., "Prevalence, clinical correlates, and longitudinal course of severe mood dysregulation in children," *Biological Psychiatry* 60, no. 9 (2006): 991-997.

23. S. Sutton Hamilton et al., "Oppositional Defiant Disorder," *American Family Physician*, 78, no. 7 (October 2008): 861-866.

24. Natasha Campbell McBride, "GAPS, the Gut and Psychology Syndrome" (lecture, The Weston A. Price Foundation, Wise Traditions Conference, San Francisco, CA, November 8, 2008).

25. Carlos Blanco MD et al., "Mental Health of College Students and Their Non–College-Attending Peers: Results From the National Epidemiologic Study on Alcohol and Related Conditions," *Archives of General Psychiatry* 65, no. 12 (2008): 1429-1437.

26. Lynn Waterhouse, "Autism Overflows: Increasing Prevalence and Proliferating Theories," *Neuropsychology Review* 18 (November 2008): 273-286.

27. Tanya E. Froehlich, MD et al., "Prevalence, Recognition, and Treatment of Attention-Deficit/Hyperactivity Disorder in a National Sample of US Children," *Archives of Pediatric and Adolescent Medicine* 161, no. 9 (2007): 857-864.

28. William E. Pelham PhD, et al., "The Economic Impact of Attention-Deficit/Hyperactivity Disorder in Children and Adolescents," *Ambulatory Pediatrics* (January/February 2007).

29. Donna Jackson Nakazawa, *The Autoimmune Epidemic* (New York: Simon & Schuster, 2008).

30. C. Jakobsen, "Incidence of ulcerative colitis and Crohn's disease in Danish children: Still rising or leveling out?" *Journal of Crohn's & Colitis* 2 (June 2008): 152-157; Johan van Limbergen et al., "A detailed investigation into epidemiological risk factors for childhood onset inflammatory bowel disease in Scotland," *Gastroenterology* 134, no. 4 (2008): A189.

31. Children's Digestive Health and Nutrition Foundation, "Pediatric Celiac Disease" www.celiachealth.org (accessed March 11, 2009).

32. MSNBC, "Celiac disease cases quadruple in the United States," *Reuters.* July 10, 2009, www.msnbc.msn.com/id/31852701/ns/health-diet_and_nutrition/ (accessed July 11, 2009).

33. Donna Jackson Nakazawa, *The Autoimmune Epidemic* (New York: Simon & Schuster, 2008): 25.

34. William E. Pelham PhD, et al., "The Economic Impact of Attention-Deficit/Hyperactivity Disorder in Children and Adolescents," *Ambulatory Pediatrics* (January/February 2007).

35. Michael L. Ganz, "The lifetime distribution of incremental societal costs of autism," *Archives of Pediatrics and Adolescent Medicine* 161 (2007): 343-349.

36. This extrapolation conservatively assumes that the prevalence of autism does <u>not</u> continue to rise, which is unlikely given recent trends. This model also assumes a constant birthrate. Thus, the costs incurred by 2065 are likely to be much higher than the given estimate.

37. Fighting Autism, "U.S. Annual Economic Cost," www.fightingautism .org (accessed August 30, 2009).

38. The Autism Society of America, "Facts and Statistics," www.autism -society.org/site/PageServer?pagename=asa_media_home (accessed August 30, 2009).

39. The National Autistic Society, "Employment," www.nas.org.uk/nas/jsp/ polopoly.jsp?d=1937 (accessed August 28, 2009).

40. E. Michael Foster et al., "The High Costs of Aggression: Public Expenditures Resulting From Conduct Disorder," *American Journal of Public Health* 95, no. 10 (October 2005): 1767.

41. Centers for Disease Control and Prevention, "Autism Information Center," www.cdc.gov/ncbddd/autism/faq_prevalence.htm (accessed March 5, 2009).

42. Chris Plauché Johnson, MD et al., "Identification and Evaluation of Children With Autism Spectrum Disorders," *Pediatrics* 120, no. 5 (November 2007).

43. PT Shattuck, "The Contribution of Diagnostic Substitution to the Growing Administrative Prevalence of Autism in US Special Education," *Pediatrics* 117, no. 4 (April 2006): 1028-1037.

44. Jacquelyn Bertrand, "Prevalence of Autism in a United States Population: The Brick Township, New Jersey, Investigation" *Pediatrics* 108, no. 5 (November 2001): 1155-116; Irva Hertz-Picciotto and Lora Delwiche, "The Rise in Autism and the Role of Age at Diagnosis," *Epidemiology* 20, no. 1 (January 2009): 84-90.

45. Mark Blaxill, "What's Going On? The Question of Time Trends in Autism," *Public Health Reports* 119, no. 5 (November 2004): 536-352.

46. Thoughtful House Center for Children, "Autism Diagnostic Substitution," FightingAutism, Austin, TX, www.fightingautism.org/idea/autism -diagnostic-substitution.php (accessed February 16, 2009).

47. Irva Hertz-Picciotto and Lora Delwiche, "The Rise in Autism and the Role of Age at Diagnosis," *Epidemiology* 20, no. 1 (January 2009): 84-90.

48. The American Academy of Pediatrics, "ADHD," www.aap.org/publiced/ br_adhd_faq.htm (accessed February 16, 2009).

49. Bruce P. Lanphear et al., "Increasing Prevalence of Recurrent Otitis Media Among Children in the United States," *Pediatrics* 99, no. 3 (March 1997): e1.

50. Dr. Robyn Cosford, "Occult Infections, Streptococcus, Biofilms, PANDAS and MINDDD in Autism," (lecture, Defeat Autism Now Conference, San Diego, CA, October 2008).

51. The American Academy of Microbiology, "Probiotic Microbes: The Scientific Basis," American Society for Microbiology, academy.asm.org/images/stories/documents/probioticmicrobesfull.pdf (accessed, March 14, 2009).

52. Jessica Snyder Sachs, *Good Germs, Bad Germs: Health and Survival in a Bacterial World* (New York: Hill and Wang, 2007): 75.

53. Ibid., 79.

54. Ibid., 87.

55. National Institutes of Mental Health, *ADHD Booklet* (2003) www.nimh.nih.gov/health/publications/attention-deficit-hyperactivity-disorder/adhd_booklet.pdf (accessed March 11, 2009).

56. Lynn Waterhouse, "Autism Overflows: Increasing Prevalence and Proliferating Theories," *Neuropsychology Review* 18 (2008) 273-286.

57. Ibid., 274. One study proposed that at least part (17 percent) of the increase in autism is due to increased television watching with the growth of cable television during the 1970 and 1980s.

58. Ibid., 274.

59. Ibid., 275. It should be noted that thimerosal has not been eliminated from all vaccines (e.g., influenza vaccines still contain thimerosal).

60. National Institutes of Mental Health, *ADHD Booklet* (2003) www.nimh.nih.gov/health/publications/attention-deficit-hyperactivity-disorder/adhd_booklet.pdf (accessed March 11, 2009).

CHAPTER TWO

1. Thomas A. Pearson et al., "Markers of Inflammation and Cardiovascular Disease," *Circulation* 107 (2003): 499.

2. Michael Camilleri, "Serotonin in the gastrointestinal tract," *Current Opinion in Endocrinology, Diabetes and Obesity* 16, no. 1 (February 2009): 53-59.

3. IN Pessah et al., "Immunologic and neurdevelopmental susceptibilities of autism," *Neurotoxicology* 29, no. 3 (May 2008): 532-45; PH Patterson, "Immune involvement in schizophrenia and autism: Etiology, pathology and animal models," *Behavioural Brain Research* 24 (Dec 2008).

4. Roland Tisch et al., "Dysregulation of T cell peripheral tolerance in type 1 diabetes," *Advances in Immunology* 100 (2008): 125-149.

5. Swiss Federal Institute of Technology, "Research," Environmental Biomedicine, www.envbiomedicine.ethz.ch/research (accessed January 19, 2009).

6. C.A. Edwards and A. M. Parrett, "Intestinal flora during the first months of life: new perspectives," *British Journal of Nutrition* 88 (2002): S11-S18.

7. One of these dysfunctions is the development of a skewed balance between Th1 and Th2 cells. White blood cells known as T-cells are central players in a body's immune system. There are different types of T-cells that serve different roles in the body. T-cells known as T helper (Th) 1 or Th2 cells secrete certain immune factors (such as interferon or interleukin) that have specific functions within the immune system, and both types of cells have been implicated in the development of chronic disease. Th1 and Th2 cells have different roles, but it has been established that a "counter-regulatory balance" between Th1 and Th2 responses is necessary for the maintenance of health and wellness. There are also T-cells known as T-regulatory cells, which help to suppress immune (Th1 and Th2) responses. When either Th1 or Th2 cells are upregulated (an increased number of cells circulating) without the presence of the other, or another regulatory response (such as the upregulation of gut-derived Th3 cells), the immune system is considered dysregulated. A skew in favor of Th1 cells (more Th1 cells circulating than Th2 or regulatory T cells, for example) has been associated with autoimmune diseases, and a skew in favor of Th2 cells has been associated with atopic (allergic) disease. In each of these cases, the immune cells are signaled to "attack" benign antigens (such as food molecules or human tissues), but critical immune suppressive or regulating responses do not occur. It is believed that disruptions to colonies of normal microflora (microorganisms) in the gastrointestinal system will result in depressed immunoregulation. For instance, the proper function of dendritic cells (which are known to direct T-cells to assume regulatory functions) is believed to be predicated upon the existence of a certain balance of commensal ("friendly") bacteria in the intestines.

8. A. Borchers et al., "Probiotics and immunity," *Journal of Gastroenterology* 44 (2009): 26-46; UG Strauch et al., "Influence of intestinal bacteria on induction of regulatory T cells: lessons from a transfer model of colitis," *Gut* 54 (2005):1546-1552; Tomas Hrncir et al., "Gut microbiota and lipopolysaccharide content of the diet influence development of regulatory T cells: studies in germ-free mice," *BMC Immunology* 9 (2008): 65; Hiroaki Kitano and Kanae Oda, "Robustness trade-offs and host-microbial symbiosis in the immune system," *Molecular Systems Biology* 2 (2006).

9. Hannah Wexler, "Bacteroides: the Good, the Bad, and the Nitty-Gritty," *Clinical Microbiology Reviews* 20, no. 4 (October 2007): 593-621.

10. Ann M. O'Hara and Fergus Shanahan, "The gut flora as a forgotten organ," *European Molecular Biology Organization Report* 7, no 7 (July 2006): 688-693.

11. Hannah Wexler, "Bacteroides: the Good, the Bad, and the Nitty-Gritty," *Clinical Microbiology Reviews* 20, no. 4 (October 2007): 593-621.

12. Jessica Snyder Sachs, *Good Germs, Bad Germs: Health and Survival in a Bacterial World* (New York: Hill and Wang, 2007).

13. Patrick Hanaway MD, "Balance of Flora, GALT, and Mucosal Integrity," *Alternative Therapies in Health and Medicine* 12, no. 5 (September/October 2006).

14. Leo Galland, MD, "The Effect of Intestinal Microbes on Systemic Immunity," Excerpted from *Power Healing* (New York: Random House, 1998) mdheal.org/microbes.htm (accessed February 12, 2009).

15. David Brady DC, CCN, DACBN, ND. "Functional Medicine," *Dynamic Chiropractic* 17, no. 8 (April 1999); G. Oliveira et al., "Mitochondrial dysfunction in autism spectrum disorders: a population-based study," *Developmental Medicine and Child Neurology* 47 (2005): 185-189.

16. Z. Liu et al., "Tight junctions, leaky intestines, and pediatric diseases," *Acta Paediatricia* 94 (2005): 386-393.

17. J.W. Bennett and M. Klich, "Mycotoxins," *Clinical Microbiology Reviews* (July 2003): 497-516.

18. Yoshinori Mine and Jie Wie Zhang, "Surfactants Enhance the Tight-Junction Permeability of Food Allergens in Human Intestinal Epithelial Caco-2 Cells," *International Archives of Allergy and Immunology* 130, no. 2 (Feb 2003); Simon Smale and Ingvar Bjarnason, "Determining small bowel integrity following drug treatment," *British Journal of Clinical Pharmacology* 56, no. 3 (September 2003): 284-291; Z. Liu et al., "Tight junctions, leaky intestines, and pediatric diseases," *Acta Paediatricia* 94 (2005): 386-393.

19. Ruchika Mohan et al., "Effects of Bifidobacterium lactis Bb12 Supplementation on Intestinal Microbiota of Preterm Infants: A Double-Blind, Placebo-Controlled, Randomized Study," *Journal of Clinical Microbiology* 44, no. 11 (November 2006): 4025-4031.

20. Samuli Rautava and Erika Isolauri, "The Development of Gut Immune Responses and Gut Microbiota: Effects of Probiotics in Prevention and Treatment of Allergic Disease," *Current Issues in Intestinal Microbiology* 3 (2002): 15-22.

21. F. Savino, "Lactobacillus reuteri (American Type Culture Collection Strain 55730) versus simethicone in the treatment of infantile colic: a prospective randomized study," *Pediatrics* 119, no. 1 (January 2007): e124-30.

22. Erica White and Caroline Sherlock, "The Effect of Nutritional Therapy for Yeast Infection (Candidiasis) in Cases of Chronic Fatigue Syndrome," *Journal of Orthomolecular Medicine* 20, no. 3 (2005).

23. Ibid.

24. *U.S. News and World Report*, "One Sweet Nation," March 28, 2005.

25. Natasha Campbell-McBride, *Gut and Psychology Syndrome* (Cambridge: Medinform Publishing, 2004).

26. Cedars-Sinai Medical Center, "Birth Control Pill: Oral Contraceptive Use May Be Safe, But Information Gaps Remain," *ScienceDaily*, January 17, 2009, www.sciencedaily.com/releases/2009/01/090114092848.htm (accessed February 26, 2009).

27. Z. Liu et al., "Tight junctions, leaky intestines, and pediatric diseases," *Acta Paediatricia* 94 (2005): 386-393.

28. Randall Fitzgerald, *The Hundred-Year Lie* (London: Plume, 2007).

29. Z. Liu et al., "Tight junctions, leaky intestines, and pediatric diseases," *Acta Paediatricia* 94 (2005): 386-393; Joanne K. Tobacman, "Review of Harmful Gastrointestinal Effects of Carrageenan in Animal Experiments," *Environmental Health Perspectives* 109, no 10 (October 2001).

30. Gail Hecht, "Microbial Pathogens That Affect Tight Junctions," in *Tight Junctions* (New York: CRC Press, 2001): 493-515; Dr. Robyn Cosford, "Occult Infections, Streptococcus, Biofilms, PANDAS and MINDDD in Autism," (lecture, Defeat Autism Now! Conference, San Diego, CA, October 2008).

31. Lindsey A. Moser et al., "Astrovirus Increases Epithelial Barrier Permeability Independently of Viral Replication," *Journal of Virology* 81, no. 21 (November 2007).

32. RC Bransfield et al., "The association between tick-borne infections, Lyme borreliosis and autism spectrum disorders," *Medical Hypotheses* 70, no. 5 (November 2007): 967-74.

33. Mark. A. Hyman, M.D, "Is the Cure for Brain Disorders Outside the Brain?" *Alternative Therapies in Health and Medicine* 13, no. 6 (November/December 2007): 6.

34. Mark Jackson, *Allergy: The History of a Modern Malady* (London: Reaktion Books, 2007).

35. Katrina J. Allen, David J. Hill and Ralf G. Heine, "Food Allergy in Childhood," *Medical Journal of Australia* 185, no 7 (October 2006).

36. William Walsh, *Food Allergies: The Complete Guide to Understanding and Relieving Your Food Allergies* (Hoboken, NJ: Wiley John and Sons Inc, 2000): 3.

37. Wikipedia, "Allergy," en.wikipedia.org/wiki/Allergy (accessed Feb 27, 2009); E. Isolauri, S.Rautava, and M. Kalliomaki, "Food allergy in irritable bowel syndrome: new facts and old fallacies," *Gut* 53, no. 10 (October 2004): 1391-1393.

38. Samuli Rautava and Erika Isolauri, "The Development of Gut Immune Responses and Gut Microbiota: Effects of Probiotics in Prevention and Treatment of Allergic Disease," *Current Issues in Intestinal Microbiology* 3 (2002):15-22.

39. C. Vael et al., "Early intestinal *Bacteroides fragilis* colonization and development of asthma," *BMC Pulmonary Medicine* 8 (September 2008): 19.

40. Dr. Robyn Cosford, "Occult Infections, Streptococcus, Biofilms, PANDAS and MINDDD in Autism," (lecture, Defeat Autism Now! Conference, San Diego, CA, October 2008).

41. Nariman Hijazi, Bahaa Abalkhail, and Anthony Seaton, "Diet and childhood asthma in a society in transition: A study in urban and rural Saudi Arabia," *Thorax* 55, no. 9 (2000): 775-779.

42. CR Morris and MC Agin, "Syndrome of allergy, apraxia, and malabsorption: characterization of a neurodevelopmental phenotype that responds to omega 3 and vitamin E supplementation," *Alternative Therapies in Health and Medicine* 15, no. 4 (July-August 2009): 34-43.

43. It is important to note that not all children display all of these characteristics. In fact, some children may only display a few of these symptoms.

44. Bernard Rimland, PhD, "The History of the Defeat Autism Now! (DAN!) Project: How it Got Started, and Why It Got Started," in *Autism: Effective Biomedical Treatments* by John Pangborn PhD and Sydney MacDonald Baker, MD (San Diego, CA: Autism Research Institute, 2005).

45. Bryan Jepson, MD, "Conference Presentations: Bryan Jepson, MD," Thoughtful House Center for Children, www.thoughtfulhouse.org/0405-conf -bjepson.htm, (accessed July 20, 2009).

46. Lynn Waterhouse, "Autism Overflows: Increasing Prevalence and Proliferating Theories," *Neuropsychology Review* 18 (November 2008): 273-286.

47. However, twin covariance rates have been estimated between 60-90 percent but never as high 100 percent, which indicates that genes may play a role, but environmental factors, at least for a subset of autistic twins, clearly play into etiology as well.

48. Lynn Waterhouse, "Autism Overflows: Increasing Prevalence and Proliferating Theories," *Neuropsychology Review* 18 (November 2008): 273-286.

49. Autism Research Institute, "Why do I pursue medical treatment for my child's autism?" www.autism.com/medical/autism_medical.pdf (accessed March 3, 2009).

50. Mark Hyman MD, "Autism: Is It All in the Head?" *Alternative Therapies in Health and Medicine* 14, no. 6 (November/December 2008): 12-15.

51. Hans Rediers et al., "Unraveling the Secret Lives of Bacteria: Use of In Vivo Expression Technology and Differential Fluorescence Induction Promoter Traps as Tools for Exploring Niche-Specific Gene Expression," *Microbiology and Molecular Biology Reviews* 69, no. 2 (June 2005): 217-261.

52. Dr. Arthur Krigsman, "Gastrointestinal Pathology in Autism: Description and Treatment," Thoughtful House Center for Children, paper adapted from

a presentation (2000), www.thoughtfulhouse.org/0405-conf-akrigsman.htm (accessed March 18, 2009).

53. Dr. Margaret Bauman, "The Autism Spectrum Disorders: Beyond Behavior—Research and Treatment Implications," (lecture, UC Davis M.I.N.D. Institute, Distinguished Lecturer Series, Sacramento, CA, January 11, 2006) www.ucdmc.ucdavis.edu/mindinstitute/events/dls_recorded_events.html#dls08. (accessed, January 21, 2009).

54. Karoly Horvath et al., "Gastrointestinal abnormalities in children with autistic disorder," *Journal of Pediatrics* 135, no. 5 (November 1999): 559-63; Karoly Horvath and JA Perman, "Autistic disorder and gastrointestinal disease," *Current Opinion in Pediatrics* 14, no. 5 (October 2002): 583-7.

55. Craig A. Erickson et al., "Gastrointestinal Factors in Autistic Disorder: A Critical Review," *Journal of Autism and Developmental Disorders* 35, no. 6, (December 2005).

56. Andrew Wakefield is considered a controversial figure because he published a study in 1998 that demonstrated the presence of measles virus in the intestinal tissue of autistic patients, which implied a link between the Measles-Mumps-Rubella vaccine and the development of regressive autism. This controversy still rages as several studies aimed to replicate Wakefield's findings have drawn different results.

57. Dr. Andrew Wakefield, "The Seat of the Soul; The Origins of the Autism Epidemic," (lecture, Carnegie Mellon University, Pittsburgh, PA, November 17, 2005, Thoughtful House Center for Children, www.thoughtfulhouse.org/awakefield_1105.pdf (accessed March 6, 2009).

58. Some of Dr. Wakefield's research is available at: www.thoughtfulhouse.org/publications.htm (accessed March 7, 2009).

59. B Thjodleifsson et al., "Effect of Pentavac and measles-mumps-rubella (MMR) vaccination on the intestine," *Gut* 51, no. 6 (December 2002): 816-7; This study, which claims to refute the findings from Andrew Wakefield's MMR study in 1998, uses only fecal calprotectin as an indicator of gastrointestinal inflammation. Fecal calprotectin is effective in determining inflammation associated with neutrophils (as seen in IBD) but may not be a reliable marker for determining all inflammatory processes in the intestine (such as inflammation associated with small intestine bacterial overgrowth). See: Massimo Montalto et al, "Fecal Calprotectin Concentrations in Patients with Small Intestinal Bacterial Overgrowth," *Digestive Diseases* 26, no. 2 (April 2008): 183-186.

60. L. Shi et al., "Activation of the maternal immune system alters cerebellar development in the offspring," *Brain, Behavior, and Immunity* 23, no. 1 (January 2009): 116-23; C. Winter et al., "Dopamine and serotonin levels following

prenatal viral infection in mouse—implications for psychiatric disorders such as schizophrenia and autism," *European Neuropsychopharmacology* 18, no. 10 (October 2008): 712-6; GL Nicolson et al., "Evidence for Mycoplasma ssp., Chlamydia pneumoniae, and human herpes virus-6 coinfections in the blood of patients with autistic spectrum disorders," *Journal of Neuroscience Research* 85, no. 5 (April 2007): 1143-8; K Lancaster et al., "Abnormal social behaviors in young and adult rats neonatally infected with Borna disease virus," *Behavioural Brain Research* 176, no. 1 (January 2007): 141-8.

61. Sidney Baker, "Canaries and Miners," *Alternative Therapies in Health and Medicine* 14, no. 6 (2008): 24-26.

62. Hans Rediers et al., "Unraveling the Secret Lives of Bacteria: Use of In Vivo Expression Technology and Differential Fluorescence Induction Promotor Traps as Tools for Exploring Niche-Specific Gene Expression," *Microbiology and Molecular Biology Reviews* 69, no. 2 (June 2005): 217-261; Fredrik Bäckhed et al., "Host-Bacterial Mutualism in the Human Intestine," *Science* 307 (March 25, 2005): 1915; Genome Alberta, "The Human Metabolome Project," www.metabolomics.ca/ (accessed March 6, 2009).

63. Jessica A. Clark and Craig M. Coopersmith, "Intestinal crosstalk—a new paradigm for understanding the gut as the 'motor' of critical illness," *Shock* 28, no. 4 (October 2007): 384-393; Ann M. O'Hara and Fergus Shanahan, "The gut flora as a forgotten organ," *European Molecular Biology Organization Reports* 7, no. 7 (2006).

64. Paul Ashwood et al., "The immune response in autism: a new frontier for autism research," *Journal of Leukocyte Biology* 80 (July 2006): 1-15.

65. M. Mary Konstantareas and Soula Homatidis, "Brief Report: Ear infections in autistic and normal children," *Journal of Autism and Developmental Disorders* 17, no. 4 (December 1987).

66. Germana Moretti, "What every psychiatrist should know about PANDAS: a review," *Clinical Practice and Epidemiology in Mental Health* 4 (May 2008): 13.

67. Harumi Jyonouchi et al., "Impact of innate immunity in a subset of children with autism spectrum disorders: a case control study," *Journal of Neuroinflammation* 5 (November 2008): 52.

68. Paul Ashwood et al., "The immune response in autism: a new frontier for autism research," *Journal of Leukocyte Biology* 80 (July 2006): 1-15.

69. Wikipedia, "Encephalitis lethargica," en.wikipedia.org/wiki/Encephalitis _lethargica (accessed February 1, 2009).

70. Russell C. Dale et al., "Encephalitis lethargica syndrome: 20 new cases and evidence of basal ganglia autoimmunity," *Brain* 127, no. 1 (October 2003).

71. Anne M. Connolly, MD et al., "Serum autoantibodies to brain in Landau-Kleffner variant, autism, and other neurologic disorders," *The Journal of Pediatrics* 134, no. 5 (May 1999): 607-13.

72. Diane L. Vargas et al., "Neuroglial activation and neuroinflammation in the brain of patients with autism," *Annals of Neurology* 57, no. 1 (January 2005): 67-81.

73. Dr. Andrew Wakefield, "The Seat of the Soul; The Origins of the Autism Epidemic," (lecture, Carnegie Mellon University, Pittsburgh, PA, November 17, 2005) www.thoughtfulhouse.org/awakefield_1105.pdf (accessed March 6, 2009).

74. Natasha Campbell-McBride, *Gut and Psychology Syndrome* (Cambridge: Medinform Publishing, 2004), 17.

75. Ibid., 18.

76. Ibid., 26.

77. R.E.O. Williams et al., "The influence of intestinal bacteria on the absorption and metabolism of foreign compounds," *Journal of Clinical Pathology* 5 Supplement (1971): 125-129.

78. Rowland et al., "Effects of diet on mercury metabolism and excretion in mice given methylmercury: role of gut flora," *Archives of Environmental Health* 39, no. 6 (1984): 401-8.

79. Center for Science in the Public Interest, "Petition to Set a Regulatory Limit for Methylmercury in Seafood that Reflects the Risk to Pregnant Women and Children From the Intake of Seafood Containing Methylmercury," Letter to Dr. Jane Henney, Commissioner, FDA, July 17, 2000 www.cspinet.org/foodsafety/methylmerc_limit.html (accessed March 8, 2009).

80. Recent studies have found unsafe levels of mercury in high fructose corn syrup, as mercury is an element used in the synthesis and manufacturing of the product; David Wallinga et al., "Not So Sweet: Missing Mercury and High Fructose Corn Syrup," *Institute for Agriculture and Trade Policy*, Minneapolis, Minnesota (January 2009).

81. James B. Adams et al., "Mercury, Lead, and Zinc in Baby Teeth of Children with Autism Versus Controls," *Journal of Toxicology and Environmental Health* 70 (2007).

82. James B. Adams et al., "Mercury in first-cut baby hair of children with autism versus typically-developing children," *Toxicological & Environmental Chemistry* 90, no. 4 (October 2008): 739-753; Also see: Amy Holmes et al., "Reduced Levels of Mercury in First Baby Haircuts of Autistic Children," *International Journal of Toxicology* 22 (March 2003): 277-285.

83. Gayle C. Windham et al., "Autism Spectrum Disorders in Relation to Distribution of Hazardous Air Pollutants in the San Francisco Bay Area," *Environmental Health Perspectives* 114, no. 9 (September 2006): 1438-44.

84. R.F. Palmer et al., "Proximity to point sources of environmental mercury release as a predictor of autism prevalence," *Health and Place* 15, no. 1 (March 2009): 18-24.

85. Richard Lathe, "Environmental factors and limbic vulnerability in childhood autism; Clinical report," *American Journal of Biochemistry and Biotechnology* 4, no. 2 (March 22, 2008).

86. Some vaccines do still contain ethylmercury (thimerosal), namely the influenza vaccine; Autism Research Institute, "The Vaccine-Autism Connection—Part I (Thimerosal)," www.autism.com/triggers/vaccine/thimerosalrefer ences.htm (accessed March 8, 2009).

87. S. Jill James et al., "Metabolic biomarkers of increased oxidative stress and impaired methylation capacity in children with autism," *American Journal of Clinical Nutrition* 80, no. 6 (December 2004): 1611-1617.

88. Ibid.

89. Arthur Allen, *Vaccine: The Controversial Story of Medicine's Greatest Lifesaver* (New York: W.W. Norton & Company, 2007), 379.

90. Doris Rapp, *Is This Your Child?*(New York: Harper Paperbacks, 1991); Donna Jackson Nakazawa, *The Autoimmune Epidemic* (New York: Simon & Schuster, 2008).

91. Kenneth Blum et al., "Attention-deficit-hyperactivity disorder and reward deficiency syndrome," *Neuropsychiatric Disease and Treatment* 4, no. 5 (2008) 893-917.

92. Physician's Postgraduate Press, "Managing ADHD in Children, Adolescents, and Adults With Comorbid Anxiety in Primary Care," *The Primary Care Companion to The Journal of Clinical Psychiatry* 9, no. 2 (2007): 129-138.

93. Richard Mackarness, *Not All in The Mind* (London: Pan, 1976).

94. Dr. William H. Philpott and Dwight K. Kalita PhD, *Brain Allergies: The Psychonutrient and Magnetic Connections* (Los Angeles: Keats Publishing, 1980) 23.

95. Paul D. Arnold and Margaret A. Richter, "Is obsessive-compulsive disorder an autoimmune disease?" *Canadian Medical Association Journal* 165, no. 10 (November 2001): 1353-1358; Daniel R. Hanson and Irving I. Gottesman, "Theories of schizophrenia: a genetic-inflammatory-vascular synthesis," *BMC Medical Genetics* 6 (February 2005): 7.

96. Hui-Li Want et al., "Case-Control Study of Blood Lead Levels and Attention Deficit Hyperactivity Disorder in Chinese Children," *Environmental Health Perspectives* 116, no. 10 (October 2008).

97. Braun et al., "Association of Environmental Toxicants and Conduct Disorder in U.S. Children," *NHANES 2001-2004* 116, no. 7 (July 2008).

98. Carol Joinson et al., "Psychological Difference Between Children With and Without Soiling Problems," *Pediatrics* 117, no. 5 (May 2006): 1575-1584.

99. M.A. Benninga et al., "Colonic transit times and behaviour profiles in children with defecation disorders," *Archives of the Diseases of Childhood* 89 (2004): 13-16.

100. Social case worker [name withheld], Massachusetts Department of Children and Families, email correspondence with author, March 1, 2009.

101. JM Swanson et al., "Etiologic subtypes of attention-deficit/hyperactivity disorder: brain imaging, molecular genetic and environmental factors and the dopamine hypothesis," *Neuropsychology Review* 17, no. 1 (March 2007): 39-59.

102. Bistra B Nankova, "Nicotinic Induction of Preproenkephalin and Tyrosine Hydroxylase Gene Expression in Butyrate-Differentiated Rat PC12 Cells: A Model for Adaptation to Gut-Derived Environmental Signals," *Pediatric Research* 53, no. 1 (January 2003): 113-118.

103. Pradeep Mally et al., "Stereospecific Regulation of Tyrosine Hydroxylase and Proenkephalin Genes by Short-Chain Fatty Acids in Rat PC12 Cells," *Pediatric Research* 55, no. 5 (May 2004): 847-854.

CHAPTER THREE

1. Abdel R. Omran, "The Epidemiologic Transition: A Theory of the Epidemiology of Population Change," *The Milbank Memorial Fund Quarterly* 49, no. 4 (1971): 509-538.

2. Stanford T. Shulman, "The History of Pediatric Infectious Diseases," *Pediatric Research* 55, no. 1 (January 2004): 163-176.

3. David Cutler and Grant Miller, "The Role of Public Health Improvements in Health Advances: The Twentieth-Century United States," *Demography* 42 (February 2005) 1.

4. Ibid.

5. Abdel R. Omran, "The Epidemiologic Transition: A Theory of the Epidemiology of Population Change," *The Milbank Memorial Fund Quarterly* 49, no. 4 (1971): 509-538.

6. S. F. Bloomfield et al., "Too clean, or not too clean: The Hygiene Hypothesis and home hygiene," *Clinical and Experimental Allergy* 36 (2006):402-425.

7. Stephen T. Holgate, "The epidemic of asthma and allergy," *Journal of the Royal Society of Medicine* 97 (March 2004).

8. N Hijazi et al., "Diet and childhood asthma in a society in transition: a study in urban and rural Saudi Arabia," *Thorax* 55 (2000): 775-6; E. von Mutius

et al., "Increasing prevalence of hay fever and atopy among children in Leipzig, East Germany," *Lancet* 351 (1998): 862-6.

9. S. F. Bloomfield et al., "'Too clean, or not too clean: The Hygiene Hypothesis and home hygiene," *Clinical and Experimental Allergy* 36 (2006): 402-425.

10. Ibid.

11. Migel Gueimonde et al., "Breast Milk: A Source of Bifidobacteria for Infant Gut Development and Maturation?" *Neonatology* 92 (2007): 64-66.

12. Natasha Campbell-McBride, *Gut and Psychology Syndrome* (Cambridge: Medinform Publishing, 2004).

13. "Contaminants in Human Milk: Weighing the Risks against the Benefits of Breastfeeding," *Environmental Health Perspectives* 116 no. 10 (October 2008): A427-A434; O. Vaarala et al., "The 'perfect storm' for type 1 diabetes: the complex interplay between intestinal microbiota, gut permeability, and mucosal immunity," *Diabetes* 57, no. 10 (October 2008): 2555-62.

14. Chana Palmer et al., "Development of the Human Infant Intestinal Microbiota," *PLoS Biology* 5, no 7 (July 2007).

15. Jason A. Hawrelak et al., "The Causes of Intestinal Dysbiosis: A Review," *Alternative Medicine Review* 9, no. 2 (2004).

CHAPTER FOUR

1. IMS Health, Top-line Industry Data, www.imshealth.com/portal/site/imshealth/menuitem.a953aef4d73d1ecd88f611019418c22a/?vgnextoid=94c0beb3a50d6110VgnVCM10000071812ca2RCRD&vgnextfmt=default (accessed March 8, 2009).

2. Maggie Mahar, *Money Driven Medicine* (New York: Collins, 2006).

3. IMS Health, Top-line Industry Data, www.imshealth.com/portal/site/imshealth/menuitem.a953aef4d73d1ecd88f611019418c22a/?vgnextoid=94c0beb3a50d6110VgnVCM10000071812ca2RCRD&vgnextfmt=default (accessed March 8, 2009); Cowen and Company, *Pharmaceuticals: Industry Overview* (New York: Cowen and Company, 2009).

4. Jason A. Hawrelak et al., "The Causes of Intestinal Dysbiosis: A Review," *Alternative Medicine Review* 9, no. 2 (2004).

5. Union of Concerned Scientists, *Hogging It!: Estimates of Antimicrobial Abuse in Livestock* (Cambridge, MA: Union of Concerned Scientists 2001) www.ucsusa.org/assets/documents/food_and_agriculture/hog_chaps.pdf (accessed March 23, 2009).

6. Martin J. Blaser, "Who are we: Indigenous microbes and the ecology of human diseases," *European Molecular Biology Organization Report* 7, no. 10 (2006).

7. Ibid.

8. Dr. Natasha Campbell-McBride, *Gut and Psychology Syndrome* (Cambridge: Medinform Publishing, 2004): 31-34.

9. Carl Erik Nord et al., "Effect of Tigecycline on Normal Oropharyngeal and Intestinal Microflora," *Antimicrobial Agents Chemotherapy* 50, no. 10 (October 2006).

10. Carl Erik Nord and C Edlund, "Impact of antimicrobial agents on human intestinal microflora," *Journal of Chemotherapy* 2 (1990): 218-237.

11. *E.R. Squibb and Sons, Inc v. Otis R. Bowen, M.D., Secretary of Health and Human Services, et al.* 85 CDC (1989) me.findacase.com/research/wfrm DocViewer.aspx/xq/fac. percent5CCDC percent5CCDC2 percent5Carchp percent5C1989 percent5C19890314_0000085.CDC.htm/qx (accessed August 28, 2009); The FDA required the Squibb company to remove this (and similar) products because of lack of perceived efficacy. It was perceived to be an ineffective drug because at the time, intestinal fungal overgrowth was not believed to be something that caused human disease. Today, opinions on this matter have changed, and many physicians treat patients for intestinal fungal overgrowth.

12. I. Williamson et al., "Consultations for middle ear disease, antibiotic prescribing and risk factors for reattendance: a case-linked cohort study," *British Journal of General Practice* 56, no. 524 (March 2006): 170-175.

13. Union of Concerned Scientists, *Hogging It!: Estimates of Antimicrobial Abuse in Livestock* (Cambridge, MA: Union of Concerned Scientists 2001) www.ucsusa.org/assets/documents/food_and_agriculture/hog_chaps.pdf (accessed March 23, 2009).

14. MJ Benotti et al., "Pharmaceuticals and endocrine disrupting compounds in U.S. drinking water," *Environmental Science Technology* 43, no. 3 (February 2009): 597-603.

15. David L. Smith et al., "Agricultural Antibiotics and Human Health," *PLoS Medicine* 2, no. 8 (August 2005).

16. Jeremy K. Nicholson et al., "Gut Microorganisms, mammalian metabolism and personalized health care," *Nature Reviews Microbiology* 3 (April 2005).

17. "Anti-inflammatory" as applied to NSAIDs is actually a misnomer in that while they may reduce inflammation in some forms, they are also known to *cause* inflammation (as in the gastrointestinal system).

18. Jack Challem, *The Inflammation Syndrome* (Hoboken, NJ: Wiley and Son, 2003).

19. D. Adebayo and I. Bjarnason, "Is non-steroidal anti-inflammatory drug (NSAID) enteropathy clinically more important than NSAID gastropathy?" *Postgraduate Medical Journal* 82, no. 965 (March 2006): 186-191.

20. Ibid.

21. Simon Smale & Ingvar Bjarnason, "Determining small bowel integrity following drug treatment," *British Journal of Clinical Pharmacology* 56 (2003): 284-291.

22. D. Adebayo and I. Bjarnason, "Is non-steroidal anti-inflammatory drug (NSAID) enteropathy clinically more important than NSAID gastropathy?" *Postgraduate Medical Journal* 82, no. 965 (March 2006): 186-191.

23. Mohammed A. S. Alem and L. Julia Douglas, "Effects of Aspirin and Other Nonsteroidal Anti-Inflammatory Drugs on Biofilms and Planktonic Cells of *Candida albicans*," *Antimicrobial Agents and Chemotherapy* 48, no. 1 (January 2004).

24. JM Hassing et al., "Acetaminophen-induced glutathione depletion in diabetic rats," *Research Communications Chemical Pathology and Pharmacology* 25, no. 1 (July 1979): 3-11.

25. "Autistic children's abnormal metabolic profile findings," *Medical News Today* April 3, 2005, www.medicalnewstoday.com/articles/22178.php (accessed August 25, 2009); James, S. Jill et al. 2004. Metabolic biomakers of increased oxidative stress and impaired methylation capacity in children with autism. *American Journal of Clinical Nutrition* 80, no. 6 (December): 1611-1617.

26. Sidney MacDonald Baker, "Canaries and Miners," *Alternative Therapies in Health and Medicine* 14 no. 6 (November/December 2008): 24-26.

27. ST Schultz et al., "Acetaminophen (paracetamol) use, measles-mumps-rubella vaccination, and autistic disorder: the results of a parent survey," *Autism* 12, no. 3 (May 2008): 293-307.

28. S. Maraki et al., "Ceftriaxone and dexamethasone affecting yeast gut flora in experimental mice," *Journal of Chemotherapy* 11, no. 5 (October 1999): 363-6; L. Arruvito et al., "NK cells expressing progesterone receptor are susceptible to progesterone-induced apoptosis," *Journal of Immunology* 180, no. 8 (April 2008): 5746-53; Margaret J. Lesmeister et al., "17beta-estradiol suppresses TLR3-induced cytokine and chemokine production in endometrial epithelial cells," *Reproductive Biology and Endocrinology* 3 (2005); A. Spinillo., "The impact of oral contraception on vulvovaginal candidiasis," *Contraception* 51, no. 5 (1995): 293-297.

29. Natasha Campbell-McBride, *Gut and Psychology Syndrome* (Cambridge: Medinform Publishing, 2004): 34.

30. BJ Vesper., "The effect of proton pump inhibitors on the human microbiota," *Current Drug Metabolism* 10, no. 1 (January 2009): 84-9.

31. Usha Stiefel et al., "Suppression of Gastric Acid Production by Proton Pump Inhibitor Treatment Facilitates Colonization of the Large Intestine by

Vancomycin-Resistant *Enterococcus* spp. And *Klebsiella pneumoniae* in Clindamycin-Treated Mice," *Antimicrobial Agents and Chemotherapy* 50, no. 11 (November 2006): 3905-3907.

32. "Children's Aching Stomachs: New Research Finds Young Children Are Increasingly Using Medications to Treat Gastrointestinal Ailments," *PR Newswire* (4 October, 2007) www.redorbit.com/news/health/1089416/childrens_aching _stomachs_new_research_finds_young_children_are_increasingly/index.html (accessed March 26, 2009).

33. Milton Silverman and Philip R. Lee, *Pills, Profits, and Politics* (Berkeley: University of California Press,1974) 6.

34. Ibid., 21.

35. Government Accounting Office, *Prescription Drugs: Improvements Needed in FDA's Oversight of Direct-to-Consumer Advertising*, GAO report number GAO-07-54, www.gao.gov/htext/d0754.html (accessed March 26, 2009).

36. John Abramson, MD, *Overdosed America: The Broken Promise of American Medicine* (New York: Harpers Collins, 2004).

37. Ibid., 149-167.

38. Ibid., 124.

39. Name withheld, former pharmaceutical sales representative, telephone interview with author, September 9, 2009.

CHAPTER FIVE

1. Donna Jackson Nakazawa, *The Autoimmune Epidemic* (New York: Simon & Schuster, 2008).

2. Ibid., 69.

3. Aisha Nazli et al., "Epithelia Under Metabolic Stress Perceive Commensal Bacteria as a Threat," *American Journal of Pathology* 164, no. 3 (March 2004): 947-957.

4. N. Johansson et al., "Flame retardant creates hyperactive mice," *Neuro-Toxicity* 29 (2008) 911-919.

5. "Levels Three Times Higher in Toddlers Than Moms," Environmental Working Group, www.ewg.org/reports/pbdesintoddlers (accessed February 14, 2009).

6. Muhammad Towhid Salam et al., "Early-Life Environmental Risk Factors for Asthma: Findings from the Children's Health Study," *Environmental Health Perspectives* 112, no 6 (May 2004).

7. Gilbert et al., "Environmental Contaminant Trichloroethylene Promotes Autoimmune Disease and Inhibits T-cell Apoptosis in MRL (+/+) Mice," *Journal of Immunotoxicology* 3, no. 4 (December 2006): 263-7.

8. Wikipedia, "Better Living Through Chemistry," en.wikipedia.org/wiki/Better_Living_Through_Chemistry (accessed March 29, 2009).

9. Randall Fitzgerald, *The Hundred-Year* Lie (New York: Penguin Group, 2006).

10. Wikipedia, "Melamine" en.wikipedia.org/wiki/Melamine (accessed March 29, 2009); Time, Inc., "Melamine," *Time Online*, www.time.com/time/health/article/0,8599,1841757,00.html (accessed March 29, 2009).

11. P. J. Osgood et al., "The sensitization of near-ultraviolet radiation killing of mammalian cells by the sunscreen agent para-aminobenzoic acid," *Journal of Investigative Dermatology* 79, no. 6 (1986): 354–357.

12. Environmental Working Group, *Sunscreen Summary—What Works and What's Safe*, www.cosmeticsdatabase.com/special/sunscreens2008/summary.php (accessed March 29, 2009).

13. Andy Arthur, "The Birth of a Cellular Nation," MRI Market Solutions www.mediamark.com/PDF/WPpercent20Thepercent20Birthpercent20of percent20apercent20Cellularpercent20Nationpercent20Revised.pdf (accessed July 31, 2009).

14. Neil Cherry, www.neilcherry.com/, Cherry Environmental Health Consulting (accessed, March 29, 2009).

15. "Rocket Fuel's Widespread, Toxic Fallout," *Environmental Working Group*, www.ewg.org/node/18901 (accessed March 29, 2009).

16. Philip and Alice Shabecoff, *Poisoned Profits* (New York: Random House, 2008): 85.

17. "Pollutants put fetuses at risk," *Environmental Working Group*, available at: www.ewg.org/node/17686, March 29, 2009.

18. Donna Jackson Nakazawa, *The Autoimmune Epidemic* (New York: Simon & Schuster, 2008): 58.

19. Robin Lee et al., "A Review of Events that Expose Children to Elemental Mercury in the United States," National Institutes of Health, U.S. Department of Health and Human Services, dx.doi.org/ (accessed January 12 2009).

20. David Wallinga, et al., "Not So Sweet: Missing Mercury and High Fructose Corn Syrup," *Institute for Agriculture and Trade Policy*, Minneapolis, Minnesota (January 2009).

21. Renee Dufault et al., "Mercury from chlor-alkali plants: measured concentrations in food product sugar," *BioMed Central*, (January 2009).

22. David J. Brenner et al. "Cancer risks attributable to low doses of ionizing radiation: Assessing what we really know," *Proceedings of the National Academy of Sciences of the United States of America* 100, no. 24 (November 2003): 13761-13766.

23. Dr. Toby Watkinson, telephone interview with author, July 26, 2009.

24. Cindy Sage et al., *The Bioinitiative Report*, The Bioinitiative Working Group, August 2007, www.bioinitiative.org (accessed August 15, 2009).

25. "Wireless Quick Facts," Cellular Telecommunications and Internet Association, www.ctia.org/advocacy/research/index.cfm/AID/10323 (accessed August 15, 2009).

26. David J. Brenner et al., "Cancer risks attributable to low doses of ionizing radiation: Assessing what we really know," *Proceedings of the National Academy of Sciences of the United States of America* 100, no. 24 (November 2003): 13761-13766.

CHAPTER SIX

1. Jack Larkin, *The Reshaping of Everyday Life: 1790-1840* (New York: HarperCollins, 1989).

2. Harvey Levenstein, *Revolution at the Table: The Transformation of the American Diet*, (Berkeley: University of California Press, 2003).

3. Ibid., 4.

4. Ibid., 5.

5. James C. Whorton, *Inner Hygiene: Constipation and the Pursuit of Health in Modern Society* (New York: Oxford University Press, 2000) 86.

6. Sally Fallon, *Nourishing Traditions* (Washington, D.C.: New Trends Publishing, 1999).

7. Claude Aubert, as quoted by Sally Fallon, *Nourishing Traditions*.

8. Carol Simontacchi, *The Crazy Makers: How the Food Industry Is Destroying Our Brains and Harming Our Children* (New York: Tarcher/Penguin, 2001) 17.

9. Ibid., 18.

10. Ibid., 18.

11. Ibid., 20-21.

12. Loren Cordain et al., "Origins and evolution of the Western diet: health implications for the 21st century," *American Journal of Clinical Nutrition* 81 (2005): 341-54.

13. AP Simopoulos, "The importance of the ratio of omega-6/omega-3 essential fatty acids," *Biomedicine & Pharmacotherapy* 56, no. 8 (October 2002):365-79.

14. Frederic Gottrand, "Long Chain Polyunsaturated Fatty Acids Influence the Immune System of Infants," *The Journal of Nutrition* 138, no. 9 (September 2008).

15. Randall Fitzgerald, *The Hundred-Year* Lie (New York: Penguin Group, 2006): 96.

16. Ibid., 99.

17. Ibid., 99.

18. Loren Cordain et al., "Origins and evolution of the Western diet: health implications for the 21st century," *American Journal of Clinical Nutrition* 81 (2005): 341-54.

19. Ibid.

20. Jason A. Hawrelak and Stephen P. Myers, "The Causes of Intestinal Dysbiosis: A Review," *Alternative Medicine Review* 9, no. 2 (2004).

21. "Organophosphate Insecticides in Children's Food," Environmental Working Group, www.ewg.org/reports/ops (accessed April 3, 2009).

22. Joanne K. Tobacman, "Review of Harmful Gastrointestinal Effects of Carrageenan in Animal Experiments," *Environmental Health Perspectives* 109, no. 10 (October 2001).

23. Yoshinori Mine and Jie Wie Zhang, "Surfactants Enhance the Tight-Junction Permeability of Food Allergens in Human Intestinal Epithelial Caco-2 Cells," *International Archives of Allergy and Immunology* 130, no. 2 (2003).

24. Felicity Lawrence, "Combining food additives may be harmful, say researchers," *The Guardian Online*, education.guardian.co.uk/higher/news/story/0,,1671821,00.html, (accessed April 3, 2009).

25. Mark Hyman, *The UltraMind Solution* (New York: Scribner, 2009).

26. "Children's Drinks Contain Ingredients that Can Form Benzene," *Environmental Working Group*, www.ewg.org/node/8773 (accessed April 3, 2009); For a list of beverages that contain both ingredients see: www.ewg.org/node/22005.

27. Karl. K. Rozman et al., "NTP-CERHR Expert Panel Report on the Reproductive and Developmental Toxicity of Soy Formula," *Birth Defects Research Part B: Developmental And Reproductive Toxicology* 77, no. 4 (August 2006): 280-397.

28. Natasha Campbell-McBride, *Gut and Psychology Syndrome* (Cambridge: Medinform Publishing, 2004): 91.

29. Andrew Kimbrell, *Your Right to Know: Genetic Engineering and the Secret Changes In Your Food* (San Rafael, CA: Earth Aware Editions, 2007).

30. Ibid.

CHAPTER SEVEN

1. Mark Jackson, *Allergy: The History of a Modern Malady* (London: Reaktion Books, 2007).

2. S. F. Bloomfield et al., "Too clean, or not too clean: The Hygiene Hypothesis and home hygiene," *Clinical and Experimental Allergy* 36 (2006): 402-425.

3. Wasim Maziak, "The asthma epidemic and our artificial habitats," *BMC Pulmonary Medicine* 5 (2005): 5.

4. The protective benefit experienced by farmers exposed to soil organisms could be outweighed by their exposure to industrial agricultural chemicals; R. Ryland, "Health effects among workers in sewage treatment plants," *Occupational Environmental Medicine* 56 (1999): 354-7.

5. Michael F. Holick, MD, PhD, "Vitamin D Deficiency," *The New England Journal of Medicine* 357, no. 3 (July 2007).

6. Sports, which accounted for approximately three hours per week, were not included in the outdoor time, as sports can be both indoors and outdoors; "To Read or Not to Read: A Question of National Consequence," *National Endowment for the Arts Research Report # 47* (November 2007), www.nea .gov/research/ToRead.PDF (accessed March 13, 2009).

7. "Indoor air pollution," *Environmental Working Group*, www.ewg.org/ node/16209 (accessed April 4, 2009).

8. Ibid.

9. Dr. Michael Hollick, "Vitamin D in Health and Disease," (lecture, Integrative Health Symposium, New York City, February 19, 2009).

10. Childbirth Connection, "What Every Pregnant Woman Needs to Know About Cesarean Section," www.childbirthconnection.org (accessed February 23, 2009); Richard W. Wertz and Dorothy C. Wertz, *Lying In: A History of Childbirth in America* (New Haven: Yale University Press, 1989) 260.

11. B. Laubereau et al., "Caesarean section and gastrointestinal symptoms, atopic dermatitis, and sensitization during the first year of life," *Archives of Disease in Childhood* 89 (2004): 993-997.

12. J. Kero et al., "Mode of delivery and asthma—is there a connection?" *Pediatric Research* 52, no. 1 (July 2002): 6-11.

13. H. Renz Polster et al., "Caesarean section delivery and the risk of allergic disorders in childhood," *Clinical and Experimental Allergy* 35, no. 11 (November 2005): 1466-72.

14. B. Laubereau et al., "Caesarean section and gastrointestinal symptoms, atopic dermatitis, and sensitization during the first year of life," *Archives of Disease in Childhood* 89 (2004):993-997.

15. M.A. Hall et al., "Factors influencing the presence of faecal lactobacilli in early infancy," *Archives of Disease in Childhood* 65 (1990): 185-188; JJ Jaakkola et al., "Preterm delivery and asthma: a systematic review and meta-analysis," *Journal of Allergy and Clinical Immunology* 118, no. 4 (October 2006): 823-30; "ADHD 'linked to premature birth,'" *BBC News Online*, news.bbc.co.uk/1/hi/health/5042308.stm (accessed, February 23, 2009).

16. Naomi Schneid-Kofman et al., "Labor Augmentation with Oxytocin Decreases Glutathione Level," *Obstetrics and Gynecology International* 2009 (2009): 1-4.

17. Will Dunham, "U.S. breast-feeding rates rise to record high," *Reuters Online* August 3, 2007, www.reuters.com/article/healthNews/idUSN0226313 220070803 (accessed April 7, 2009); Stanley Ip et al., "Breastfeeding and Maternal and Infant Health Outcomes in Developed Countries," U.S. Department of Health and Human Services, 2007, www.ncbi.nlm.nih.gov/books/ bv.fcgi?rid=hstat1b.chapter.106732 (accessed April 7, 2009).

18. Laura M'Rabet et al., "Breast-feeding and its role in early development of the immune system in infants: consequences for health later in life," *The Journal of Nutrition* 138, no. 9 (September 2008).

19. de Moreno et al., "Effect of the administration of a fermented milk containing Lactobacillus casei DN-114001 on intestinal microbiota and gut associated immune cells of nursing mice and after weaning until immune maturity," *BMC Immunology* 9 (June 2008): 27

20. Harvey Levenstein, *Revolution at the Table: The Transformation of the American Diet,* (Berkeley: University of California Press, 2003).

21. American Psychological Association, "APA Poll Finds Women Bear Brunt of Nation's Stress, Financial Downturn," *Stress in America Annual Report,* 2008, apahelpcenter.mediaroom.com/index.php?s=pageC (accessed April 8, 2009).

22. Jason A. Hawrelak et al., "The Causes of Intestinal Dysbiosis: A Review," *Alternative Medicine Review* 9, no. 2 (2004).

23. PR Saunders et al., "Acute stressors stimulate ion secretion and increase epithelial permeability in rat intestine," *American Journal of Physiology* 267, no. 5 (1994): G794-9; JB Meddings and MG Swain, "Environmental stress-induced gastrointestinal permeability is mediated by endogenous glucocorticoids in the rat" *Gastroenterology* 119 (2000):1019-1028.

24. Martin J. Blaser, "Who are we: Indigenous microbes and the ecology of human diseases," *European Molecular Biology Organization Report* 7, no. 10 (2006).

CHAPTER EIGHT

1.Professor of Physiology (name withheld) at a large Southern Medical School, telephone interview with author, February 24, 2009.

2. Dr. Paul Offit, *The Cutter Incident: How America's First Polio Vaccine Led to the Growing Vaccine Crisis* (New Haven: Yale University Press, 2005).

3. Arthur Allen, *Vaccine: The Controversial Story of Medicine's Greatest Life-saver* (New York: W.W. Norton & Company, 2007) 198.

4. Ibid., 232.

5. U.S. Department of Health and Human Services, *National Vaccine Injury Compensation Program Statistics Report*, April 3, 2009, www.hrsa.gov/vaccine compensation/statistics_report.htm (accessed April 3, 2009).

6. U.S. Department of Health and Human Services, *National Vaccine Injury Compensation Program—Omnibus Autism Proceeding*, www.hrsa.gov/vaccine compensation/omnibusproceeding.htm (accessed April 3, 2009).

7. Alberto Eugenio Tozzi et al., "Neuropsychological Performance 10 Years After Immunization in Infancy With Thimerosal-Containing Vaccines," *Pediatrics* 123, no. 2 (February 2009): 475-482.

8. "Vaccine case draws new attention to autism debate," *CNNhealth.com* www.cnn.com/2008/HEALTH/conditions/03/06/vaccines.autism/index.html (accessed August 22, 2009).

9. Generation Rescue, "Fourteen Studies," www.fourteenstudies.org (accessed April 14, 2009).

10. Dr. Bernadine Healy, "The Vaccines-Autism War: Détente Needed," *U.S. News and World Report* health.usnews.com/blogs/heart-to-heart/2009/04/14/the-vaccines-autism-war-dtente-needed.html (accessed April 14, 2009). Copyright 2009 U.S. News & World Report, L.P. Reprinted with permission.

11. U.S. Department of Health and Human Services, "Recommended Childhood Immunization Schedule," Centers for Disease Control, www .cdc.gov/nip/acip (accessed April 14, 2009).

12. Generation Rescue, "Autism and Vaccines around the World: Vaccine Schedules, Autism Rates, and Under 5 Mortality," www.generationrescue .org/documents/SPECIALpercent20REPORTpercent20AUTISMpercent 202.pdf (accessed April 14, 2009).

13. Dr. Sherri Tenpenny, *Saying No to Vaccines*, (Cleveland, OH: NMA Media Press, 2008); Deirdre Imus, *Growing Up Green: Baby and Childcare*, (New York: Simon & Schuster, 2008).

14. The oral polio vaccine, which is no longer routinely used in children, is the exception to this rule.

15. Daniel P. Stites et al., *Medical Immunology* (Stamford, CT: Appleton & Lange, 1997) 75.

16. Julie Rowe et al., "Th2-Associated Local Reactions to the Accellular Diphtheria-Tetanus-Pertussis Vaccine in 4-to 6-Year-Old Children," *Infectious Immunology* 73, no. 12 (December 2005): 8130-8135; Jessica Strid et al., "Epicutaneous immunization converts subsequent and established antigen-specific

T helper type 1 (Th1) to Th2-type responses," *Immunology* 119, no. 1 (September 2006): 27-35.

17. Mansour Mohamadzadeh et al., "Lactobacilli activate human dendritic cells that skew T cells toward T helper polarization," *Proceedings of the National Academy of Sciences USA*, 102, no. 8 (February 2005): 2880-2885.

18. Laura M'Rabet et al., "Breast-feeding and its role in early development of the immune system in infants: consequences for health later in life," *The Journal of Nutrition* 138, no. 9 (September 2008).

19. Dr. Kenneth Bock, *Healing the New Childhood Epidemics: Autism, ADHD, Asthma, and Allergies* (New York: Ballantine Books, 2007).

20. Arthur Allen, *Vaccine: The Controversial Story of Medicine's Greatest Lifesaver* (New York: W.W. Norton & Company, 2007).

21. E. Fuenzalida et al., "Antirabies Antibody Response in Main to Vaccine Made from Infected Suckling-Mouse Brains," *Bulletin of The World Health Organization* 30 (1964): 431-436.

22. Itzchak Samina et al., "An inactivated West Nile virus vaccine for domestic geese-efficacy study and a summary of 4 years of field application," *Vaccine* 23, no. 41 (September 2005): 4955-4958.

23. Neil Z. Miller, *Vaccine Safety Manual: For Concerned Families and Health Practitioners* (Santa Fe, NM: New Atlantean Press, 2003).

24. Marc Fischer et al., "Promise of new Japanese encephalitis vaccines," *The Lancet* 370, no 9602 (December 2007): 1806; Etsuo Ohtaki et al., "Acute disseminated encephalomyelitis after treatment with Japanese B encephalitis vaccine (Nakayama-Yoken and Beijing strains)," *Journal of Neurology, Neurosurgery, and Psychiatry* 59 (September 1995): 316-317.

25. Neil Z. Miller, *Vaccine Safety Manual: For Concerned Families and Health Practitioners* (Santa Fe, NM: New Atlantean Press, 2003).

26. Arthur M. Silverstein, *Pure Politics and Impure Science: The Swine Flu Affair* (Baltimore: Johns Hopkins University Press, 1981): 116-123.

27. Arthur Allen, *Vaccine: The Controversial Story of Medicine's Greatest Lifesaver* (New York: W.W. Norton & Company, 2007): 261.

28. Donna Jackson Nakazawa, *The Autoimmune Epidemic* (New York: Simon & Schuster, 2008): 142.

29. Ibid., 143.

30. Sherri Tenpenny, "Gardasil and the History of Mandatory Vaccination," (lecture, Integrative Healthcare Symposium, New York City, February 20, 2009); Vaccine Adverse Event Reporting System, vaers.hhs.gov/ (accessed February 27, 2009).

31. Arthur Allen, *Vaccine: The Controversial Story of Medicine's Greatest Lifesaver* (New York: W.W. Norton & Company, 2007): 240.

32. Anabel Aharon-Maor and Yehuda Shoenfeld, "The Good, the Bad and the Ugly of Vaccination," *Israel Medical Association Journal* 2 (2000): 225-227.

33. JF de Carvalho and Y. Shoenfeld, "Status epilepticus and lymphocytic pneumonitis following hepatitis B vaccination," *European Journal of Internal Medicine* 19, no. 5 (July 2008): 383-5.

34. Havarinasab S et al., "Immunosuppressive and autoimmune effects of thimerosal in mice," *Toxicology and Applied Pharmacology* 204 (2005): 109-121; Anshu Agrawal et al., "Thimerosal induces Th2 responses via influencing cytokine secretion by human dendritic cells," *Journal of Leukocyte Biology* 81 (2007): 474-482.

35. Yann Mikaeloff MD, PhD et al., "Hepatitis B Vaccine and the risk of CNS inflammatory demyelination in childhood," *Neurology* 72 (March 2009): 873-880.

36. François-Jérôme Authier, MD, PhD, et al., "Chronic Fatigue Syndrome in Patients with Macrophagic Myofasciitis," *Arthritis and Rheumatism* 48, no. 2 (February 2003): 569-572; RK Gherardi, "Lessons from macrophagic myofasciitis: towards definition of a vaccine adjuvant-related syndrome," *Revue Neurologique (Paris)* 159, no. 2 (February 2003): 162-4.

KL McDonald et al., "Delay in diphtheria, pertussis, tetanus vaccination is associated with a reduced risk of childhood asthma," *Journal of Allergy and Clinical Immunology* 121, no 3 (March 2008): 626-31.

37. Y Kuroda et al., "Autoimmunity induced by adjuvant hydrocarbon oil components of vaccine," *Biomedicine and Pharmacotherapy* 58, no 5, (June 2004): 325-37.

38. Barbro C. Carlson et al., "The Endogenous Adjuvant Squalene Can Induce a Chronic T-Cell Mediated Arthritis in Rats," *The American Journal of Pathology* 156 (2000): 22057-2065.

39. Yehuda Shoenfeld and Noel R. Rose, ed., *Infection and Autoimmunity* (Amsterdam: Elsevier Science, 2004): 87-105.

40. Autoimmune Technologies, "Gulf War Syndrome: Anti-Squalene Antibodies Link Gulf War Syndrome to Anthrax Vaccine," www.autoimmune.com/GWSGen.html (accessed August 22, 2009).

41. BD Poole et al., "Lupus-like autoantibody development in rabbits and mice after immunization with EBNA-1 fragments," *Journal of Autoimmunity* 31, no. 4 (December 2008): 362-71.

42. BD Poole et al., "Epstein-Barr virus and molecular mimicry in systemic lupus erythematosus," *Autoimmunity* 39, no. 1 (February 2006): 63-70.

43. Carolyn Gallagher and Melody Goodman, "Hepatitis B triple series vaccine and developmental disability in US children aged 1-9 years," *Toxicological & Environmental Chemistry* 90, no. 5 (September/October 2008): 997-1008.

44. Laura Hewitson et al., "Delayed acquisition of neonatal reflexes in newborn primates receiving a thimerosal-containing hepatitis B vaccine: influence of gestational age and birth weight," *NeuroToxicology* 31 no. 5 (October 2009).

45. CM Gallagher et al., "Hepatitis B vaccination of male neonates and autism," *Annals of Epidemiology* 19 no. 9 (September 2009) 659.

46. Generation Rescue, "Cal-Oregon Vaccinated vs. Unvaccinated Study," www.generationrescue.org/survey.html (accessed May 3, 2009).

47. Dan Olmstead, "The Age of Autism: 'A pretty big secret'" *UPI* (December 7, 2005) www.upi.com/Health_News/2005/12/07/The-Age-of-Autism-A-pretty-big-secret/UPI-68291133982531/ (accessed May 3, 2009).

48. Dr. Mayer Eisenstein, Vaccine Webinar, May 3, 2009.

49. M-M-R II (Measles, Mumps, and Rubella Virus Vaccine Live) Prescribing Information, www.merck.com/product/usa/pi_circulars/m/mmr_ii/mmr_ii_pi.pdf (accessed May 3, 2009).

50. Centers for Disease Control and Prevention "Guide to Vaccine Contraindications and Precautions," www.cdc.gov/vaccines/recs/vac-admin/downloads/contraindications-guide-508.pdf (accessed May 3, 2009).

51. Paul Ashwood et al., "The immune response in autism: a new frontier for autism research," *Journal of Leukocyte Biology* 80, no. 1 (July 2006): 1-15.

52. Luke Heuer et al., "Reduced Levels of Immunoglobulin in Children with Autism Correlates With Behavioral Symptoms," *Autism Research* 1, no. 5 (October 2008): 275-283.

53. Natasha Campbell-McBride, *Gut and Psychology Syndrome* (Cambridge: Medinform Publishing, 2004): 25-26.

54. A. Bitnun et al., "Measles inclusion-body encephalitis caused by the vaccine strain of measles virus," *Clinical Infectious Diseases* 29, no. 4 (1999): 855-61.

55. Andrew J. Wakefield et al., "MMR vaccination and autism," *Lancet* 354, no. 9182 (September 1999): 949-50

56. Mireille T.M. Vossen et al.,"Persistent Detection of Varicella-Zoster Virus DNA in a Previously Healthy Child after Severe Chickenpox," *Journal of Clinical Microbiology* 43, no. 11 (November 2005): 5614-5621.

57. Henk Van Loveren et al., "Vaccine-Induced Antibody Responses as Parameters of the Influence of Endogenous and Environmental Factors," *Environmental Health Perspectives* 109 (2001): 757-764.

58. Laura M'Rabet et al., "Breast-feeding and its role in early development of the immune system in infants: consequences for health later in life," *The Journal of Nutrition* 138, no. 9 (September 2008).

59. Patrick G. Holt and Julie Rowe, ed., Donald Y.M. Leung et al., "The Developing Immune System and Allergy," *Pediatric Allergy: Principles and Practice* (St. Louis, Missouri: Mosby, 2003): 74.

60. The Jordan Report 2007, www3.niaid.nih.gov/about/organization/dmid/PDF/Jordan2007.pdf. (accessed May 3, 2009).

61. Arthur Allen, *Vaccine: The Controversial Story of Medicine's Greatest Lifesaver* (New York: W.W. Norton & Company, 2007): 425.

62. Ibid., 426-432.

63. Anh Dai K. Nguyen and Robert F. Lemanske Jr., "Atopy in Children of Families with an Anthroposophic Lifestyle," *Pediatrics* (August 2000): 433.

64. JS Alm et al., "An anthroposophic lifestyle and intestinal microflora in infancy," *Pediatric Allergy and Immunology* 13, no. 6 (December 2002): 402-11.

CHAPTER NINE

1. "Marketplace Report: Singulair Suicide Link?" *NPR* (March 28, 2008) www.npr.org/templates/story/story.php?storyId=89186918 (accessed August 22, 2009).

2. GL Nicolson et al., "Evidence for Mycoplasma ssp, Chlamydia pneunomiae, and human herpes virus-6 coinfections in the blood of patients with autism spectrum disorders," *Journal of Neuroscience Research* 85, no. 5 (April 2007): 1143-8.

CHAPTER TEN

1. Environmental Working Group, "Executive Summary: Body Burden-The Pollution in Newborns" July 14, 2005, www.ewg.org/reports/bodyburden2/execsumm.php (accessed July 20, 2009).

2. Nancy Pelosi, then House Democratic Leader, now Speaker of the House, "Infants Biological Systems are Being Disrupted by Synthetic Chemicals We are Exposed to Every Day," July 14, 2005, www.house.gov/pelosi/press/releases/July05/infants.html (accessed August 21, 2009).

3. HJ Tsai et al., "Familial Aggregation of Food Allergy and Sensitization to Food Allergens: a Family-Based Study," *Clinical and Experimental Allergy*, 39, no.1 (January 2009):101-9; DA Watts and J Satsangi J, "The Genetic Jigsaw of Inflammatory Bowel Disease," *Gut* 50 (May 2002): Suppl 3:III31-6; H Bisgaard

et al., "Risk Analysis of Early Childhood Eczema," *Journal of Allergy and Clinical Immunology* 123, no.6 (June 2009): 1355-60; J Biederman, et al., "Further Evidence for Family-Genetic Risk Factors in Attention Deficit Hyperactivity Disorder. Patterns of Comorbidity in Probands and Relatives Psychiatrically and Pediatrically Referred Samples," *Archives of General Psychiatry* 49, no. 9 (September 1992): 728-38.

4. H Autrup, "Transplacental Transfer of Genotoxins and Transplacental Carcinogenesis," *Environmental Health Perspectives* 101, Suppl 2 (July 1993): 33-8; M Hooiveld, et al., "Adverse Reproductive Outcomes Among Male Painters with Occupational Exposure to Organic Solvents," *Journal of Occupational and Environmental Medicine* 63 (June 2006): 538-544.

5. V Rondeau et al., "Aluminum and Silica in Drinking Water and the Risk of Alzheimer's Disease or Cognitive Decline: Findings from 15-year Follow-up of the PAQUID Cohort," *American Journal of Epidemiology* 169, no. 4 (June 2009): 489-96.

6. GM Whitford, "The Physiological and Toxicological Characteristics of Fluoride," *Journal of Dental Research* 69 (February 1990): 539-549.

7. SC Freni, "Exposure to High Fluoride Concentrations in Drinking Water is Associated with Decreased Birth Rates" *Journal of Toxicological and Environmental Health* 42, no. 1 (May 1994): 109-21.

8. QQ Tang et al., "Fluoride and Children's Intelligence: a Meta-analysis," *Biological Trace Element Research* 126, no. 1-3 (Winter 2008): 115-20.

9. JA Varner et al., "Chronic Administration of Aluminum-Fluoride or Sodium-Fluoride to Rats in Drinking Water: Alterations in Neuronal and Cerebrovascular Integrity," *Brain Research* 784, no. 1-2 (February 1998): 284-98.

10. Environmental Working Group, "Citizen Petition to Cease Unlawful Sale of Misbranded and Adulterated Cosmetics" (2004), www.cosmeticsdatabase.com/research/fdapetition.php (accessed August 2, 2009).

11. M Allmyr et al., "Triclosan in Plasma and Milk from Swedish Nursing Mothers and Their Exposure via Personal Care Products," *The Science of the Total Environment* 372, no. 1 (December 2006): 87-93.

12. N Veldhoen et al., "The Bactericidal Agent Triclosan Modulates Thyroid Hormone-Associated Gene Expression and Disrupts Postembryonic Anuran Development," *Aquatic Toxicology* 80, no. 3 (December 2006): 217-27.

13. SB Levy, "Antibacterial Household Products: Cause for Concern," *Emerging Infectious Diseases* 7, no 3 (2001): 512-515.

14. RH Gee et al., "Oestrogenic and Androgenic Activity of Triclosan in Breast Cancer Cells," *Journal of Applied Toxicology* 28, no. 1 (2008): 78-91.

15. M Mezcua et al., "Evidence of 2,7/2,8-dibenzodichloro-p-dioxin as a Photodegradation Product of Triclosan in Water and Wastewater Samples," *Analytica Chimica Acta* 524, no. 1-2 (2004): 241-247.

16. Environmental Working Group, Skin Deep Cosmetic Database, www.cosmeticsdatabase.com/ingredient.php?ingred06=700740 (accessed July 24, 2009).

17. California Office of Environmental Health Hazard Assessment, "Chronic Toxicity Summary Toluene," CAS Registry Number: 108-88-3, www.oehha.ca.gov/air/chronic_rels/pdf/108883.pdf (accessed August 9, 2009).

18. The Environment Agency, "Nonylphenol Ethoxylate," www.environ ment-agency.gov.uk/business/topics/pollution/39187.aspx (accessed August 9, 2009).

19. P Eriksson, E Jakobsson, and A Frederiksson, "Brominated Flame Retardants: a Novel Class of Developmental Neurotoxicants in our Environment?" *Environmental Health Perspectives* 109 no 9 (September 2001): 903-908.

20. New Jersey Department of Health and Senior Services, "Hazardous Substance Fact Sheet Tetracholroethylene," CAS 127-18-4 Rev., March 2002.

21. Ibid.

22. PE Stackelberg et al., "Persistence of Pharmaceutical Compounds and Other Organic Wastewater Contaminants in a Conventional Drinking-Water Treatment Plant," *The Science of the Total Environment* 329, no 1-3 (August 2004): 99-113.

23. RD Morris et al., "Chlorination, Chlorination By-products and Cancer: a Meta-analysis," *American Journal of Public Health* 82 (September 1993): 955–963.

24. F Bove, Y Shim and P Zeitz, "Drinking Water Contaminants and Adverse Pregnancy Outcomes: A Review," *Environmental Health Perspectives* 110, suppl. 1 (February 2002): 61-74.

25. HW Kuo, et al., "Estimates of Cancer Risk from Chloroform Exposure During Showering in Taiwan," *The Science of the Total Environment* 218, no.10 (July 1998): 1-7.

26. PE Stackelberg et al., "Persistence of Pharmaceutical Compounds and Other Organic Wastewater Contaminants in a Conventional Drinking-Water Treatment Plant," *The Science of the Total Environment* 329, no 1-3 (August 2004): 99-113.

27. C Lu et al., "Dietary Intake and Its Contribution to Longitudinal Organophosphorus Pesticide Exposure in Urban/Suburban Children," *Environmental Health Perspectives* 116, no. 4, (April 2008).

28. V Worthington, "Nutritional Quality of Organic Versus Conventional Fruits, Vegetables, and Grains," *The Journal of Alternative and Complementary Medicine* 7, no. 2 (November 2001): 161-173; DK Asami et al., "Comparison of the Total Phenolic and Ascorbic Acid Content of Freeze-Dried and Air-Dried Marionberry, Strawberry, and Corn Grown Using Conventional, Organic, and Sustainable Agricultural Practices," *Journal of Agricultural and Food Chemistry* 51, no.5 (February 2003): 1237-41.

29. CJ Lopez-Bote, et al., "Effect of Free-range Feeding on Omega-3 Fatty Acids and Alpha-tocopherol Content and Oxidative Stability of Eggs," *Animal Feed Science and Technology* 72 (1998): 33-40.

30. A Tolan, et al., "Studies on the Composition of Food. 5. The chemical Composition of Eggs Produced Under Battery, Deep Litter and Free-range Conditions," *British Journal of Nutrition* 31 (1974):185.

31. SK Duckett et al, "Effects of Winter Stocker Growth Rate and Finishing System on: III. Tissue Proximate, Fatty acid, Vitamin and Cholesterol Content," *Journal of Animal Science* 87, no. 9 (2009): 2961-8; G.C. Smith, "Dietary supplementation of vitamin E to cattle to improve shelf life and case life of beef for domestic and international markets," Colorado State University, Fort Collins, Colorado 80523-1171.

32. C Ip, et al., "Conjugated linoleic acid. A Powerful Anti-Carcinogen from Animal Fat Sources," *Cancer* 74, suppl. 3 (1994): 1050-4.

33. J Banu, "Beneficial Effects of Conjugated Linoleic Acid and Exercise on Bone of Middle Aged Female Mice," *Journal of Bone and Mineral Metabolism* 26, no.5 (September 2008): 436-45.

34. TR Dhiman et al., "Conjugated Linoleic Acid Content of Milk From Cows Fed Different Diets," *Journal of Dairy Science* 82, no. 10 (1999): 2146-56.

35. R Hites, et al., "Global Assessment of Organic Contaminants in Farmed Salmon," *Science* 303, no.5655 (January 2004): 226-229.

36. R Williams, *"The Relationship Between the Composition of Milk and the Properties of Bulk Milk Properties,"* Australian Journal of Dairy Technology 57 no.1 (2002): 30-44.

37. T Saukkonen et al., "Significance of Cow's Milk Protein Antibodies as Risk Factor for Childhood IDDM: Interactions with Dietary Cow's Milk Intake and HLA-DQB1 Genotype. Childhood Diabetes in Finland Study Group," *Diabetologia* 41, no.1 (January 1998): 72-8.

38. D Gunnell, "Are Diet-Prostate Cancer Associations Mediated by the IGF Axis? A Cross-Sectional Analysis of Diet, IGF-I and IGFBP-3 in Healthy Middle-Aged Men," *British Journal of Cancer* 88, no.11 (June 2003): 1682-6.

39. I Kimber and RJ Dearman, "Factors Affecting the Development of Food Allergy," *The Proceedings of the Nutrition Society* 61, no. 4 (November 2002): 435-9.

40. G Caramia, "The Essential Fatty Acids Omega-6 and Omega-3: From their Discovery to their Use in Therapy," *Minerva Pediatrica* 60, no. 2 (April 2008): 219-33. Italian.

41. D Mozaffarian, A Aro, and W Willett, "Health Effects of Trans-Fatty Acids: Experimental and Observational Evidence," *European Journal of Clinical Nutrition* 63, suppl. 2 (May 2009): S5-21.

42. S Angell et al., "Cholesterol Control Beyond the Clinic: New York City's Trans Fat Restriction," *Annals of Internal Medicine* 151, no. 2 (July 2009): 129-34.

43. Do Ogbolu et al., "In Vitro Antimicrobial Properties of Coconut Oil on Candida Species in Ibadan, Nigeria," *Journal of Medicinal Food* 10, no. 2 (June 2007): 384-7.

44. Mark Hyman, *The UltraMind Solution* (New York, NY: Scribner, 2009).

45. E Somer, "Minerals," in *The Essential Guide to Vitamins and Minerals* (New York, NY: Harper Perennial, 1995): 89-94; LK Mahan and S Escott-Stump, "Minerals" in *Krause's Food, Nutrition and Diet Therapy*, 9th ed, (Philadelphia, PA: WB. Saunders Company, 1996): 124-130.

46. J Miller, et al., "Calcium Absorption from Calcium Carbonate and a New Form of Calcium (CCM) in Healthy Male and Female Adolescents." *American Journal of Clinical Nutrition* 48 (November 1988): 1291–4; KT Smith et al., "Calcium Absorption From a New Calcium Delivery System (CCM)" *Calcified Tissue International* 41 (December 1987): 351–2.

47. GM Scelfo and AR Flegal, "Lead in Calcium Supplements," *Environmental Health Perspectives* 108, no.4 (April 2000): 309-13.

48. R Lucas et al., "Future Health Implications of Prenatal and Early Life Vitamin D Status," *Nutrition Reviews* 66, no. 12 (December 2008): 710 – 720; A Lapillone, "Vitamin D Deficiency During Pregnancy May Impair Maternal and Fetal Outcomes," *Medical Hypotheses* (August 2009).

49. C Bender-Gotze, "Therapy of Juvenile Iron Deficiency with Bivalent Iron Dragees (Fe2-fumarate, succinate, sulfate). Controlled Double-Blind Study," *Fortschritte der Medizen* 98 (April 1980): 590–3 [German]; D Casparis et al., "Effectiveness and Tolerability of Oral Liquid Ferrous Gluconate in Iron-Deficiency Anemia in Pregnancy and in the Immediate Post-Partum Period: Comparison with Other Liquid or Solid Formulations Containing Bivalent or Trivalent Iron," *Minerva Ginecologica* 48 (November 1996): 511–8 [Italian].

50. F Stonek et al., "Methylenetetrahydrofolate reductase C677T polymorphism and pregnancy complications," *Obstetrics and Gynecology* 110, no.2 (August 2007): 363-8.

51. K Rothman et al., "Teratogenicity of High Vitamin A Intake," *New England Journal of Medicine* 333 (November 1995):1369–73.

52. P Mastroiacovo et al., "High Vitamin A Intake in Early Pregnancy and Major Malformations: a Multicenter Prospective Controlled Study," *Teratology* 59 (January 1999): 7–11.

53. Q Li et al., "Dietary Prenatal Choline Supplementation Alters Postnatal Hippocampal Structure and Function," *Journal of Neurophysiology* 91, no. 4 (April 2004): 1545-55.

54. GM Shaw et al., "Choline and Risk of Neural Tube Defects in a Folate-Fortified Population," *Epidemiology* 20, no.5 (September 2009): 714-9.

55. A Simopolous, "Omega 3 Fatty Acids in Inflammation and Autoimmune Disease," *Journal of the American College of Nutrition* 21, no. 6 (2002): 495-505.

56. EF Verdu, "Probiotics Effects on Gastrointestinal Function: Beyond the Gut?" *Neurogastroenterology and Motility* 21, no.5 (May 2009): 477-80.

57. S Halken, "Prevention of Allergic Disease in Childhood: Clinical and Epidemiological Aspects of Primary and Secondary Allergy Prevention," *Pediatric Allergy and Immunology* 15, suppl. 16 (June 2004): 4-5.

58. A Marini et al., "Effects of a Dietary and Environmental Prevention Programme on the Incidence of Allergic Symptoms in High Atopic Risk Infants: Three Years' Follow-up," *Acta Paediatrica* 414 (May 1996): 1-21.

59. Ibid.

60. RK Bush, "Indoor Allergens, Environmental Avoidance, and Allergic Respiratory Disease," *Allergy and Asthma Proceedings* 29, no.6 (November/December 2008): 575-9.

61. M Pesonen et al., "Prolonged Exclusive Breastfeeding is Associated With Increased Atopic Dermatitis: a Prospective Follow-up Study of Unselected Healthy Newborns From Birth to Age 20 Years," *Clinical and Experimental Allergy* 36, no. 8 (August 2006):1011-8.

62. JD Smith et al., "Relief of Fibromyalgia Symptoms Following Discontinuation of Dietary Excitotoxins," *Annals of Pharmacotherapy* 35, no. 6 (June 2001): 702-6.

63. M Soffritti et al., "First Experimental Demonstration of the Multipotential Carcinogenic Effects of Aspartame Administered in the Feed to Sprague-Dawley Rats," *Environmental Health Perspectives* 114, no.3 (March 2006): 379-85.

64. Melanie Warner, "The Lowdown on Sweet," *New York Times*, February 12, 2006.

65. D Geier, J Kern and M Geier, "A Prospective Study of Prenatal Mercury Exposure from Maternal Dental Amalgams and Autism Severity," *Acta Neurobiologiae Experimentalis (Wars)* 69, no. 20 (2009): 189-97; J Vas and M Monestier, "Immunology of Mercury," *Annals of the New York Academy of Science* 1143 (November 2008): 240-67. Review.

66. B Michalke, S Halbach, and V Nischwitz, "JEM Spotlight: Metal Speciation Related to Neurotoxicity in Humans," *Journal of Environmental Monitoring* 5 (2009): 939-54.

67. MJ Vimy et al., "Mercury from Maternal 'Silver' Tooth Fillings in Sheep and Human Breast Milk. A Source of Neonatal Exposure," *Biological Trace Element Research* 56, no. 2 (February 1997): 143-52.

68. MJ Vimy, Y Takahashi, and F Lorscheider, "Maternal-Fetal Distribution of Mercury (203Hg) Released from Dental Amalgam Fillings," *The American Journal of Physiology* 258, no. 4 (1990): R939-45.

69. D Geier, J Kern, and M Geier, "A Prospective Study of Prenatal Mercury Exposure from Maternal Dental Amalgams and Autism Severity," *Acta Neurobiologiae Experimentalis (Wars)* 69 no. 20 (2009): 189-97.

70. Federal Trade Commission, "FTC Report Sheds New Light on Food Marketing to Children and Adolescents," July 29, 2008, www.ftc.gov/opa/2008/07/foodmkting.shtm (accessed July 20, 2009).

71. Center for Science in the Public Interest, "Guidelines for Marketing Foods to Kids," proposed January 5, 2005, www.cspinet.org/new/200501051 .html (accessed July 30, 2009).

72. B Starfield et al., "The Concept of Prevention: a Good Idea Gone Astray?" *Journal of Epidemiology and Community Health* 62 (July 2008): 580-83.

73. G Welch, "Campaign Myth: Prevention as Cure-all," *New York Times*, October 6, 2008.

CONCLUSION

1. "Skin Scourge," *Current Health* 2 31, no. 4 (December 2004): 2.

2. Devra Davis, *The Secret History of the War on Cancer* (New York: Basic Books, 2007).

3. SH Ibrahim et al., "Incidence of gastrointestinal symptoms in children with autism: a population based study," *Pediatrics* 124, no. 2 (August 2009): 796-8.

4. (Nancy Snyderman, interview by Natalie Morales, *The Today Show*, NBC, July 2009.)

5. SH Ibrahim et al., "Incidence of gastrointestinal symptoms in children with autism: a population based study," *Pediatrics* 124, no. 2 (August 2009): 796-8.

6. Duff Wilson, "Harvard Medical School in Ethics Quandry," *The New York Times*, March 2, 2009.

7. Ibid.

8. Autism Society of America, "Facts and Statistics," www.autism-society.org/site/PageServer?pagename=about_whatis_factsstats (accessed August 17, 2009).

INDEX

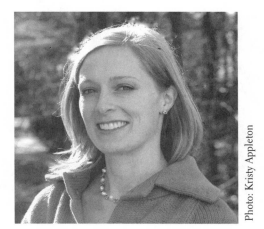

Photo: Kristy Appleton

Beth Lambert is a former healthcare consultant and teacher. She attended Oxford University and graduated with honors from Williams College. She holds an M.A. in American Studies, with a concentration in American Healthcare, from Fairfield University.

Beth worked for a number of healthcare consulting firms in New York City including The Wilkerson Group, IBM Healthcare Consulting, and Easton Associates. She was also involved in market research and business development for an e-health company. She has worked with physicians, scientific and medical researchers, and corporate executives to assess products, business strategies, and emerging trends in pharmaceuticals, biotech, diagnostics, medical devices and healthcare delivery.

She taught and coached at secondary schools in Massachusetts, New Jersey and New York City. As an educator, she worked closely with students who struggled with learning disabilities. She has traveled extensively throughout the United States, networking and collaborating with other educators through the National Endowment for the Humanities Landmarks of American History and Culture Program.

Beth is the Executive Director of PEACE: *Parents Ending America's Childhood Epidemic*, a 501c3 non-profit organization dedicated to educating the public about the epidemic of chronic illness affecting our youth, and helping parents connect with other parents and appropriate healthcare providers. In 2009, she launched ANSWERS *for an Epidemic* (www.epidemicanswers.org), an educational website with a healthcare provider directory for parents looking for practitioners that specialize in recovering children from chronic illnesses. Beth is the mother of three, and is passionate about preventing chronic illnesses in children. Her website is www.acompromisedgeneration.com.

Sentient Publications, LLC publishes books on cultural creativity, experimental education, transformative spirituality, holistic health, new science, ecology, and other topics, approached from an integral viewpoint. Our authors are intensely interested in exploring the nature of life from fresh perspectives, addressing life's great questions, and fostering the full expression of the human potential. Sentient Publications' books arise from the spirit of inquiry and the richness of the inherent dialogue between writer and reader.

Our Culture Tools series is designed to give social catalyzers and cultural entrepreneurs the essential information, technology, and inspiration to forge a sustainable, creative, and compassionate world.

We are very interested in hearing from our readers. To direct suggestions or comments to us, or to be added to our mailing list, please contact:

SENTIENT PUBLICATIONS, LLC
1113 Spruce Street
Boulder, CO 80302
303-443-2188
contact@sentientpublications.com
www.sentientpublications.com